T0293391

Mitochondrial Dysfunction: A Functional Medicine Approach to Aging and Diseases

Mitochondrial Dysfunction: A Functional Medicine Approach to Aging and Diseases

Editor: John Binnington

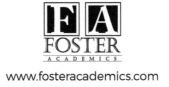

www.fosteracademics.com

www.fosteracademics.com

Cataloging-in-Publication Data

Mitochondrial dysfunction : a functional medicine approach to aging and diseases / edited by John Binnington.
   p. cm.
Includes bibliographical references and index.
ISBN 978-1-64646-559-0
1. Mitochondrial pathology. 2. Aging. 3. Metabolism--Disorders. I. Binnington, John.
RB147.5 .M58 2023
616.07--dc23

© Foster Academics, 2023

Foster Academics,
118-35 Queens Blvd., Suite 400,
Forest Hills, NY 11375, USA

ISBN 978-1-64646-559-0 (Hardback)

This book contains information obtained from authentic and highly regarded sources. Copyright for all individual chapters remain with the respective authors as indicated. All chapters are published with permission under the Creative Commons Attribution License or equivalent. A wide variety of references are listed. Permission and sources are indicated; for detailed attributions, please refer to the permissions page and list of contributors. Reasonable efforts have been made to publish reliable data and information, but the authors, editors and publisher cannot assume any responsibility for the validity of all materials or the consequences of their use.

Trademark Notice: Registered trademark of products or corporate names are used only for explanation and identification without intent to infringe.

Contents

Preface

Mitochondria are double-membrane-bound organelles found in eukaryotic cells. They build cable-like structures and deliver energy to cells with the help of oxidative phosphorylation (OXPHOS) process. Aging causes a wide range of interrelated conditions and is also a leading cause of various human diseases. The age-associated changes in mitochondria are linked with deterioration in mitochondrial function. The accumulation of oxidative damage and mutations caused by reactive oxygen species (ROS), mitochondrial functionality, and DNA volume and integrity decline with age. Mitochondrial dysfunction includes an increase in oxidative damage and a reduction in oxidative capacity, and plays a significant role in biological aging. The accumulation of dysfunctional mitochondria occurs in all the tissues with aging, including brain, liver and skeletal muscle. These dysfunctional mitochondria are marked and removed through an autophagic process named mitophagy. Mitochondrial dysfunction occurs in many neurodegenerative diseases such as Huntington's disease (HD), amyotrophic lateral sclerosis (ALS), Parkinson's disease (PD), Friedreich's ataxia (FRDA) and Alzheimer's disease (AD). This book explores all the important aspects of mitochondrial dysfunction and its impact on aging and diseases. Experts and students actively engaged in researches on mitochondrial dysfunction will find it full of crucial and unexplored concepts.

This book has been the outcome of endless efforts put in by authors and researchers on various issues and topics within the field. The book is a comprehensive collection of significant researches that are addressed in a variety of chapters. It will surely enhance the knowledge of the field among readers across the globe.

It gives us an immense pleasure to thank our researchers and authors for their efforts to submit their piece of writing before the deadlines. Finally in the end, I would like to thank my family and colleagues who have been a great source of inspiration and support.

Editor

Unlocking the Door to Neuronal Woes in Alzheimer's Disease: Aβ and Mitochondrial Permeability Transition Pore

Heng Du [1] and Shirley ShiDu Yan [1,2,3,*]

[1] Department of Surgery, Physicians & Surgeons College of Columbia University, New York, NY 10032, USA

[2] Department of Pathology & Cell Biology, Physicians & Surgeons College of Columbia University, New York, NY 10032, USA

[3] The Taub institute for Research on Alzheimer's Disease and the Aging Brain, Columbia University, New York, NY 10032, USA

* Author to whom correspondence should be addressed; E-Mail: sdy1@columbia.edu;

Abstract: Mitochondrial dysfunction occurs early in the progression of Alzheimer's disease. Amyloid-β peptide has deleterious effects on mitochondrial function and contributes to energy failure, respiratory chain impairment, neuronal apoptosis, and generation of reactive oxygen species in Alzheimer's disease. The mechanisms underlying amyloid-β induced mitochondrial stress remain unclear. Emerging evidence indicates that mitochondrial permeability transition pore is important for maintenance of mitochondrial and neuronal function in aging and neurodegenerative disease. Cyclophilin D (Cyp D) plays a central role in opening mitochondrial permeability transition pore, ultimately leading to cell death. Interaction of amyloid-β with cyclophilin D triggers or enhances the formation of mitochondrial permeability transition pores, consequently exacerbating mitochondrial and neuronal dysfunction, as shown by decreased mitochondrial membrane potential, impaired mitochondrial respiration function, and increased oxidative stress and cytochrome c release. Blockade of cyclophilin D by genetic abrogation or pharmacologic inhibition protects mitochondria and neurons from amyloid-β induced toxicity, suggesting that cyclophilin D dependent mitochondrial transition pore is a therapeutic target for Alzheimer's disease.

Keywords: amyloid beta; mitochondrial permeability transition; cyclophilin D; therapy

1. Introduction

Amyloid beta (Aβ), a major component of amyloid plaque, is a neurotoxic peptide, the accumulation of which leads to neuronal degeneration relevant to the pathogenesis of Alzheimer's disease (AD) [1-5]. Aβ accumulates in the extracellular and intracellular compartments, including mitochondria. Notably, recent studies from several independent groups including our laboratory demonstrate the accumulation of Aβ in mitochondria of brains from AD patients and AD mouse models [1,6-12]. It is known that progressive accumulation of mitochondrial Aβ is significantly related to the mitochondrial and neuronal dysfunction in an Aβ rich environment [1,6,7,11-14]. Predominant mitochondrial pathological changes in AD include mitochondrial membrane potential dissipation [15-17], respiration defect [6,7,18], oxidative stress [1,14,19-21], Aβ accumulation in mitochondria [1,5,6,10,11], impaired calcium buffering capacity [22-25], altered mitochondrial dynamics and trafficking [26-28], mtDNA mutation [29-31] and mitochondrial permeability transition [7,13,32]. Mitochondria are essential for provision of energy by oxidative phosphorylation; this organelle also modulates intra-neuronal calcium homeostasis necessary to sustain neuronal function and survival. Dysregulation of mitochondrial function leads to synaptic stress, disruption of synaptic transmission, apoptosis and ultimately neuronal death [6,15,33-35]. Thus, it is highly important to unravel the mechanism(s) of Aβ-associated mitochondrial alterations to enhance our understanding of the pathophysiological process of AD.

Recent studies emphasize that mitochondrial permeability transition pore (mPTP) is involved in Aβ induced mitochondrial perturbation [7,13,25,32,36-38]. The formation of mPTP is closely related to Aβ superimposition and perturbation of mitochondrial structure and function. Inhibition of mPTP formation in an AD animal model and in Aβ-insulted cells results in enhanced protection of neurons from Aβ toxicity and oxidative stress. Here, we review the role of mPTP in mitochondrial pathology relevant to the pathogenesis of AD, particularly related to the involvement of Cyclophilin D (Cyp D) in mPTP.

2. mPTP and Alzheimer's Disease

Mitochondrial permeability transition, or MPT, is an increase in permeability of the mitochondrial membranes to molecules of less than 1,500 Daltons in molecular weight. MPT results from opening of mitochondrial permeability transition pores, known as MPT pores or mPTP. mPTP is a protein pore that is formed in mitochondrial membranes under certain pathological conditions such as oxidative stress, ischemia, traumatic brain injury and stroke. Induction of the permeability transition pore can lead to mitochondrial swelling and cell death. The deleterious impact of mitochondrial permeability transition on mitochondrial function has long been proposed [39-41].

Mitochondria are two-membrane encapsulated organelles with strict regulation of the uptake and release of substances. Disruptions in this regulation lead to mitochondrial and cellular perturbation. For example, the release of cytochrome c from mitochondria triggers a signal transduction cascade and apoptosis. mPTP is one among several factors that interfere with the integrity of mitochondrial membrane. The formation of mPTP in a mitochondrial membrane opens a nonselective portal that results in abnormal exchange of solutes and molecules > 1,500 Daltons between mitochondria and cytoplasm [42].

Though the exact structure of the mPTP is still unknown, it is postulated that several proteins come together to form the pore, including the outer membrane voltage-dependent anion channel (VDAC), adenine nucleotide translocase (ANT) located in the mitochondrial inner membrane, and cyp D residing in mitochondrial matrix [43-46]. A recent study suggests that phosphate carrier (PiC) in mitochondrial inner membrane is also a possible component of mPTP [47]. It is known that formation of mPTP relies on the translocation of cyp D to inner mitochondrial membrane and the intra-mitochondrial perturbations of calcium, phosphate and oxidative stress are strong inducers of the cyp D translocation [39,42,47-49]. Mitochondria undergoing mPTP show dissipated membrane potential, perturbed mitochondrial respiration chain, decreased ATP production, increased free radical generation, and disruption of calcium modulation [7,40,50]. Calcium effluxes from mitochondria while cytoplasm solutes flow into mitochondria; thereby causing mitochondrial swelling that in turn leads to ruptures in mitochondrial membrane. Importantly, pre-apoptotic molecules such as cytochrome c are released from the mPTP afflicted mitochondria through these ruptures, which then trigger apoptosis [43,50]. Obviously, mPTP formation is a detrimental process that significantly contributes to mitochondrial and cellular malfunction.

Involvement of mPTP in neurodegeneration has been reported in neurodegenerative diseases, including AD [7], ALS (amyotrophic lateral sclerosis) [51,52], HD (Huntington's disease) [53] and PD (Parkinson's disease) [54,55], as evidenced by increased CypD expression, decreased mitochondrial calcium handling capacity and mitochondrial oxidative stress in disease-affected brain regions. In our published studies, we demonstrated that CypD levels were elevated in mitochondria isolated from the hippocampus and temporal pole of AD patients. Increased Cyp D expression is predominantly localized in neurons in these specific areas of AD patients [7]. Given the positive correlation of Cyp D expression to mPTP opening [7,43,52,56], neurons with increased expression of CypD in AD-affected brain regions would be more susceptible to mPTP formation and the resultant consequences. Similarly, AD mice overexpressing amyloid precursor protein (APP) and Aβ (APP mice) demonstrated up-regulation of CypD expression in cortical mitochondria. As expected, cortical mitochondria containing Aβ undergo increased mitochondrial swelling in the presence of calcium. In addition, APP mice demonstrate increased CypD translocation to mitochondrial inner membrane and decreased mitochondrial calcium buffering capacity, suggesting that mitochondria enriched for Aβ environment are susceptible to mPTP formation, which is consistent with increased CypD expression also seen in this strain [7,13].

Transgenic AD mouse models show age-dependent accumulation of cerebral/mitochondrial Aβ as well as neuronal and mitochondrial stress. In APP mice (J-20 line), Aβ accumulation in the brain occurs by 4-5 months and progresses with age. By the age of 10-12 months, there are plentiful amyloid deposits in the brain [57,58]. Consistent with this observation, impaired mPTP function and calcium buffering capacity correlate with age-related Aβ accumulation in APP mouse brain and mitochondria. Cortical mitochondria from transgenic and nonTg mice showed swelling in response to Ca^{2+}, although APP mitochondria show greater swelling compared to nonTg mitochondria at the ages of 12-24 months. Cortical mitochondria of both nonTg and APP mice exhibited an age-dependent increased swelling in response to Ca^{2+}. Similarly, brain mitochondria isolated from APP mice demonstrated an age-related mitochondrial respiration defect, mitochondrial oxidative stress, and decreased ATP production [7,13]. Another study showed that the inhibition of ANT substantially attenuated apoptosis and autophagy in a mouse model for cerebral amyloid angiopathy, lending further credence to the involvement of mPTP in AD [59]. Taken together, these data indicate that mitochondrial permeability transition pore is sensitized in the Aβ milieu.

3. The Interplay of Aβ and mPTP

Aβ has been shown to directly perturb mPTP function. Moreira and colleagues demonstrated that Aβ directly induces mitochondrial swelling, cytochrome c release and mitochondrial membrane potential decrease in isolated brain mitochondria [37, 60]. Administration of Aβ 25-35 triggers mPTP formation accompanying mitochondrial oxidative stress [38]. We observed in isolated brain, that the addition of Aβ to mitochondria in the presence of mPTP inducers (e.g. phosphate) enhances mitochondrial swelling in a dose-dependent manner [7]. It has been demonstrated that Aβ treatment significantly sequestrates Cyp D translocation to mitochondrial inner membrane and reduces mitochondrial calcium buffering capacity. These data indicate that Aβ is responsible for mPTP formation.

An indirect effect of Aβ on mPTP is due to the ability of Aβ to elevate intra-cellular calcium and free radical levels. Aβ, a peptide cleaved from its precursor protein (APP), causes severe intra-neuronal free radical injury and calcium dysregulation, leading to accelerated neuronal damage [22,61-63]. Calcium and free radicals are strong inducers of mPTP and conversely mPTP formation further exacerbates calcium perturbation and oxidative stress. Thus, it is proposed that deregulated neuronal calcium metabolism and accumulation/production of reactive oxygen species (ROS) are possible mechanisms underlying Aβ-induced mPTP formation. Aβ treatment in cells or primary cultured neurons induces oxidative stress, calcium perturbation, increased cobalt quenching of intra-mitochondrial calcein intensity and mitochondrial cytochrome c release, suggesting the involvement of mPTP formation in an Aβ-induced disturbance of calcium and free radical production [60,64-70]. Thus, Aβ mediates ROS accumulation and stimulates intracellular and intra-mitochondrial calcium accumulation, thereby triggering the formation of mPTP, which, in turn, leads to further mitochondrial calcium efflux and free radical generation from mitochondria.

Mechanistically, we know that Aβ enhances translocation of CypD to mitochondrial inner membrane to trigger mPTP formation and forming Aβ-Cyp D complex. Using co-immunoprecipitation of Aβ and Cyp D, Aβ-Cyp D complex was found in mitochondrial fractions from brains of AD subjects and APP mice as well as in neurons and isolated brain mitochondria exposed to Aβ. These findings indicate the presence of Aβ-CypD interaction *in vivo* in brain mitochondria. Using surface plasmon resonance (SPR), different species of Aβ, including monomeric and oligomeric Aβ, were found to have high affinity for binding to Cyp D *in vitro*, confirming interaction of Aβ with Cyp D [7,13]. In addition, a recent report using molecular docking experiments postulates that Aβ binds with ANT [71]. However, we are not aware of any conclusive report regarding interaction of Aβ with ANT.

Although Aβ or oxidative stress could directly or indirectly affect mitochondrial function, such as mPTP formation, enhancement of mPTP formation by Aβ might be due to synergistic action of the two. Given that mPTP is critical for mitochondrial pathology and neuronal dysfunction in the pathogenesis of AD, blocking or limiting mPTP formation holds potential as a therapeutic strategy for AD.

4. Blockage of mPTP Attenuates Aβ-Mediated Neuronal and Mitochondrial Malfunction

Several studies have shown that the blockage of mPTP by either genetic depletion of the mPTP key component, Cyp D or through use of the Cyp D or VDAC inhibitors protects neurons against oxidative stress- or Aβ-induced injury [7, 72-74]. Genetic depletion of Cyp D decreases mitochondrial swelling induced by calcium. Cyp D deficient cells show less oxidative stress and apoptosis and maintain mitochondrial membrane potential even in the presence of stress inducers [7,43,50]. Further, Cyp D depletion attenuates cardiac ischemia and reperfusion injuries in mice [7,75,76] and ameliorates axonal degeneration and movement disorders in a multiple sclerosis (MS) mouse model [77]. To investigate the protective effect of blockading mPTP by genetic depletion of Cyp D in an Aβ milieu, we generated Cyp D deficient APP mice by crossing APP/Aβ overexpressing mice (APP mice) to Cyp D-deficient mice and then investigated the effect of Cyp D depletion on Aβ-induced toxicity. Cyp D-deficient APP mice preserve mitochondrial function including mitochondrial cytochrome c oxidase activity, mitochondrial respiration control ratio and mitochondrial ATP production. Furthermore, the protective effects of CypD deficiency were observed even in aged AD mice (22–24 months), suggesting that abrogation of CypD results in persistent life-long protection against Aβ toxicity in an Alzheimer's disease mouse model [7,13]. Cyp D depletion also results in improved synaptic function and spatial learning memory, even in aged 22-24-month-old APP mice.

Pharmaceutical inhibition of Cyp D is another approach to inhibit mPTP formation. There are several known Cyp D inhibitors: cyclosporin A, sanglifehrin A, FK506 and FK1706. Administration of these inhibitors results in significant protection against mPTP-associated mitochondrial pathology in several animal models of neurodegenerative diseases, as follows. Cyclosporin A injection ameliorated the moving disorders in an ALS mouse models [78]. Cyclosporin A, FK506 or FK1706 treatment attenuated the symptoms of MS mouse models [79]. Administration of cyclosporin A or FK506 also had protective effects on HD mouse model [80]; the protective effects of these Cyp D inhibitors are proposed to be, at least in part, due to the inhibition of mPTP formation. Notably, treatment with Cyp D inhibitors at experimental dosages did not show detectable adverse effects in the mice, suggesting probable safety of these drugs in clinical translation.

The effect of Cyp D inhibitors on Aβ toxicity has also been investigated. We and other groups have demonstrated that cyclosporin A significantly inhibited apoptosis and production of oxidative stress induced by Aβ accumulation [7,13,32,81]. Cyclosporin A treatment attenuated Aβ- induced mitochondrial swelling and increased mitochondrial calcium buffering capacity. In addition, the addition of cyclosporin A to the hippocampal CA1 region completely rescued Aβ-induced long term potentiation (LTP) reduction. These data indicate that pharmaceutical inhibition of Cyp D is a potential strategy to protect neurons from Aβ toxicity [7]. It remains to be determined whether the protective effects of CypD inhibitors are present in animal model studies.

VDAC is another key component of mPTP. A recent report using a VDAC inhibitor, cholest-4-en-3-one oxime (TRO19622), showed results of significantly extended lifespan as well as attenuation of symptoms in G93A SOD1 ALS mice [82]. TRO19622 has not yet been tested in AD mouse or cell models. 4,4'-Diisothiocyanatostilbene-2,2'-disulfonic acid (DIDS) is a VDAC blocker and has been shown to protect cells from VDAC -potentiated cell apoptosis [73]. Small and his colleagues demonstrated that DIDS protected against neurotoxicity induced by Aβ25-35 or staurosporine on primary cultured neurons as evidenced by significantly less cell death upon the application of DIDS. These findings implicate that inhibiting VDAC-mediated mPTP might be a potential therapeutic option for the protection of neurodegeneration in AD [74].

In summary, interventions affecting mPTP formation such as genetic Cyp D depletion or use of Cyp D or VDAC inhibitors have been proven experimentally to be effective in counteracting the detrimental effects of Aβ or oxidative stress on mitochondrial and neuronal perturbation, suggesting that targeting mPTP may result in the rescue of neurons from Aβ-induced damage.

5. Conclusions

We reviewed here the recent studies eliciting the involvement of mPTP in the pathogenesis of AD and the effects of inhibiting mPTP on mitochondrial and neuronal dysfunction. The interplay of Aβ with mPTP may be a novel mechanism underlying Aβ-associated mitochondrial pathology. CypD-dependent mitochondrial permeability transition contributes significantly to Aβ-induced neuronal and mitochondrial injury relevant to the pathogenesis of Alzheimer's disease. In an Aβ-rich environment, Aβ gains access to the mitochondrial matrix by the translocase of the outer membrane (TOM) machinery [10] or an as yet unknown mechanism, and forms a complex with CypD, promoting its translocation to the inner mitochondrial membrane and formation of mPTP. In addition, CypD-Aβ interaction enhances generation of ROS and triggers signal transduction. These events eventually lead to cell death relevant to the AD pathogenesis (Figure 1). Thus, decreasing CypD dependent mPTP formation through pharmacologic inhibition on cyp D is an important therapeutic target for prevention and treatment of Alzheimer disease and other neurodegenerative diseases. There is also potential benefit in the development of new inhibitors of other mitochondrial transition pore components (e.g. VDAC) as therapeutic approaches to treat AD and other diseases.

Figure 1. Cyclophilin D-Aβ interaction: implications for mitochondrial function.

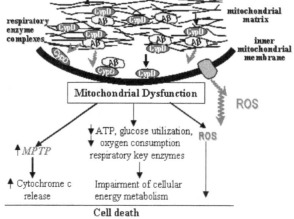

Acknowledgements

This study is supported by National Institutes of Health Grant PO1AG17490 and the Alzheimer's Association.

References and Notes

1. Lustbader, J.W.; Cirilli, M.; Lin, C.; Xu, H.W.; Takuma, K.; Wang, N.; Caspersen, C.; Chen, X.; Pollak, S.; Chaney, M.; Trinchese, F.; Liu, S.; Gunn-Moore, F.; Lue, L.F.; Walker, D.G.; Kuppusamy, P.; Zewier, Z.L.; Arancio, O.; Stern, D.; Yan, S.S.; Wu, H. ABAD directly links Abeta to mitochondrial toxicity in Alzheimer's disease. *Science* **2004**, *304*, 448-452.

2. Selkoe, D.J. Alzheimer's disease is a synaptic failure. *Science* **2002**, *298*, 789-791.

3. Cummings, B.J.; Pike, C.J.; Shankle, R.; Cotman, C.W. Beta-amyloid deposition and other measures of neuropathology predict cognitive status in Alzheimer's disease. *Neurobiol. Aging* **1996**, *17*, 921-933.

4. Gu, Z.; Liu, W.; Yan, Z. {beta}-Amyloid impairs AMPA receptor trafficking and function by reducing Ca2+/calmodulin-dependent protein kinase II synaptic distribution. *J. Biol. Chem.* **2009**, *284*, 10639-10649.

5. Takuma, K.; Fang, F.; Zhang, W.; Yan, S.; Fukuzaki, E.; Du, H.; Sosunov, A.; McKhann, G.; Funatsu, Y.; Nakamichi, N.; Nagai, T.; Mizoguchi, H.; Ibi, D.; Hori, O.; Ogawa, S.; Stern, D.M.; Yamada, K.; Yan, S.S. RAGE-mediated signaling contributes to intraneuronal transport of amyloid-beta and neuronal dysfunction. *Proc. Natl. Acad. Sci. USA* **2009**, *106*, 20021-20026.

6. Caspersen, C.; Wang, N.; Yao, J.; Sosunov, A.; Chen, X.; Lustbader, J.W.; Xu, H.W.; Stern, D.; McKhann, G.; Yan, S.D. Mitochondrial Abeta: a potential focal point for neuronal metabolic dysfunction in Alzheimer's disease. *FASEB J.* **2005**, *19*, 2040-2041.

7. Du, H.; Guo, L.; Fang, F.; Chen, D.; Sosunov, A.A.; McKhann, G.M.; Yan, Y.; Wang, C.; Zhang, H.; Molkentin, J.D.; Gunn-Moore, F.J.; Vonsattel, J.P.; Arancio, O.; Chen, J.X.; Yan, S.D. Cyclophilin D deficiency attenuates mitochondrial and neuronal perturbation and ameliorates learning and memory in Alzheimer's disease. *Nat. Med.* **2008**, *14*, 1097-1105.

8. Wang, X.; Su, B.; Perry, G.; Smith, M.A.; Zhu, X. Insights into amyloid-beta-induced mitochondrial dysfunction in Alzheimer disease. *Free Radical Biol. Med.* **2007**, *43*, 1569-1573.

9. Eckert, A.; Hauptmann, S.; Scherping, I.; Rhein, V.; Muller-Spahn, F.; Gotz, J.; Muller, W.E. Soluble beta-amyloid leads to mitochondrial defects in amyloid precursor protein and tau transgenic mice. *Neuro-Degenerative Dis.* **2008**, *5*, 157-159.

10. Hansson Petersen, C.A.; Alikhani, N.; Behbahani, H.; Wiehager, B.; Pavlov, P.F.; Alafuzoff, I.; Leinonen, V.; Ito, A.; Winblad, B.; Glaser, E.; Ankarcrona, M. The amyloid beta-peptide is imported into mitochondria via the TOM import machinery and localized to mitochondrial cristae. *Proc. Natl. Acad. Sci. USA* **2008**, *105*, 13145-13150.

11. Manczak, M.; Anekonda, T.S.; Henson, E.; Park, B.S.; Quinn, J.; Reddy, P.H. Mitochondria are a direct site of A beta accumulation in Alzheimer's disease neurons: implications for free radical generation and oxidative damage in disease progression. *Hum. Mol. Genet.* **2006**, *15*, 1437-1449.

12. Yao, J.; Irwin, R.W.; Zhao, L.; Nilsen, J.; Hamilton, R.T.; Brinton, R.D. Mitochondrial bioenergetic deficit precedes Alzheimer's pathology in female mouse model of Alzheimer's disease. *Proc. Natl. Acad. Sci. USA* **2009**.

13. Du, H.; Guo, L.; Zhang, W.; Rydzewska, M.; Yan, S. Cyclophilin D deficiency improves mitochondrial function and learning/memory in aging Alzheimer disease mouse model. *Neurobiol. Aging* **2009**.

14. Takuma, K.; Yao, J.; Huang, J.; Xu, H.; Chen, X.; Luddy, J.; Trillat, A.C.; Stern, D.M.; Arancio, O.; Yan, S.S. ABAD enhances Abeta-induced cell stress via mitochondrial dysfunction. *FASEB J.* **2005**, *19*, 597-598.

15. Cardoso, S.M.; Santana, I.; Swerdlow, R.H.; Oliveira, C.R. Mitochondria dysfunction of Alzheimer's disease cybrids enhances Abeta toxicity. *J. Neurochem.* **2004**, *89*, 1417-1426.

16. Hauptmann, S.; Scherping, I.; Drose, S.; Brandt, U.; Schulz, K.L.; Jendrach, M.; Leuner, K.; Eckert, A.; Muller, W.E. Mitochondrial dysfunction: an early event in Alzheimer pathology accumulates with age in AD transgenic mice. *Neurobiol. Aging* **2009**, *30*, 1574-1586.

17. Qiao, H.; Koya, R.C.; Nakagawa, K.; Tanaka, H.; Fujita, H.; Takimoto, M.; Kuzumaki, N. Inhibition of Alzheimer's amyloid-beta peptide-induced reduction of mitochondrial membrane potential and neurotoxicity by gelsolin. *Neurobiol. Aging* **2005**, *26*, 849-855.

18. Casley, C.S.; Canevari, L.; Land, J.M.; Clark, J.B.; Sharpe, M.A. Beta-amyloid inhibits integrated mitochondrial respiration and key enzyme activities. *J. Neurochem.* **2002**, *80*, 91-100.

19. Swerdlow, R.H.; Parks, J.K.; Cassarino, D.S.; Binder, D.R.; Bennett, J.P., Jr.; Di Iorio, G.; Golbe, L.I.; Parker, W.D., Jr. Biochemical analysis of cybrids expressing mitochondrial DNA from Contursi kindred Parkinson's subjects. *Exp. Neurol.* **2001**, *169*, 479-485.

20. Dumont, M.; Wille, E.; Stack, C.; Calingasan, N.Y.; Beal, M.F.; Lin, M.T. Reduction of oxidative stress, amyloid deposition, and memory deficit by manganese superoxide dismutase overexpression in a transgenic mouse model of Alzheimer's disease. *FASEB J.* **2009**, *23*, 2459-2466.

21. Butterfield, D.A.; Galvan, V.; Lange, M.B.; Tang, H.; Sowell, R.A.; Spilman, P.; Fombonne, J.; Gorostiza, O.; Zhang, J.; Sultana, R.; Bredesen, D.E. *In vivo* oxidative stress in brain of Alzheimer disease transgenic mice: Requirement for methionine 35 in amyloid beta-peptide of APP. *Free Radic. Biol. Med.* *48*, 136-144.

22. Ferreiro, E.; Oliveira, C.R.; Pereira, C.M. The release of calcium from the endoplasmic reticulum induced by amyloid-beta and prion peptides activates the mitochondrial apoptotic pathway. *Neurobiol. Dis.* **2008**, *30*, 331-342.

23. Reddy, P.H. Amyloid beta, mitochondrial structural and functional dynamics in Alzheimer's disease. *Exp. Neurol.* **2009**, *218*, 286-292.

24. Suen, K.C.; Lin, K.F.; Elyaman, W.; So, K.F.; Chang, R.C.; Hugon, J. Reduction of calcium release from the endoplasmic reticulum could only provide partial neuroprotection against beta-amyloid peptide toxicity. *J. Neurochem.* **2003**, *87*, 1413-1426.

25. Sanz-Blasco, S.; Valero, R.A.; Rodriguez-Crespo, I.; Villalobos, C.; Nunez, L. Mitochondrial Ca2+ overload underlies Abeta oligomers neurotoxicity providing an unexpected mechanism of neuroprotection by NSAIDs. *PLoS One* **2008**, *3*, e2718.

26. Wang, X.; Su, B.; Lee, H.G.; Li, X.; Perry, G.; Smith, M.A.; Zhu, X. Impaired balance of mitochondrial fission and fusion in Alzheimer's disease. *J. Neurosci.* **2009**, *29*, 9090-9103.

27. Wang, X.; Su, B.; Siedlak, S.L.; Moreira, P.I.; Fujioka, H.; Wang, Y.; Casadesus, G.; Zhu, X. Amyloid-beta overproduction causes abnormal mitochondrial dynamics via differential modulation of mitochondrial fission/fusion proteins. *Proc. Natl. Acad. Sci. USA* **2008**, *105*, 19318-19323.

28. Rui, Y.; Tiwari, P.; Xie, Z.; Zheng, J.Q. Acute impairment of mitochondrial trafficking by beta-amyloid peptides in hippocampal neurons. *J. Neurosci.* **2006**, *26*, 10480-10487.

29. Mancuso, M.; Orsucci, D.; Siciliano, G.; Murri, L. Mitochondria, mitochondrial DNA and Alzheimer's disease. What comes first? *Curr. Alzheimer Res.* **2008**, *5*, 457-468.

30. Swerdlow, R.H. Mitochondrial DNA--related mitochondrial dysfunction in neurodegenerative diseases. *Arch. Pathol. Lab. Med.* **2002**, *126*, 271-280.

31. Bozner, P.; Grishko, V.; LeDoux, S.P.; Wilson, G.L.; Chyan, Y.C.; Pappolla, M.A. The amyloid beta protein induces oxidative damage of mitochondrial DNA. *J. Neuropathol. Exp. Neurol.* **1997**, *56*, 1356-1362.

32. Moreira, P.I.; Santos, M.S.; Moreno, A.; Rego, A.C.; Oliveira, C. Effect of amyloid beta-peptide on permeability transition pore: a comparative study. *J. Neurosci. Res.* **2002**, *69*, 257-267.

33. Billups, B.; Forsythe, I.D. Presynaptic mitochondrial calcium sequestration influences transmission at mammalian central synapses. *J. Neurosci.* **2002**, *22*, 5840-5847.

34. Li, Z.; Okamoto, K.; Hayashi, Y.; Sheng, M. The importance of dendritic mitochondria in the morphogenesis and plasticity of spines and synapses. *Cell* **2004**, *119*, 873-887.

35. Reddy, P.H.; Beal, M.F. Amyloid beta, mitochondrial dysfunction and synaptic damage: implications for cognitive decline in aging and Alzheimer's disease. *Trends Mol. Med.* **2008**, *14*, 45-53.

36. Li, G.; Zou, L.Y.; Cao, C.M.; Yang, E.S. Coenzyme Q10 protects SHSY5Y neuronal cells from beta amyloid toxicity and oxygen-glucose deprivation by inhibiting the opening of the mitochondrial permeability transition pore. *Biofactors* **2005**, *25*, 97-107.

37. Moreira, P.I.; Santos, M.S.; Moreno, A.; Oliveira, C. Amyloid beta-peptide promotes permeability transition pore in brain mitochondria. *Biosci. Rep.* **2001**, *21*, 789-800.

38. Shevtzova, E.F.; Kireeva, E.G.; Bachurin, S.O. Effect of beta-amyloid peptide fragment 25-35 on nonselective permeability of mitochondria. *Bull. Exp. Biol. Med.* **2001**, *132*, 1173-1176.

39. Baumgartner, H.K.; Gerasimenko, J.V.; Thorne, C.; Ferdek, P.; Pozzan, T.; Tepikin, A.V.; Petersen, O.H.; Sutton, R.; Watson, A.J.; Gerasimenko, O.V. Calcium elevation in mitochondria is the main Ca2+ requirement for mitochondrial permeability transition pore (mPTP) opening. *J. Biol. Chem.* **2009**, *284*, 20796-20803.

40. Halestrap, A. Biochemistry: a pore way to die. *Nature* **2005**, *434*, 578-579.

41. Kowaltowski, A.J.; Castilho, R.F.; Vercesi, A.E. Opening of the mitochondrial permeability transition pore by uncoupling or inorganic phosphate in the presence of Ca2+ is dependent on mitochondrial-generated reactive oxygen species. *FEBS Lett.* **1996**, *378*, 150-152.

42. Clarke, S.J.; Khaliulin, I.; Das, M.; Parker, J.E.; Heesom, K.J.; Halestrap, A.P. Inhibition of mitochondrial permeability transition pore opening by ischemic preconditioning is probably

mediated by reduction of oxidative stress rather than mitochondrial protein phosphorylation. *Circ. Res.* **2008**, *102*, 1082-1090.

43. Baines, C.P.; Kaiser, R.A.; Purcell, N.H.; Blair, N.S.; Osinska, H.; Hambleton, M.A.; Brunskill, E.W.; Sayen, M.R.; Gottlieb, R.A.; Dorn, G.W.; Robbins, J.; Molkentin, J.D. Loss of cyclophilin D reveals a critical role for mitochondrial permeability transition in cell death. *Nature* **2005**, *434*, 658-662.

44. Connern, C.P.; Halestrap, A.P. Chaotropic agents and increased matrix volume enhance binding of mitochondrial cyclophilin to the inner mitochondrial membrane and sensitize the mitochondrial permeability transition to [Ca2+]. *Biochemistry* **1996**, *35*, 8172-8180.

45. Zheng, Y.; Shi, Y.; Tian, C.; Jiang, C.; Jin, H.; Chen, J.; Almasan, A.; Tang, H.; Chen, Q. Essential role of the voltage-dependent anion channel (VDAC) in mitochondrial permeability transition pore opening and cytochrome c release induced by arsenic trioxide. *Oncogene* **2004**, *23*, 1239-1247.

46. Pestana, C.R.; Silva, C.H.; Pardo-Andreu, G.L.; Rodrigues, F.P.; Santos, A.C.; Uyemura, S.A.; Curti, C. Ca(2+) binding to c-state of adenine nucleotide translocase (ANT)-surrounding cardiolipins enhances (ANT)-Cys(56) relative mobility: a computational-based mitochondrial permeability transition study. *Biochim. Biophys. Acta* **2009**, *1787*, 176-182.

47. Leung, A.W.; Varanyuwatana, P.; Halestrap, A.P. The mitochondrial phosphate carrier interacts with cyclophilin D and may play a key role in the permeability transition. *J. Biol. Chem.* **2008**, *283*, 26312-26323.

48. Li, V.; Brustovetsky, T.; Brustovetsky, N. Role of cyclophilin D-dependent mitochondrial permeability transition in glutamate-induced calcium deregulation and excitotoxic neuronal death. *Exp. Neurol.* **2009**, *218*, 171-182.

49. Nakagawa, T.; Shimizu, S.; Watanabe, T.; Yamaguchi, O.; Otsu, K.; Yamagata, H.; Inohara, H.; Kubo, T.; Tsujimoto, Y. Cyclophilin D-dependent mitochondrial permeability transition regulates some necrotic but not apoptotic cell death. *Nature* **2005**, *434*, 652-658.

50. Schinzel, A.C.; Takeuchi, O.; Huang, Z.; Fisher, J.K.; Zhou, Z.; Rubens, J.; Hetz, C.; Danial, N.N.; Moskowitz, M.A.; Korsmeyer, S.J. Cyclophilin D is a component of mitochondrial permeability transition and mediates neuronal cell death after focal cerebral ischemia. *Proc. Natl. Acad. Sci. USA* **2005**, *102*, 12005-12010.

51. Martin, L.J.; Gertz, B.; Pan, Y.; Price, A.C.; Molkentin, J.D.; Chang, Q. The mitochondrial permeability transition pore in motor neurons: involvement in the pathobiology of ALS mice. *Exp. Neurol.* **2009**, *218*, 333-346.

52. Karlsson, J.; Fong, K.S.; Hansson, M.J.; Elmer, E.; Csiszar, K.; Keep, M.F. Life span extension and reduced neuronal death after weekly intraventricular cyclosporin injections in the G93A transgenic mouse model of amyotrophic lateral sclerosis. *J. Neurosurg.* **2004**, *101*, 128-137.

53. Brustovetsky, N.; Brustovetsky, T.; Purl, K.J.; Capano, M.; Crompton, M.; Dubinsky, J.M. Increased susceptibility of striatal mitochondria to calcium-induced permeability transition. *J. Neurosci.* **2003**, *23*, 4858-4867.

54. Gandhi, S.; Wood-Kaczmar, A.; Yao, Z.; Plun-Favreau, H.; Deas, E.; Klupsch, K.; Downward, J.; Latchman, D.S.; Tabrizi, S.J.; Wood, N.W.; Duchen, M.R.; Abramov, A.Y. PINK1-associated

Parkinson's disease is caused by neuronal vulnerability to calcium-induced cell death. *Mol. Cell* **2009**, *33*, 627-638.

55. Wang, H.L.; Chou, A.H.; Yeh, T.H.; Li, A.H.; Chen, Y.L.; Kuo, Y.L.; Tsai, S.R.; Yu, S.T. PINK1 mutants associated with recessive Parkinson's disease are defective in inhibiting mitochondrial release of cytochrome c. *Neurobiol. Dis.* **2007**, *28*, 216-226.

56. Brown, M.R.; Sullivan, P.G.; Geddes, J.W. Synaptic mitochondria are more susceptible to Ca2+overload than nonsynaptic mitochondria. *J. Biol. Chem.* **2006**, *281*, 11658-11668.

57. Rockenstein, E.M.; McConlogue, L.; Tan, H.; Power, M.; Masliah, E.; Mucke, L. Levels and alternative splicing of amyloid beta protein precursor (APP) transcripts in brains of APP transgenic mice and humans with Alzheimer's disease. *J. Biol. Chem.* **1995**, *270*, 28257-28267.

58. Mucke, L.; Masliah, E.; Johnson, W.B.; Ruppe, M.D.; Alford, M.; Rockenstein, E.M.; Forss-Petter, S.; Pietropaolo, M.; Mallory, M.; Abraham, C.R. Synaptotrophic effects of human amyloid beta protein precursors in the cortex of transgenic mice. *Brain Res.* **1994**, *666*, 151-167.

59. Soskic, V.; Klemm, M.; Proikas-Cezanne, T.; Schwall, G.P.; Poznanovic, S.; Stegmann, W.; Groebe, K.; Zengerling, H.; Schoepf, R.; Burnet, M.; Schrattenholz, A. A connection between the mitochondrial permeability transition pore, autophagy, and cerebral amyloidogenesis. *J. Proteome Res.* **2008**, *7*, 2262-2269.

60. Moreira, A.E.; Hueb, W.A.; Soares, P.R.; Meneghetti, J.C.; Jorge, M.C.; Chalela, W.A.; Martinez Filho, E.E.; Oliveira, S.A.; Jatene, F.B.; Ramires, J.A. Comparative study between the therapeutic effects of surgical myocardial revascularization and coronary angioplasty in equivalent ischemic situations: analysis through myocardial scintigraphy with 99mTc-Sestamibi. *Arq. Bras. Cardiol.* **2005**, *85*, 92-99.

61. Chin, J.H.; Tse, F.W.; Harris, K.; Jhamandas, J.H. Beta-amyloid enhances intracellular calcium rises mediated by repeated activation of intracellular calcium stores and nicotinic receptors in acutely dissociated rat basal forebrain neurons. *Brain Cell Biol.* **2006**, *35*, 173-186.

62. Brewer, G.J.; Lim, A.; Capps, N.G.; Torricelli, J.R. Age-related calcium changes, oxyradical damage, caspase activation and nuclear condensation in hippocampal neurons in response to glutamate and beta-amyloid. *Exp. Gerontol.* **2005**, *40*, 426-437.

63. Schoneich, C.; Pogocki, D.; Hug, G.L.; Bobrowski, K. Free radical reactions of methionine in peptides: mechanisms relevant to beta-amyloid oxidation and Alzheimer's disease. *J. Am. Chem. Soc.* **2003**, *125*, 13700-13713.

64. Morais Cardoso, S.; Swerdlow, R.H.; Oliveira, C.R. Induction of cytochrome c-mediated apoptosis by amyloid beta 25-35 requires functional mitochondria. *Brain Res.* **2002**, *931*, 117-125.

65. Celsi, F.; Svedberg, M.; Unger, C.; Cotman, C.W.; Carri, M.T.; Ottersen, O.P.; Nordberg, A.; Torp, R. Beta-amyloid causes downregulation of calcineurin in neurons through induction of oxidative stress. *Neurobiol. Dis.* **2007**, *26*, 342-352.

66. Montiel, T.; Quiroz-Baez, R.; Massieu, L.; Arias, C. Role of oxidative stress on beta-amyloid neurotoxicity elicited during impairment of energy metabolism in the hippocampus: protection by antioxidants. *Exp. Neurol.* **2006**, *200*, 496-508.

67. Parks, J.K.; Smith, T.S.; Trimmer, P.A.; Bennett, J.P., Jr.; Parker, W.D., Jr. Neurotoxic Abeta peptides increase oxidative stress *in vivo* through NMDA-receptor and nitric-oxide-synthase

mechanisms, and inhibit complex IV activity and induce a mitochondrial permeability transition *in vitro*. *J. Neurochem.* **2001**, *76*, 1050-1056.

68. Kim, H.S.; Lee, J.H.; Lee, J.P.; Kim, E.M.; Chang, K.A.; Park, C.H.; Jeong, S.J.; Wittendorp, M.C.; Seo, J.H.; Choi, S.H.; Suh, Y.H. Amyloid beta peptide induces cytochrome C release from isolated mitochondria. *Neuroreport* **2002**, *13*, 1989-1993.

69. Rodrigues, C.M.; Sola, S.; Brito, M.A.; Brondino, C.D.; Brites, D.; Moura, J.J. Amyloid beta-peptide disrupts mitochondrial membrane lipid and protein structure: protective role of tauroursodeoxycholate. *Biochem. Biophys. Res. Commun.* **2001**, *281*, 468-474.

70. Zhang, S.; Zhang, Z.; Sandhu, G.; Ma, X.; Yang, X.; Geiger, J.D.; Kong, J. Evidence of oxidative stress-induced BNIP3 expression in amyloid beta neurotoxicity. *Brain Res.* **2007**, *1138*, 221-230.

71. Singh, P.; Suman, S.; Chandna, S.; Das, T.K. Possible role of amyloid-beta, adenine nucleotide translocase and cyclophilin-D interaction in mitochondrial dysfunction of Alzheimer's disease. *Bioinformation* **2009**, *3*, 440-445.

72. Vlachos, P.; Nyman, U.; Hajji, N.; Joseph, B. The cell cycle inhibitor p57(Kip2) promotes cell death via the mitochondrial apoptotic pathway. *Cell Death Differ.* **2007**, *14*, 1497-1507.

73. Vale, C.; Nicolaou, K.C.; Frederick, M.O.; Vieytes, M.R.; Botana, L.M. Cell volume decrease as a link between azaspiracid-induced cytotoxicity and c-Jun-N-terminal kinase activation in cultured neurons. *Toxicol Sci.* *113*, 158-168.

74. Xia, Z.; Tauskela, J.; Small, D.L. Disulfonic stilbenes prevent beta-amyloid (25-35) neuronal toxicity in rat cortical cultures. *Neurosci. Lett.* **2003**, *340*, 53-56.

75. Clarke, S.J.; McStay, G.P.; Halestrap, A.P. Sanglifehrin A acts as a potent inhibitor of the mitochondrial permeability transition and reperfusion injury of the heart by binding to cyclophilin-D at a different site from cyclosporin A. *J. Biol. Chem.* **2002**, *277*, 34793-34799.

76. Halestrap, A.P.; Connern, C.P.; Griffiths, E.J.; Kerr, P.M. Cyclosporin A binding to mitochondrial cyclophilin inhibits the permeability transition pore and protects hearts from ischaemia/reperfusion injury. *Mol. Cell Biochem* **1997**, *174*, 167-172.

77. Forte, M.; Gold, B.G.; Marracci, G.; Chaudhary, P.; Basso, E.; Johnsen, D.; Yu, X.; Fowlkes, J.; Rahder, M.; Stem, K.; Bernardi, P.; Bourdette, D. Cyclophilin D inactivation protects axons in experimental autoimmune encephalomyelitis, an animal model of multiple sclerosis. *Proc. Natl. Acad. Sci. USA* **2007**, *104*, 7558-7563.

78. Keep, M.; Elmer, E.; Fong, K.S.; Csiszar, K. Intrathecal cyclosporin prolongs survival of late-stage ALS mice. *Brain Res.* **2001**, *894*, 327-331.

79. Gold, B.G.; Voda, J.; Yu, X.; McKeon, G.; Bourdette, D.N. FK506 and a nonimmunosuppressant derivative reduce axonal and myelin damage in experimental autoimmune encephalomyelitis: neuroimmunophilin ligand-mediated neuroprotection in a model of multiple sclerosis. *J. Neurosci. Res.* **2004**, *77*, 367-377.

80. Kumar, P.; Kumar, A. Neuroprotective effect of cyclosporine and FK506 against 3-nitropropionic acid induced cognitive dysfunction and glutathione redox in rat: possible role of nitric oxide. *Neurosci. Res.* **2009**, *63*, 302-314.

81. Van Den Heuvel, C.; Donkin, J.J.; Finnie, J.W.; Blumbergs, P.C.; Kuchel, T.; Koszyca, B.; Manavis, J.; Jones, N.R.; Reilly, P.L.; Vink, R. Downregulation of amyloid precursor protein

(APP) expression following post-traumatic cyclosporin-A administration. *J. Neurotrauma* **2004**, *21*, 1562-1572.

82. Bordet, T.; Buisson, B.; Michaud, M.; Drouot, C.; Galea, P.; Delaage, P.; Akentieva, N.P.; Evers, A.S.; Covey, D.F.; Ostuni, M.A.; Lacapere, J.J.; Massaad, C.; Schumacher, M.; Steidl, E.M.; Maux, D.; Delaage, M.; Henderson, C.E.; Pruss, R.M. Identification and characterization of cholest-4-en-3-one, oxime (TRO19622), a novel drug candidate for amyotrophic lateral sclerosis. *J. Pharmacol. Exp. Ther.* **2007**, *322*, 709-720.

Mitochondria-Derived Reactive Oxygen Species Play an Important Role in Doxorubicin-Induced Platelet Apoptosis

Zhicheng Wang [1,†,*], Jie Wang [1,†], Rufeng Xie [2], Ruilai Liu [1] and Yuan Lu [1,*]

[1]   Department of Laboratory Medicine, Huashan Hospital, Shanghai Medical College,
     Fudan University, Shanghai 200040, China; E-Mails: Jiewang2015@126.com (J.W.);
     liuruilai88@163.com (R.L.)

[2]   Blood Engineering Laboratory, Shanghai Blood Center, Shanghai 200051, China;
     E-Mail: xierufeng555@163.com

†   These authors contributed equally to this work.

*   Authors to whom correspondence should be addressed;
    E-Mails: ahwzc@126.com (Z.W.); yuanlu@hsh.stn.sh.cn (Y.L.)

Academic Editors: Lars Olson, Jaime M. Ross and Giuseppe Coppotelli

---

Abstract: Doxorubicin (DOX) is an effective chemotherapeutic agent; however; its use is limited by some side effects; such as cardiotoxicity and thrombocytopenia. DOX-induced cardiotoxicity has been intensively investigated; however; DOX-induced thrombocytopenia has not been clearly elucidated. Here we show that DOX-induced mitochondria-mediated intrinsic apoptosis and glycoprotein (GP)Ibα shedding in platelets. DOX did not induce platelet activation; whereas; DOX obviously reduced adenosine diphosphate (ADP)- and thrombin-induced platelet aggregation; and impaired platelet adhesion on the von Willebrand factor (vWF) surface. In addition; we also show that DOX induced intracellular reactive oxygen species (ROS) production and mitochondrial ROS generation in a dose-dependent manner. The mitochondria-targeted ROS scavenger Mito-TEMPO blocked intracellular ROS and mitochondrial ROS generation. Furthermore; Mito-TEMPO reduced DOX-induced platelet apoptosis and GPIbα shedding. These data indicate that DOX induces platelet apoptosis; and impairs platelet function. Mitochondrial ROS play a pivotal role in DOX-induced platelet apoptosis and GPIbα shedding. Therefore; DOX-induced platelet apoptosis might contribute to DOX-triggered thrombocytopenia; and mitochondria-targeted

ROS scavenger would have potential clinical utility in platelet-associated disorders involving mitochondrial oxidative damage.

Keywords: platelets; mitochondria; reactive oxygen species; doxorubicin; apoptosis

---

1. Introduction

Doxorubicin (DOX) has been used for the treatment of solid tumors and hematologic malignancy. However, DOX therapy has some side effects, such as thrombocytopenia [1,2]. Up to now, the pathogenesis of DOX-induced thrombocytopenia is not completely understood. Recently, several studies have reported that DOX can induce platelet cytotoxicity and procoagulant activity [2,3]. It has been generally accepted the anticancer effects of DOX via inducing apoptosis of malignant cell [4,5]. Platelet apoptosis induced by either physiological or chemical compounds occurs widely *in vitro* or *in vivo* [6–10], which might play important roles in controlling the number of circulating platelets or in the development of platelet-related diseases. Accumulating evidences indicate that platelet apoptosis might play a key role in chemotherapeutic agents induced-thrombocytopenia [8,9].

DOX localizes to the mitochondria and is highly susceptible to enzymatic reduction to generate ROS, which can cause mitochondrial swelling and ultrastructural changes and alter mitochondrial function [11]. Recently, most studies supported that the major mechanism of DOX-induced apoptosis was related to excessive generation of intracellular ROS [11–16]. Mitochondria are considered the main intracellular source of ROS [17]. ROS are produced at very low levels during mitochondrial respiration under normal physiological conditions. The formation of ROS occurs when unpaired electrons escape the electron transport chain and react with molecular oxygen, generating ROS. Complexes I, II, and III of the electron transport chain are the major potential loci for ROS generation [18,19]. Recently, several studies reported that NADPH oxidase 4 (NOX4) localizes to mitochondria, and NOX4 is a novel source of ROS produced in the mitochondria [20,21]. ROS degradation is performed by endogenous enzymatic antioxidants, such as superoxide dismutase, catalase, and non-enzymatic antioxidants, such as glutathione, ascorbic acid [17]. Under physiological conditions, ROS are maintained at proper levels by a balance between its synthesis and its elimination. An increase in ROS generation, a decrease in antioxidant capacity, or a combination both will lead to oxidative stress [17].

In recent years, mitochondria-targeted ROS antagonists and mitochondrial ROS detection probes have been developed. Thus, with the advent of such tools, the importance of mitochondrial ROS in cell signaling, proliferation and apoptosis gradually attracted much attention. For example, Cheung *et al.* [12] recently reported that SIRT3 prevents DOX-induced mitochondrial ROS production in H9c2 cardiomyocytes. Increased mitochondrial ROS is a significant contributor to the development of DOX-induced myopathy in both cardiac and skeletal muscle fibers [13].

We recently reported that mitochondrial ROS play important roles in hyperthermia-induced platelets [7]. In the present study, using mitochondria-targeted ROS scavenger and mitochondrial ROS detection probe, we explored whether DOX induces mitochondrial ROS production, and whether mitochondria-targeted ROS scavenger has a protective effect on DOX-induced platelet apoptosis.

2. Results

2.1. Doxorubicin (DOX) Dose-Dependently Induces $\Delta\Psi m$ Depolarization and Phosphatidylserine (PS) Exposure in Platelets

In order to investigate whether DOX could induce platelet apoptosis, platelets were incubated with different concentrations of DOX. The effect of DOX on platelet $\Delta\Psi m$ depolarization and PS exposure is analyzed by flow cytometry. We found that DOX dose-dependently induced $\Delta\Psi m$ depolarization and PS exposure (Figure 1A,B). In order to investigate the effect of incubation time on apoptosis, platelets were incubated with DOX for different times. The data indicate that DOX time-dependently induced $\Delta\Psi m$ depolarization and PS exposure (Figure 1C,D). Therefore, in order to obtain obvious apoptotic events, 3 h incubation was selected for the following experiments.

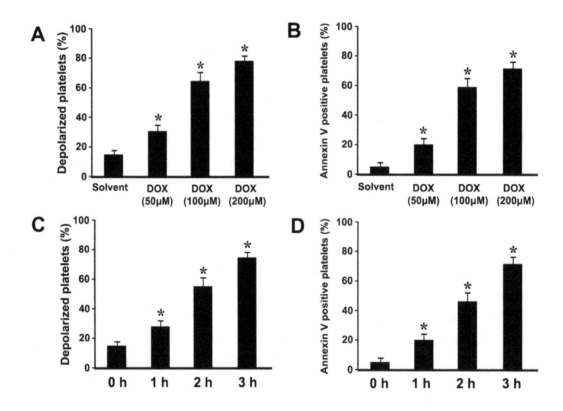

Figure 1. Doxorubicin (DOX) induced mitochondrial inner transmembrane potential ($\Delta\Psi m$) depolarization and PS exposure. (**A–D**) Platelets were incubated with different concentrations of DOX or solvent control (**A,B**), or incubated with DOX (200 μM) at 37 °C for different times (**C,D**). Treated platelets were incubated with tetramethylrhodamine ethyl ester (TMRE) (**A,C**), or fluorescein isothiocyanate (FITC)-conjugated annexin V (**B,D**), and analyzed by flow cytometry. $\Delta\Psi m$ depolarization was quantified as the percentage of depolarized platelets. Means ± SEM from three independent experiments are shown (**A,C**). PS exposure was quantified as the percentage of PS positive platelets. Means ± SEM of the percentage of PS positive platelets from three independent experiments are shown (**B,D**). * $p < 0.017$ (after a Bonferroni correction) compared with solvent control.

2.2. DOX Dose-Dependently Induces Mitochondrial Translocation of Bax, Cytochrome C Release, and Caspase-3 Activation in Platelets

Pro-apoptotic protein Bax translocation to the mitochondria is a key event that regulates the release of apoptogenic factors like cytochrome C from the mitochondria, which leads to activation of caspases such as executioner caspase-3 [22]. Thus, to further explore whether DOX could induce mitochondrial translocation of Bax and cytochrome C release, platelets were incubated with different concentrations of DOX and subjected to isolation and analysis of cytosolic and mitochondrial fractions. We found that DOX dose-dependently promoted mitochondrial translocation of Bax and cytochrome C release (Figure 2A,B). Meanwhile, caspase-3 activation was examined in DOX-treated platelets. Compared with the control, the 17-kDa caspase-3 fragment, which indicated the activation of caspase-3, dose-dependently increased in platelets treated with DOX (Figure 2C). Taken together, these data suggested that DOX induced apoptotic cascades leading to platelet apoptosis.

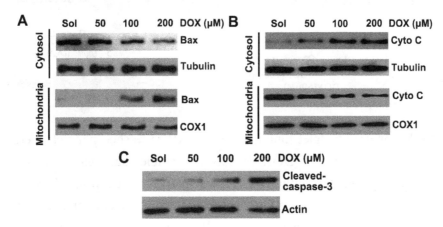

Figure 2. DOX induced mitochondrial translocation of Bax, cytochrome C release, and caspase-3 activation. (**A,B**) Platelets were incubated with different concentrations of DOX or solvent. Treated platelets were lysed, and cytosol and mitochondrial fractions were isolated and analyzed by Western blot with anti-Bax (**A**), and anti-cytochrome C antibodies (**B**), COX1 and tubulin were used as internal controls; (**C**) Platelets were incubated with different concentrations of DOX or solvent. Treated platelets were lysed and analyzed by Western blot with anti-caspase-3 antibody. Actin levels were assayed to demonstrate equal protein loading. Representative data of three independent experiments are presented. Cytochrome C is labeled as Cyto C.

2.3. DOX Impairs Platelet Function

Platelets play a central role in maintaining integrity of endothelium and biological hemostasis. To investigate the effect of DOX on platelet function, platelets were treated with different concentrations of DOX or solvent control, and then examined for platelet aggregation and adhesion. ADP- and thrombin-induced platelet aggregations were reduced in DOX-treated platelets in a dose-dependent manner (Figure 3A,B). Furthermore, compared with solvent control, DOX-treated platelets displayed a significant decrease in adhering on the vWF surface in dose-dependent manner (Figure 3C). Taken together, these data indicate that platelet functions are impaired by DOX.

The interaction of GPIbα with vWF at sites of injured blood vessel walls initiates platelet adhesion under flow conditions [23]. GPIbα shedding is a physiological regulatory mechanism leading to platelet dysfunction [23]. In order to investigate whether GPIbα shedding is involved in DOX-induced platelet dysfunction, GPIbα shedding was examined in platelets incubated with DOX. We found that glycocalicin, which is a cleaved production of GPIbα, gradually increased with increasing concentration of DOX (Figure 3D).

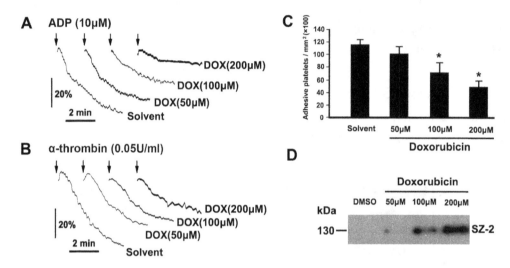

Figure 3. DOX impaired platelet function. (**A**,**B**) PRP or washed platelets were incubated with different concentrations of DOX or solvent. Platelet aggregation was induced by addition of ADP (**A**) or thrombin (**B**); representative traces from three independent experiments are shown; (**C**) Platelets were incubated with different concentrations of DOX or solvent. Treated platelets were perfused into vWF-coated glass capillary. The results from three independent experiments are shown as the means ± SEM of cell number/mm^2. * $p < 0.017$ (after Bonferroni correction) as compared with solvent; (**D**) Platelets were incubated with different concentrations of DOX or solvent. Treated platelets were centrifuged, and the supernatants were analyzed by Western blot with SZ-2. Representative data of three independent experiments are presented.

2.4. DOX Dose-Dependently Increases Intracellular ROS and Mitochondrial ROS Production in Platelets

In order to investigate whether DOX augments intracellular ROS levels in platelets, we determined platelet ROS levels using DCFDA. As shown in Figure 4A, DOX dose-dependently induced ROS production. As a positive control, A23187 significantly induces intracellular ROS production (Figure 4A). Several potential sources of ROS have been suggested, including the mitochondria and NADPH oxidase. Several reports support a role for NADPH oxidase in DOX-induced nuclear cell apoptosis [15,16]. In order to investigate the sources of ROS in DOX-treated anuclear platelets, apocynin, which is an inhibitor of NADPH oxidase, and Mito-TEMPO, which is a mitochondria-targeted ROS antagonist, were used. We found that DOX-induced ROS production was partly inhibited by apocynin, and was obviously inhibited by Mito-TEMPO (Figure 4B). These data demonstrate that mitochondria are a major source of ROS in DOX-treated platelets.

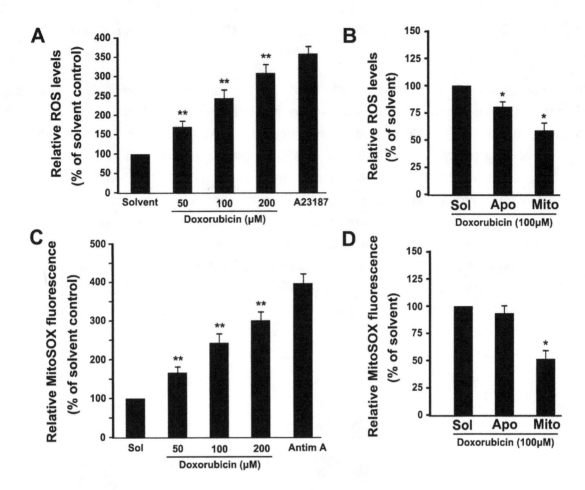

Figure 4. DOX increased intracellular ROS and mitochondrial ROS production. (**A–D**) Platelets were loaded with 2'7'-dichlorofluorescin diacetate (DCFDA) (**A,B**) or MitoSOX™ Red (**C,D**), and incubated with various concentrations of DOX or solvent (**A,C**), or pre-incubated with apocynin, Mito-TEMPO, and then incubated with DOX (**B,D**). As a positive control, loaded platelets were incubated with A23187 (3 µM) or antimycin A (50 µM) at 37 °C for 30 min. Treated platelets were analyzed for intracellular ROS or mitochondrial ROS levels by flow cytometry. The relative ROS levels are expressed as a percentage of platelets, which were incubated with solvent. Data are expressed as a percentage of platelets that were incubated with solvent control. Percentage is presented as means ± SEM from three independent experiments. ** $p < 0.017$ (after Bonferroni correction) as compared with solvent control. * $p < 0.025$ (after Bonferroni correction) as compared with solvent control. Solvent, apocynin, Mito-TEMPO and Antimycin A are labeled as Sol, Apo, Mito and Antim A, respectively.

To assist in confirming that mitochondria were a major site of ROS production in DOX-treated platelets, we used MitoSOX™ Red fluorescence, which detects superoxide synthesis, to quantify mitochondrial ROS [7]. We found that DOX dose-dependently induced mitochondrial superoxide production (Figure 4C). In addition, Mito-TEMPO significantly inhibited DOX-induced mitochondrial ROS generation as compared with the solvent control (Figure 4D). Together, these observations further confirm that DOX can induce mitochondrial ROS production in platelets. As a positive control, we found that antimycin A markedly induced mitochondrial ROS production in platelets (Figure 4C).

2.5. DOX Dose-Dependently Increases Malonyldialdehyde (MDA) Production and Cardiolipin Peroxidation in Platelets

Phospholipids are rich in unsaturated fatty acids that are particularly susceptible to ROS attack, which promotes lipid peroxidation. In order to demonstrate whether DOX treatment induces lipid peroxidation in platelets, we detected the production of MDA, which is a sensitive indicator of ROS-mediated lipid peroxidation. Production of MDA was increased in a dose-dependent manner (Figure 5A), suggesting that DOX induces platelet lipid peroxidation. Mito-TEMPO partly inhibited DOX-induced MDA production (Figure 5B). Mitochondria are the primary site of ROS generation and the major target of ROS. Cardiolipin, a unique phospholipid located at the level of the inner mitochondrial membrane, contains polyunsaturated fatty acid residues, and are thus highly prone to oxidation. In order to demonstrate whether DOX treatment induces cardiolipin peroxidation in platelets, we used the fluorescent dye NAO to estimate cardiolipin peroxidation. NAO binds to cardiolipin with high affinity, and the fluorochrome loses its affinity for peroxidized cardiolipin [7]. As shown in Figure 5C, cardiolipin peroxidation was increased in a dose-dependent manner. Mito-TEMPO obviously inhibited DOX-induced cardiolipin peroxidation (Figure 5D).

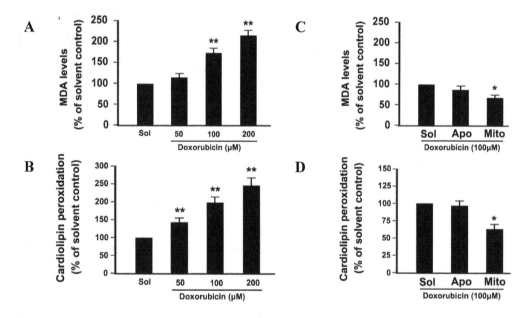

Figure 5. DOX increased malonyldialdehyde (MDA) production and cardiolipin peroxidation. (**A,B**) Platelets were incubated with different concentrations of DOX or solvent (**A**), or pre-incubated with apocynin, Mito-TEMPO, and then incubated with DOX (**B**). MDA levels were measured using an MDA assay kit. The MDA levels are expressed as a percentage of platelets that were incubated with solvent; (**C,D**) Platelets were incubated with different concentrations of DOX or solvent (**C**), or pre-incubated with apocynin, Mito-TEMPO, and then incubated with DOX (**D**). Cardiolipin peoxidation was detected as described in Methods. Data are expressed as a percentage of platelets that were incubated with solvent. Percentage is presented as means ± SEM from three independent experiments. ** $p < 0.017$ (after Bonferroni correction) as compared with solvent. * $p < 0.025$ (after Bonferroni correction) as compared with solvent control. Solvent, apocynin and Mito-TEMPO and are labeled as Sol, Apo and Mito, respectively.

2.6. Mitochondrial ROS Mediates DOX-Induced Platelet Apoptosis

The above observations confirmed that DOX treatment enhanced mitochondrial ROS levels in platelets. To investigate whether mitochondria-derived ROS were involved in DOX-induced platelet apoptotic events, Mito-TEMPO was pre-incubated with platelets before to DOX treatment. We found that Mito-TEMPO significantly inhibited DOX-induced platelets apoptosis, including $\Delta\Psi$m dissipation, PS exposure, caspase-3 activation, mitochondrial translocation of Bax, and cytochrome C release (Figure 6A–E). Together, these data indicate that mitochondrial-derived ROS play a pivotal role in DOX-induced platelet apoptosis. In addition, Mito-TEMPO also partly inhibited DOX-induced GPIbα shedding (Figure 6F).

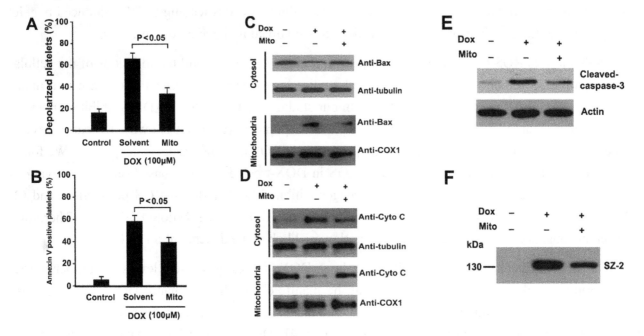

Figure 6. Mitochondria-targeted ROS scavenger attenuated DOX- induced platelet apoptosis. (**A,B**) Platelets were pre-incubated with Mito-TEMPO or solvent, and then incubated with DOX; Treated platelets were incubated with TMRE (**A**), or annexin V-FITC (**B**), and analyzed by flow cytometry. $\Delta\Psi$m depolarization and PS exposure was quantified as the percentage of depolarized platelets. Means ± SEM from three independent experiments are shown; (**C,D**) Platelets were pre-incubated with Mito-TEMPO or solvent, and then incubated with DOX. Treated platelets were lysed, and cytosol and mitochondrial fractions were isolated and analyzed by Western blot with anti-Bax (**C**), and anti-cytochrome C antibodies (**D**); Representative results of three independent experiments are presented; (**E**) Platelets were pro-incubated with Mito-TEMPO or solvent, and then incubated with DOX. Treated platelets were lysed and analyzed by Western blot with anti-caspase-3 antibody. Actin levels were assayed to demonstrate equal protein loading. Representative results of three independent experiments are presented; (**F**) Platelets were pre-incubated with Mito-TEMPO or solvent, and then incubated with DOX. Treated platelets were centrifuged, and supernatants were analyzed by Western blot with SZ-2. Representative results of three independent experiments are presented. Mito-TEMPO is labeled as Mito.

3. Discussion

DOX is a highly effective chemotherapeutic agent that is widely used to treat a variety of cancers, however, its use is limited by some side effects, such as cardiotoxicity and thrombocytopenia [1,2,11,12]. Although it has been generally accepted that DOX exerts its anticancer effect by inducing different kinds of malignant cells apoptosis, it still remains unclear whether DOX incurs platelet apoptosis. In the current observation, DOX dose-dependently induces $\Delta\Psi m$ depolarization, PS exposure, mitochondrial translocation of Bax, cytochrome C release and caspase-3 activation, providing sufficient evidence to indicate that DOX incurs mitochondria-mediated intrinsic platelet apoptosis. We also found that DOX did not induce platelet activation through examining P-selectin expression and PAC-1 binding (data not shown). In addition, we have tried to explore the signaling cascades leading to DOX-induced platelet apoptosis, and the data indicate mitochondrial ROS is involved in the apoptotic process.

DOX induces ROS generation and apoptosis in various cell types, and the identities of the cellular sources of ROS remain controversial. Several studies have shown that NADPH oxidase is a major source of ROS in DOX-treated cells [15,16]. In our studies, we found that NADPH inhibitor apocynin did not significantly inhibited DOX-induced platelet apoptosis (data not shown). Recently, several studies have shown that mitochondria are major source of ROS in DOX-treated cells [12,13]. We found that mitochondria are the primary source of ROS in DOX-treated platelets based on our observations that (1) the mitochondria-targeted ROS scavenger inhibited DOX-induced ROS production; and (2) DOX-induced ROS was detected by the mitochondrial ROS probe MitoSOX™ Red. Therefore, different sources of DOX-induced ROS generation are likely to be dependent on cell type.

The precise mechanisms responsible for how DOX causes increased levels of mitochondrial ROS remain undetermined. The reasons may be manifold. On the one hand, DOX might increase mitochondrial ROS production. It has been reported that DOX could induce mitochondrial dysfunction, and thus augment mitochondrial ROS generation [14]. On the other hand, DOX might provoke decreased antioxidant capacity in mitochondria. Li *et al.* reported that myocardial MnSOD mRNA was not significantly changed, but its protein levels were significantly decreased in rats treated with DOX [24].

The functional role of mitochondrial ROS in DOX-induced platelet apoptosis was determined by pre-treating platelets with a mitochondria-targeted ROS scavenger before DOX treatment and then analyzing apoptotic markers. The mitochondria-targeted ROS scavenger was found to be effective in inhibiting DOX-induced platelet apoptosis. These observations indicate that mitochondrial ROS are key mediators of DOX-induced platelet apoptosis. However, the question remains, how does mitochondrial ROS triggers platelet apoptosis? It has been previously reported that mitochondria-derived ROS plays a pivotal role in triggering apoptosis in various cell types. Several studies have shown that mitochondrial ROS easily oxidizes cardiolipin, and oxidized cardiolipin appears to be essential for mitochondrial membrane permeabilization and releases of pro-apoptotic factors into the cytosol [25]. Conversely, prevention of cardiolipin peroxidation leads to inhibition of apoptosis [26]. These findings suggest that cardiolipin might be a crucial molecule that regulates the initiation of apoptosis. Our recent data demonstrated that hyperthermia increased cardiolipin peroxidation and that mitochondrial ROS plays an important role in hyperthermia-induced cardiolipin peroxidation [7]. Future work will be necessary to define how mitochondrial ROS regulates platelet apoptosis in DOX-treated platelets.

The reasons of Dox-induced thrombocytepenia may be manifold. On the one hand, DOX might increase platelet clearance. On the other hand, DOX might inhibit megakaryocyte function and decrease platelet generation. Up to now, the effect of DOX on megakaryocyte has not been clearly elucidated. Future work will be necessary to explore how DOX influence megakaryocyte function by *in vitro* or *in vivo* experiment.

In summary, our study provides direct evidence that DOX increases mitochondria-derived ROS generation in platelets, which in turn, induces platelet apoptosis. DOX does not incur platelet activation, whereas, it impairs platelet function. These findings may reveal a mechanism for platelet clearance and dysfunction *in vivo* or *in vitro*, and also suggest a possible pathogenesis of thrombocytopenia in some patients treated with DOX.

4. Experimental Section

4.1. Reagents and Antibodies

Anti-cleaved p17 fragment of caspase-3 antibody was obtained from Millipore (Billerica, MA, USA). Mito-TEMPO was obtained from Enzo Life Sciences (Plymouth Meeting, PA, USA). A23187, DOX, adenosine diphosphate (ADP), tetramethylrhodamine ethyl ester (TMRE), apocynin, 2', and 7'-dichlorofluorescin diacetate (DCFDA) were obtained from Sigma (St. Louis, MO, USA). Monoclonal antibodies against Bax, cytochrome C, tubulin, cytochrome C oxidase subunit 1 (COX1), actin, SZ-2, and HRP-conjugated goat anti-mouse IgG were obtained from Santa Cruz Biotechnology (Santa Cruz, CA, USA). FITC-conjugated annexin V was obtained from Bender Medsystem (Vienna, Austria). MitoSOX™ Red was obtained from Invitrogen/Molecular Probes (Eugene, OR, USA). Mitochondria isolation kit was obtained from Pierce (Rockford, IL, USA).

4.2. Preparation of Platelet-Rich Plasma (PRP) and Washed Platelets

For studies involving human subjects, approval was obtained from the Huashan Hospital institutional review board, China. Informed consent was provided in accordance with the Declaration of Helsinki. PRP and washed platelets were prepared as described previously [7]. Briefly, fresh blood from healthy volunteers (7 males and 5 females; age range: 24–35 years) was anti-coagulated with one-seventh volume of acid-citratedextrose (ACD, 2.5% trisodium citrate, 2.0% D-glucose and 1.5% citric acid). Anti-coagulated blood was separated by centrifuging, and the supernatant was PRP. Platelets were washed twice with CGS buffer (123 mM NaCl, 33 mM D-glucose, 13 mM trisodium citrate, pH 6.5) and re-suspended in modified Tyrode's buffer (MTB) (2.5 mM Hepes, 150 mM NaCl, 2.5 mM KCl, 12 mM NaHCO$_3$, 5.5 mM D-glucose, pH 7.4) to a final concentration of 3×10^8/mL, and incubated at room temperature (RT) for 1 h to recover to resting state.

4.3. Measurement of Mitochondrial Inner Transmembrane Potential ($\Delta\Psi m$)

Washed platelets were incubated with different concentrations of DOX (50, 100, 200 μM) or solvent control at 37 °C for indicated time. TMRE was added according to a previously described method [7]. For the inhibition experiments, washed platelets were pre-incubated with Mito-TEMPO (10 μM) or solvent control at 37 °C for 15 min, and then incubated with DOX at 37 °C for 3 h.

4.4. Phosphatidylserine (PS) Externalization Assay

Washed platelets were incubated with different concentrations of DOX or solvent control at 37 °C for indicated time. Annexin V binding buffer was mixed according to a previously described method [7]. For the inhibition experiments, washed platelets were pre-incubated with Mito-TEMPO (10 μM) or solvent control at 37 °C for 15 min, and then incubated with DOX at 37 °C for 3 h.

4.5. Measurement of Intracellular ROS and Mitochondrial ROS Levels

Intracellular ROS and mitochondrial ROS levels were examined using DCFDA and MitoSOX™ Red, respectively, according to a previously described method [7]. Briefly, washed platelets were loaded with DCFDA (10 μM) or MitoSOX™ Red (5 μM) at 37 °C for 20 min in the dark and washed three times with modified Tyrode's buffer (MTB). Pre-loaded platelets were incubated with different concentrations of DOX or solvent control at 37 °C for different time. For the inhibition experiments, pre-loaded platelets were incubated with apocynin (100 μM), Mito-TEMPO (10 μM), or solvent control at 37 °C for 15 min, and then treated with DOX at 37 °C for 3 h. A23187-treated and antimycin A-treated platelets were used as positive controls for intracellular cellular ROS and mitochondrial ROS levels, respectively.

4.6. Assessment of Malonyldialdehyde (MDA) Levels

Washed platelets were incubated with different concentrations of DOX or solvent control at 37 °C for 3 h. Samples were treated according to a previously described method [7]. For the inhibition experiments, washed platelets were pre-incubated with Mito-TEMPO, apocynin or solvent control at 37 °C for 15 min and then incubated with DOX at 37 °C for 3 h.

4.7. Assessment of Cardiolipin Peroxidation

Washed platelets were incubated with different concentrations of DOX or solvent control at 37 °C for 3 h, and then loaded with NAO according to a previously described method [7]. For the inhibition experiments, platelets were pre-incubated with Mito-TEMPO, apocynin or solvent control at 37 °C for 15 min and then incubated with DOX at 37 °C for 3 h.

4.8. Subcellular Fractionation

Washed platelets were incubated with different concentrations of DOX or solvent control at 37 °C for 3 h. Samples were suspended according to a previously described method [7]. For inhibition experiments, platelets were pre-incubated with Mito-TEMPO or solvent control at 37 °C for 15 min, and then further incubated with DOX at 37 °C for 3 h.

4.9. Western Blot Analysis

After subcellular fractionation Bax and cytochrome C were detected by Western blot using anti-Bax, and anti-cytochrome C antibodies. COX1 and tubulin were used as mitochondrial and cytosolic internal controls, respectively. Caspase-3 activation and GPIbα shedding was assessed with platelet whole lysates and supernatant, respectively. Washed platelets were incubated with different concentrations of

DOX or solvent control at 37 °C for 3 h. One part treated platelets were lysed with an equal volume of lysis buffer on ice for 30 min. The samples were subjected to Western blot analysis using anti-cleaved p17 fragment of caspase-3 antibody. Anti-actin antibody was used as an equal protein loading control. Another part treated platelets were centrifuged at 4000 rpm for 5 min, and the supernatants were analyzed by Western blot with anti-GPIbα N-terminal antibody SZ-2. In the inhibition experiments, platelets were pre-incubated with Mito-TEMPO or solvent control at 37 °C for 15 min, and incubated with DOX at 37 °C for 3 h.

4.10. Platelet Aggregation

PRP or washed platelets were incubated with different concentrations of DOX or solvent control at 37 °C for 3 h. Platelet aggregation was induced by addition of ADP or thrombin at 37 °C with a stirring speed of 1000 rpm.

4.11. Platelet Adhesion under Flow Condition

The glass capillary was coated according to a previously described method [7]. Washed platelets were incubated with different concentrations of DOX or solvent control at 37 °C for 3 h, then perfused into the glass capillary by a syringe pump at a flow shear rate of 250 s^{-1} for 5 min, and then washed with MTB for 5 min. The number of adherent platelets was counted in 10 randomly selected fields of 0.25 mm^2 and at randomly selected time points.

4.12. Statistical Analysis

The experimental data were expressed as means ± SEM. Each experiment was carried out at least three times. Statistical analysis for multiple group comparisons were performed by one-way analysis of variance (ANOVA), followed by *post-hoc* Dunnett's test. A *p*-value of less than 0.05 was considered statistically significant.

5. Conclusions

In the current study, the data show that DOX induces mitochondria-mediated intrinsic apoptosis and GPIbα shedding. Dox does not incur platelet activation, however, it obviously impair platelet aggregation and adhesion. Meanwhile, DOX induces mitochondrial ROS generation, and mitochondria-targeted ROS scavenger obviously reduces DOX-induced platelet apoptosis and GPIbα shedding. Thus, mitochondria-targeted ROS scavenger would have potential clinical utility in platelet-associated disorders involving mitochondrial oxidative damage.

Acknowledgments

This study was supported by grants from the National Natural Science Foundation of China (NSFC 81270650), the Natural Science Foundation of Shanghai (12ZR1429900, 15ZR1438300).

Author Contributions

Zhicheng Wang and Yuan Lu contributed to the manuscript concept and design, and critical review of the literature; Zhicheng Wang and Jie Wang contributed to perform the experiments and data analysis; Rufeng Xie and Ruilai Liu contributed to interpretation of results and language revision. All authors wrote the manuscript.

References

1. Wasle, I.; Gamerith, G.; Kocher, F.; Mondello, P.; Jaeger, T.; Walder, A.; Auberger, J.; Melchardt T.; Linkesch, W.; Fiegl, M.; *et al.* Non-pegylated liposomal DOX in lymphoma: Patterns of toxicity and outcome in a large observational trial. *Ann. Hematol.* **2015**, *94*, 593–601.

2. Kim, E.J.; Lim, K.M.; Kim, K.Y.; Bae, O.N.; Noh, J.Y.; Chung, S.M.; Shin, S.; Yun, Y.P.; Chung, J.H. DOX-induced platelet cytotoxicity: A new contributory factor for DOX-mediated thrombocytopenia. *J. Thromb. Haemost.* **2009**, *7*, 1172–1183.

3. Kim, S.H.; Lim, K.M.; Noh, J.Y.; Kim, K.; Kang, S.; Chang, Y.K.; Shin, S.; Chung, J.H. DOX-induced platelet procoagulant activities: An important clue for chemotherapy-associated thrombosis. *Toxicol. Sci.* **2011**, *124*, 215–224.

4. Mendivil-Perez, M.; Velez-Pardo, C.; Jimenez-Del-Rio, M. DOX induces apoptosis in Jurkat cells by mitochondria-dependent and mitochondria-independent mechanisms under normoxic and hypoxic conditions. *Anticancer Drugs* **2015**, in press.

5. Wang, H.; Lu, C.; Li, Q.; Xie, J.; Chen, T.; Tan, Y.; Wu, C.; Jiang, J. The role of Kif4A in DOX-induced apoptosis in breast cancer cells. *Mol. Cells* **2014**, *37*, 812–818.

6. Leytin, V. Apoptosis in the anucleate platelet. *Blood Rev.* **2012**, *26*, 51–63.

7. Wang, Z.; Cai, F.; Chen, X.; Luo, M.; Hu, L.; Lu, Y. The role of mitochondria-derived reactive oxygen species in hyperthermia-induced platelet apoptosis. *PLoS ONE* **2013**, *8*, e75044.

8. Zhang, J.; Chen, M.; Zhang, Y.; Zhao, L.; Yan, R.; Dai, K. Carmustine induces platelet apoptosis. *Platelets* **2014**, *23*, 1–6.

9. Thushara, R.M.; Hemshekhar, M.; Kemparaju, K.; Rangappa, K.S.; Devaraja, S.; Girish, K.S. Therapeutic drug-induced platelet apoptosis: An overlooked issue in pharmacotoxicology. *Arch. Toxicol.* **2014**, *88*, 185–198.

10. Zhang, W.; Liu, J.; Sun, R.; Zhao, L.; Du, J.; Ruan, C.; Dai, K. Calpain activator dibucaine induces platelet apoptosis. *Int. J. Mol. Sci.* **2011**, *12*, 2125–2137.

11. Danz, E.D.; Skramsted, J.; Henry, N.; Bennett, J.A.; Keller, R.S. Resveratrol prevents DOX cardiotoxicity through mitochondrial stabilization and the Sirt1 pathway. *Free Radic. Biol. Med.* **2009**, *46*, 1589–1597.

12. Cheung, K.G.; Cole, L.K.; Xiang, B.; Chen, K.; Ma, X.; Myal, Y.; Hatch, G.M.; Tong, Q.; Dolinsky, V.W. SIRT3 attenuates DOX-induced oxidative stress and improves mitochondrial respiration in H9c2 cardiomyocytes. *J. Biol. Chem.* **2015**, in press.

13. Min, K.; Kwon, O.S.; Smuder, A.J.; Wiggs, M.P.; Sollanek, K.J.; Christou, D.D.; Yoo, J.K.; Hwang, M.H.; Szeto, H.H.; Kavazis, A.N.; *et al.* Increased mitochondrial emission of reactive

oxygen species and calpain activation are required for DOX-induced cardiac and skeletal muscle myopathy. *J. Physiol.* **2015**, in press.

14. Shokoohinia, Y.; Hosseinzadeh, L.; Moieni-Arya, M.; Mostafaie, A.; Mohammadi-Motlagh, H.R. Osthole attenuates DOX-induced apoptosis in PC12 cells through inhibition of mitochondrial dysfunction and ROS production. *Biomed. Res. Int.* **2014**, *2014*, doi:10.1155/2014/156848.

15. Zhao, Y.; McLaughlin, D.; Robinson, E.; Harvey, A.P.; Hookham, M.B.; Shah, A.M.; McDermott, B.J.; Grieve, D.J. Nox2 NADPH oxidase promotes pathologic cardiac remodeling associated with DOX chemotherapy. *Cancer Res.* **2010**, *70*, 9287–9297.

16. Gilleron, M.; Marechal, X.; Montaigne, D.; Franczak, J.; Neviere, R.; Lancel, S. NADPH oxidases participate to DOX-induced cardiac myocyte apoptosis. *Biochem. Biophys. Res. Commun.* **2009**, *388*, 727–731.

17. Balaban, R.S.; Nemoto, S.; Finkel, T. Mitochondria, oxidants, and aging. *Cell* **2005**, *120*, 483–495.

18. Schulz, E.; Wenzel, P.; Munzel, T.; Daiber, A. Mitochondrial redox signaling: Interaction of mitochondrial reactive oxygen species with other sources of oxidative stress. *Antioxid. Redox Signal.* **2014**, *20*, 308–324.

19. Quinlan, C.L.; Orr, A.L.; Perevoshchikova, I.V.; Treberg, J.R.; Ackrell, B.A.; Brand, M.D. Mitochondrial complex II can generate reactive oxygen species at high rates in both the forward and reverse reactions. *J. Biol. Chem.* **2012**, *32*, 27255–27264.

20. Block, K.; Gorin, Y.; Abboud, H.E. Subcellular localization of Nox4 and regulation in diabetes. *Proc. Natl. Acad. Sci. USA* **2009**, *106*, 14385–14390.

21. Koziel, R.; Pircher, H.; Kratochwil, M.; Lener, B.; Hermann, M.; Dencher, N.A.; Jansen-Durr, P. Mitochondrial respiratory chain complex I is inactivated by NADPH oxidase Nox4. *Biochem. J.* **2013**, *452*, 231–239.

22. Renault, T.T.; Manon, S. Bax: Addressed to kill. *Biochimie* **2011**, *93*, 1379–1391.

23. Wang, Z.; Shi, Q.; Yan, R.; Liu, G.; Zhang, W.; Dai, K. The role of calpain in the regulation of ADAM17-dependent GPIbα ectodomain shedding. *Arch. Biochem. Biophys.* **2010**, *495*, 136–143.

24. Li, T.; Danelisen, I.; Singal, P.K. Early changes in myocardial antioxidant enzymes in rats treated with adriamycin. *Mol. Cell. Biochem.* **2002**, *232*, 19–26.

25. Kagan, V.E.; Bayir, A.; Bayir, H.; Stoyanovsky, D.; Borisenko, G.G.; Tyurina, Y.Y.; Wipf, P.; Atkinson, J.; Greenberger, J.S.; Chapkin, R.S.; *et al.* Mitochondria-targeted disruptors and inhibitors of cytochrome c/cardiolipin peroxidase complexes: A new strategy in anti-apoptotic drug discovery. *Mol. Nutr. Food Res.* **2009**, *53*, 104–114.

26. Tyurina, Y.Y.; Tyurin, V.A.; Kaynar, A.M.; Kapralova, V.I.; Wasserloos, K.; Li, J.; Mosher, M.; Wright, L.; Wipf, P.; Watkins, S.; *et al.* Oxidative lipidomics of hyperoxic acute lung injury: Mass spectrometric characterization of cardiolipin and phosphatidylserine peroxidation. *Am. J. Physiol. Lung Cell Mol. Physiol.* **2010**, *299*, L73–L85.

3

Mitochondrial and Ubiquitin Proteasome System Dysfunction in Ageing and Disease: Two Sides of the Same Coin?

Jaime M. Ross *, Lars Olson and Giuseppe Coppotelli *

Department of Neuroscience, Karolinska Institutet, Retzius väg 8, Stockholm 171 77, Sweden;
E-Mail: lars.olson@ki.se

* Authors to whom correspondence should be addressed;
  E-Mails: jaime.ross@ki.se (J.M.R.); giuseppe.coppotelli@ki.se (G.C.)

Academic Editor: Irmgard Tegeder

Abstract: Mitochondrial dysfunction and impairment of the ubiquitin proteasome system have been described as two hallmarks of the ageing process. Additionally, both systems have been implicated in the etiopathogenesis of many age-related diseases, particularly neurodegenerative disorders, such as Alzheimer's and Parkinson's disease. Interestingly, these two systems are closely interconnected, with the ubiquitin proteasome system maintaining mitochondrial homeostasis by regulating organelle dynamics, the proteome, and mitophagy, and mitochondrial dysfunction impairing cellular protein homeostasis by oxidative damage. Here, we review the current literature and argue that the interplay of the two systems should be considered in order to better understand the cellular dysfunction observed in ageing and age-related diseases. Such an approach may provide valuable insights into molecular mechanisms underlying the ageing process, and further discovery of treatments to counteract ageing and its associated diseases. Furthermore, we provide a hypothetical model for the heterogeneity described among individuals during ageing.

Keywords: ageing; mitochondria; ubiquitin; proteasome; ROS

1. Introduction

An increase in the average age of the world population has heightened the interest in ageing research in order to find treatments to improve health in old age. However, despite vast scientific efforts, the mechanisms that regulate ageing remain poorly understood. Outstanding questions include when the process starts and how it proceeds, why different species age at different rates, and why even individuals within the same species age differently. Ageing is a complex process, including genetic and environmental factors, both with stochastic components, all concurring and integrating in a manner difficult to predict. In a recent review, López-Otín and colleagues underlined nine hallmarks of ageing: genomic instability, telomere attrition, epigenetic alterations, loss of proteostasis, deregulated nutrient-sensing, mitochondrial dysfunction, cellular senescence, stem cell exhaustion, and altered intercellular communication [1]. Notably, such putative hallmarks are not isolated cellular processes but are highly interconnected. In order to properly understand the ageing process and to identify therapies to combat ageing, the role and interconnectedness of the putative hallmarks must be further dissected.

Impairment of the ubiquitin proteasome system (UPS) and mitochondrial dysfunction are two hallmarks of ageing and both have been implicated in a plethora of ageing-associated diseases, such as Alzheimer's and Parkinson's disease and certain cancers [1–6]. UPS is part of the "proteostasis network" (PN), and together with the autophagy lysosome system (ALS) and the molecular chaperone network contribute to maintaining cellular protein homeostasis by removing unwanted or damaged proteins that could aggregate and become toxic for the cell [7–10]. Mitochondria are the main source of energy production, generating ATP through oxidative phosphorylation (OXPHOS), and are also involved in many other important cellular processes, such as calcium buffering, apoptosis, steroid synthesis, and reactive oxygen species (ROS) production [11–13]. Although mitochondria are equipped with several mechanisms to quench free radicals, they are still subject to oxidative damage and thus rely on the UPS along with other quality control mechanisms to remove damaged mitochondrial proteins. Hence, an efficient UPS is crucial to preserve healthy mitochondria, and *vice versa*, healthy mitochondria are needed to maintain an efficient UPS system, since excessive ROS production could not only overflow the proteasome by increasing the amount of damaged proteins to be removed, but could also oxidize and damage the proteasomal subunits themselves and thereby decrease their catalytic activities. Once either mitochondrial dysfunction or proteasomal impairment develops, a vicious cycle may start, leading to progressive failure of both systems. Here, we summarize current knowledge of the interplay between the two systems, underlining how they affect each other in health, ageing, and disease, as well as how therapies targeting one deficiency might also benefit the other.

2. The Ubiquitin Proteasome System

The discovery of the ubiquitin-mediated protein degradation system earned Aaron Ciechanover, Avram Hershko, and Irwin Rose the 2004 Nobel Prize in Chemistry. Before uncovering the UPS, protein degradation was thought to occur mainly in the lysosome, an organelle filled with hydrolytic enzymes with an optimal proteolytic activity at a low pH [14]. Proteasome-mediated protein degradation differs from lysosomal-mediated proteolysis by operating at a neutral pH, mainly degrading short-lived proteins, taking place in a protein complex, and by not involving intracellular compartmentalization.

The conjugation of a polyubiquitin chain is an essential step to target unwanted or damaged proteins for proteasomal degradation [9]. Proteasome activity generates small peptides that are further digested into amino acids by the abundant cytosolic endopeptidases and aminopeptidases, while lysosomal degradation directly produces single amino acids [15]. The UPS is a highly selective system and operates in both nuclear and cytoplasmic compartments. Conversely, lysosomes are present only in the cytoplasm and are able to remove a wide range of substrates, ranging from a single protein delivered to it via chaperone-mediated autophagy (CMA) to large aggregates and whole organelles (e.g., mitochondria) engulfed via macroautophagy [16,17].

Ubiquitin [Ub] is a 76 amino acid ≈8 kDa protein that is highly conserved among Eukaryota [18,19]. Protein ubiquitination is an ATP dependent process that occurs through a three-step sequential enzymatic cascade performed by the ubiquitin-activating enzyme (E1), ubiquitin-conjugating enzyme (E2), and ubiquitin ligase (E3). The result generates an isopeptidyl bond between ubiquitin at glycine 76 and either the ε-amino group of an internal lysine residue on the protein substrate or its amino terminus. Subsequently, multiple rounds of ubiquitination extend the ubiquitin chain by adding more ubiquitins on one of the seven internal lysine residues (Lys 6, 11, 27, 29, 33, 48 and 63) of the previously added ubiquitin, which generates polyubiquitin chains with different linkages (e.g., K48, K63, *etc.*) [20]. The length and type of the ubiquitin chain determine the fate of the ubiquitinated protein; the K48-linked polyubiquitin chain is the main signal that targets substrates for 26S proteasome degradation, while other types of linkages have been shown to play a role in receptor signaling, endocytosis, transcription, DNA repair, and autophagy [21]. The E3 ligase enzyme confers specificity to the ubiquitination system by recognizing the target's substrate; indeed, while there is one type of ubiquitin-activating E1 enzyme (ubiquitin-like modifier-activating enzyme 1, UBA1) present in all cells and a second E1 type (Ubiquitin-activating Enzyme 1-like 2, UBE1L2) with seemingly more tissue specificity [22], there are about 30 E2 enzymes and more than 600 members of the E3 family. E3 ligase enzymes can be grouped into two classes: those that are homologous to the E6-AP carboxyl terminus (HECT) and the really interesting new gene [RING] ligases. The two classes differ not only in their structure but also in the way they catalyze the last step of ubiquitination. The HECT ligases accept the activated ubiquitin from an E2 enzyme on a cysteine residue in the active domain and then transfer it to the substrate, whereas the RING ligases act as scaffold proteins by bringing together an E2 conjugating enzyme and the substrate [23].

Ubiquitination is a reversible post-translational modification, and a family of proteases, the deubiquitinating enzymes (DUBs), can remove ubiquitin from substrates, thereby regulating the ubiquitination process and recycling ubiquitin. DUBs are highly specific and have been grouped into five subfamilies: Ub carboxyl-terminal hydrolases (UCH), Ub-specific proteases (Usp), ovarian tumor like proeases, JAB1/MPN/Mov34 (JAMM/MPN) metalloproteases, and the Machado–Jakob disease proteases. Removal of ubiquitin adducts from the substrate is a critical step for proteasomal degradation [24,25].

The 26S proteasome is a multi-subunit holoenzyme of ≈2.5 MDa, with two distinct subdomains, a 20S core particle (CP) and, in the classical conformation, either one or two 19S (PA 700) regulatory particles (RP) on either side of the CP. The CP is a barrel-shaped complex made by two α- and two β-rings, each containing seven subunits ($α_{1-7}$ and $β_{1-7}$), and arranged with two β-rings in the middle and two α-rings on either side. The proteolytic activity is carried out by three β subunits (β1, β2, β5), each with different amino acid specificity, caspase-, trypsin-, and chymotrypsin-like activity, respectively [26].

The α subunits seem to have a regulatory function, allowing only unfolded substrates access to the inner chamber, where the proteolytic activities are located, thus avoiding non-specific degradation of cellular proteins. Ubiquitinated substrates are docked and unfolded by the 19S RP, which can be functionally subdivided into a base and a lid [27]. The base consists of six AAA-ATPase rings (Rpt1-6) and three non-ATPase subunits (Rpn1, Rpn2, Rpn13), while another subunit, Rpn10, seems to associate with the base and the lid after their assembly. The AAA-ATPases use energy to unfold the substrate and translocate it through the central pore of the 20S chamber, while two of the non-ATPase subunits (Rpn10, Rpn13) serve as ubiquitin receptors [28–32]. The lid has more than nine proteins, including the deubiquinating enzyme Rpn11, which is essential for efficient substrate degradation [33]. Other regulatory particles have also been described, such as 11S (PA 28) and PA 200, with different functions and activations as compared to the 19S RP. The 11S RP is involved in the immune-proteasome and is regulated by γ-interferon, whereas PA 200 RP is only present in the nucleus, although little is known about its specific function [26].

3. Mitochondria

The endosymbiotic origin of mitochondria explains some of the unique biological aspects of these organelles [34], which form a dynamic network, often referred to as the mitochondrial network [35]. Mitochondria are regulated by fusion and fission, processes that are crucial to maintain functional mitochondria and energetic homeostasis. These processes, for example, enable small mitochondria to move along the cytoskeleton and relocate to areas where energy delivery is needed, such as the presynaptic terminals of an axon. In mammals, several proteins have been implicated in the regulation of fusion and fission of mitochondria. Mitofusin-1 and -2 (MFN1, MFN2) together with the optic atrophy 1 protein (OPA1) are required for mitochondrial fusion, while dynamin-related protein 1 (DRP1) is indispensable for fission [36,37]. All mitochondria contain two lipid bi-layers, an outer membrane (OMM) and an inner membrane (IMM), leading to the intermembrane space (IMS), chemically equivalent to the cytoplasm, and the matrix, an internal space that contains enzymes important for fatty acid oxidation as well as for the tricarboxylic acid (TCA), or Krebs cycle, as well as mtDNA. The IMM is highly impermeable, and by folding in a convoluted manner, forms the *cristae*, a large surface area where the respiratory chain (RC) complexes I–V are located (Figure 1).

Mitochondria are the only organelles that contain their own DNA. In humans, mitochondrial DNA (mtDNA) is a circular molecule that encodes 13 proteins, all of which are involved in OXPHOS, 22 transfer RNA species (tRNAs), and two ribosomal RNA types (16S, 12S). Each cell can contain several hundred copies of mtDNA (10^3–10^4 copies per cell) depending on the energy demand of the tissue, the differentiation stage of the cell, hormonal balance, and exercise level [38,39]. The vast majority of the ≈1000 mitochondrial proteins are encoded by nuclear genes [40], synthetized in the cytoplasm, and imported into the mitochondria in an unfolded state. During this process, cellular and mitochondrial chaperones (mtHSP70, mtHSP60, mtHSP10, *etc.*) assist the folding of imported proteins to ensure that they reach their destination to execute their function [41,42]. Mitochondria are the main source of reactive oxygen species (ROS), a natural by-product of OXPHOS. If not properly regulated, ROS can be extremely harmful to DNA, lipids and proteins, especially matrix proteins, which are not accessible by the cellular quality control machinery. In this regard, mitochondria possess their own quality control system consisting of several proteases, such as Lon, ClpXP, *i*-AAA, and *m*-AAA, to ensure that damaged or unfolded proteins that cannot be rescued and refolded by the mitochondrial chaperons are turned-over, thereby avoiding toxicity. Several reviews have been published on this topic [43–45]. The UPS is also an integral component of the mitochondrial protein quality control system, and mediates degradation not only of outer membrane embedded proteins, but also matrix proteins, implicating the existence of retro-translocation mechanisms of proteins from the mitochondrial matrix to the cytoplasm for proteasomal degradation [46].

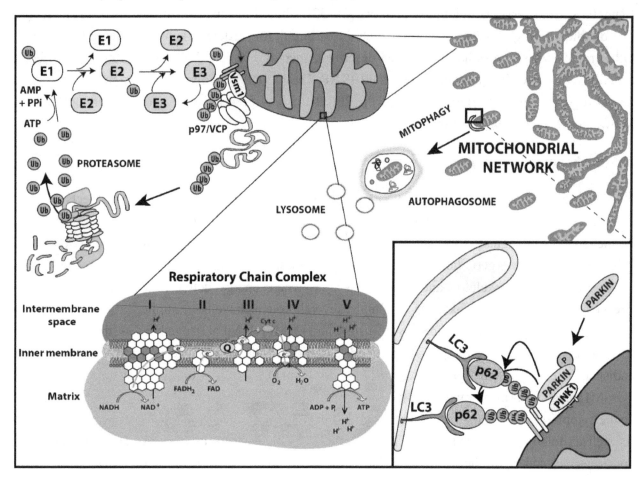

Figure 1. UPS and mitochondrial quality control. Polyubiquitination of mitochondrial proteins by the catalyzed reaction of E1, E2 and E3 enzymes in this depiction leads to the recruitment of the p97/VCP complex to the mitochondrial outer membrane (**upper left**). p97/VCP can extract a ubiquitinated protein in an ATP-dependent process that facilitates its proteasomal degradation. The UPS is also needed for the autophagic degradation of damaged mitochondria, a process known as mitophagy. Loss of mitochondrial membrane polarization stabilizes PINK1, which relocalizes to the outer membrane where it recruits and activates the E3 ligase PARKIN by phosphorylation. Once activated, PARKIN ubiquitinates several mitochondrial proteins, which flag the mitochondria for autophagic degradation (**lower right**). A schematic representation of the mitochondrial respiratory chain (complexes I, II, III, IV and V) is shown, with nuclear-encoded subunits depicted as white hexagons and the mitochondrial-encoded subunits as orange (**lower left**).

4. Role of the Ubiquitin Proteasome System in Mitochondrial Protein Quality Control

The involvement of the UPS in the quality control of mitochondrial proteins started to emerge after several studies found components of the UPS in the mitochondria as well as ubiquitination of numerous mitochondrial proteins. In an early study conducted in yeast, the SCF ubiquitin ligase complex subunit Mdm30 (mitochondrial distribution and morphology protein 30) was shown to affect mitochondrial shape by regulating the steady-state level of Fzo1, an ortholog of mammalian mitofusin-1 and -2; thus connecting the ubiquitin proteasome system with mitochondria [47]. While attempting to determine the mitochondrial proteome of *Saccharomyces cerevisiae*, numerous E3 ligases and DUBs were found to be associated with the mitochondrial compartment [48]. In another study, the purification of total ubiquitinated proteins from mouse heart expressing 8xHis/Flag-Ubiquitin (HisF-Ub) under the α-myosin heavy chain (α-MHC) promoter, led to the finding that 38% of all ubiquitinated proteins were mitochondrial and found in all compartments, including the matrix [49]. One possible explanation for such findings could be that nuclear encoded mitochondrial proteins that are not properly folded during translation are directly targeted for degradation. In this regard, it has been estimated that one third of all synthetized proteins are defective ribosomal products (DRiPs), due to errors in transcription and/or translation, and are turned-over by the proteasome before reaching their final destination [50]. However, an interesting alternative possibility has been proposed: the existence of a mechanism to retro-translocate mitochondrial proteins into the cytosol for degradation, akin to the endoplasmic reticulum-associated degradation (ERAD) pathway, and thus named the mitochondria-associated degradation (MAD) system, also referred to as the outer mitochondrial membrane-associated degradation (OMMAD) system [51–53].

In support of the MAD process, it has been shown that colon cancer cells (COLO 205) treated with inhibitors of the chaperone protein, heat shock protein 90 (HSP90), undergo apoptotic cell death preceded by dramatic changes in the mitochondrial compartment [54]. The most prominent change was an accumulation of mitochondrial proteins due to an increase in protein half-life, as determined by ^{35}S-methionine/cysteine pulse-chase. The authors found that one protein in particular, oligomycin-sensitivity-conferring protein (OSCP), which is a component of the mitochondrial membrane ATP synthase (F1F0-ATP synthase or complex V) and located in the IMM, was ubiquitinated and degraded by the proteasome in an HSP90-dependent manner [54]. Additionally, a role for ubiquitination and proteasome degradation has been described for the mitochondrial uncoupling protein 1 and 2 (UCP1, 2) as well as for the endonuclease G (endoG) protein [55–57]. Similarly with what has been described in the ERAD pathway, the Cdc48/p97 complex (cdc48: cell division control protein 48) seems to be required for the extraction of mitochondrial proteins in the MAD system [58]. In fact, it has been shown in yeast treated with mitochondrial stressors that the cytoplasmic protein Vms1 (valosin-containing protein (VCP)/Cdc48-associated mitochondrial stress-responsive 1) re-localizes to mitochondria and recruits the Cdc48/p97–Npl4 (Npl4: nuclear protein localization protein 4) complex (Figure 1) [52]. Interestingly, Vms1 overexpression in yeast has been shown to counteract the mitochondrial damage and cell death induced by the expression of UBB+1, a frame-shift variant of ubiquitin B, which is associated with Alzheimer's disease [59]. Complex p97, known as VCP in mammals and Cdc48 in yeast, belongs to the ATPases associated with diverse cellular activities (AAA+) protein family, and is a barrel-shaped hexameric complex that uses ATP to unfold and extract proteins from membranes and protein complexes [23]. Notably, Cdc48/VCP mutations have been shown to induce a decrease in mitochondrial membrane potential and to increase mitochondrial oxygen consumption leading to mitochondrial damage and cell death both in yeast and human-derived fibroblasts [60,61].

Among the numerous E3 ligases associated with mitochondria, PARKIN is by far the most studied. Mutations in the PARK2 locus, where the *PARKIN* gene is located, were initially associated with autosomal recessive juvenile Parkinson's disease (AR-JP) [62]. Further studies have contributed to understanding the function of PARKIN and the possible mechanism by which it might promote disease [63]. PARKIN has been described as an hybrid E3 ubiquitin ligase that possesses both RING and HECT E3 ligase characteristics [64]. Upon mitochondrial depolarization, the self-inactivated enzyme is thought to be recruited to the mitochondrial membrane where it is phosphorylated and activated by PTEN-induced putative kinase 1 (PINK1) [65]. PINK1 is constantly imported and degraded in healthy mitochondria; however, when perturbations of mitochondrial homeostasis affect the mitochondrial membrane potential, PINK1 escapes degradation and accumulates on the outer membrane. There, it recruits and activates PARKIN by phosphorylating the Ser65 residue of the PARKIN ubiquitin-like domain; however, its full activation also requires the phosphorylation of Ser65 on the ubiquitin molecule [66–68]. Once activated, PARKIN induces the removal of depolarized mitochondria by mitophagy through a poorly understood mechanism, which requires the poly-ubiquitination of several other outer membrane mitochondrial proteins, including MFN1 and 2, Mitochondrial Rho GTPase (RHOT)-1 and 2, and voltage-dependent anion channel (VDAC)-1, 2, and 3 [69–72]. Notably, up-regulation of Parkin in *Drosophila* resulted in increased mean and maximal lifespan, and was associated with reduced protein aggregation and improved mitochondrial activity in aged flies [73]. Although the PINK1/PARKIN pathway has been shown to be involved in the removal of depolarized mitochondria induced by stressors, such as carbonyl cyanide 3-chlorophenylhydrazone (CCCP), an uncoupler of oxidative phosphorylation, its involvement in the physiological removal of mitochondria seems to be nonessential, as demonstrated by the absence of striking phenotypes in Parkin and Pink1 knockout mice, thus suggesting the presence of additional mechanisms for the removal of mitochondria, independent of the PINK1/PARKIN pathway (reviewed in [74]). In fact, a study from our group showed that dysfunctional mitochondria in a mouse model for Parkinson's disease generated by knocking out the mitochondrial transcription factor A (TFAM) in dopaminergic neurons, did not recruit PARKIN. Neither removal of defective mitochondria nor the neurodegenerative phenotype was affected by the absence of PARKIN in these mice [75].

Another RING/E3 ubiquitin ligase that seems to regulate mitochondrial dynamics is MITOL/MARCH-V (mitochondrial ubiquitin ligase), a membrane protein located in the OMM where it interacts with and ubiquitinates several substrates [76]. One such substrate is Drp1, which is degraded upon MITOL-mediated ubiquitination; thus, MITOL might affect mitochondrial fission by regulating Drp1 levels [77,78]. Furthermore, MITOL seems to be involved in the ubiquitination and degradation of misfolded proteins located in mitochondria, such as a mutated form of superoxide dismutase 1 (SOD1), an antioxidant enzyme that has been implicated in amyotrophic lateral sclerosis (ALS, or Lou Gehrig's disease) [79]. Additionally, several DUBs have been localized to mitochondria, such as ataxin-3, a deubiquitinating enzyme that is associated with Machado-Joseph disease and seems to interact with PARKIN in order to counteract self-ubiquitination [80].

Taken together, these studies support a central role for the UPS in the maintenance of mitochondrial homeostasis by regulating organelle dynamics (fission and fusion), the proteome, and mitophagy.

Thus, it is not surprising that disturbances affecting UPS activity might also have an effect on mitochondrial function. With that said, studies also support that the converse is also true.

5. Effect of Mitochondrial Dysfunction on the Ubiquitin Proteasome System

Evidence that mitochondrial dysfunction might affect proteasomal activity has been reported in different systems, including yeast, *C. elegans*, and mammalian cells. It has been shown that inhibition of OXPHOS in rat-derived cortical neurons also affects proteasomal activity and protein ubiquitination [81]. Two recent reports have helped to shed light on the possible molecular mechanisms underlying such an effect [82,83]. Stimulation of ROS production in a respiration-deficient yeast mutant (*Δfzo1*) was shown to induce proteasome disassembly, with the complete detachment of the 20S CP and 19S RPs, similar to what was observed in yeast and mammalian cells treated with either hydrogen peroxide (H_2O_2) or antimycin A, a cytochrome *c* reductase inhibitor. Proteasome disassembly was associated with proteasomal substrate accumulation and was reversed upon treatment with antioxidants or dithiothreitol (DTT), a strong reducing agent [82]. Comparable results were obtained in a different study, using a short-lived ubiquitin fused protein expressed in *C. elegans* as a reporter, to screen for factors involved in regulating protein turnover. Screening revealed reporter accumulation in two worm mutants carrying mutations in proteins involved in mitochondrial processes: IVD-1 and ACS-19. IVD-1 is the ortholog of a human mitochondrial enzyme (isovaleryl-CoA dehydrogenase) involved in the leucin catabolism pathway, while ACS-19 is predicted to be the ortholog of a human enzyme (ACSS2, acetyl-CoA synthetase) involved in fatty acid metabolism in the mitochondrial matrix. In both cases, the effect of mitochondrial dysfunction on proteasomal function was due to an increase in ROS production, which was prevented by treatment with the antioxidant *N*-acetylcysteine (NAC) [83].

ROS is a group of potentially harmful compounds that can damage all cellular components, including proteins, DNA, and lipids. Oxidation can affect protein structure, thus impairing function, and might also render proteins prone to aggregation, which could result in toxicity. The complete disassembly of the proteasome, resulting in an increase of 20S CPs, could be a protective mechanism to counteract a temporary rise in oxidative damage. It has been shown that 20S CP is more resistant to oxidative damage, compared to 19S RP, and is able to bind and degrade mis-folded oxidized proteins without the need for ubiquitination and ATP expenditure [84–86]. Thus, a temporary disassembly of the proteasome holoenzyme together with an up-regulation of an antioxidant stress response, heat shock proteins, and autophagic flux could be seen as part of a cellular strategy to counteract an acute increase in oxidative damage. Hence, through the uncapping of the 20S CP, cells might redirect the degradation capability of the proteasome from the removal of ubiquitinated substrates to the removal of oxidized proteins. However, since oxidative stress is a hallmark of ageing and age-related diseases, chronic exposure to oxidative stress could result in proteasome disassembly, which could further aggravate these conditions (Figure 2).

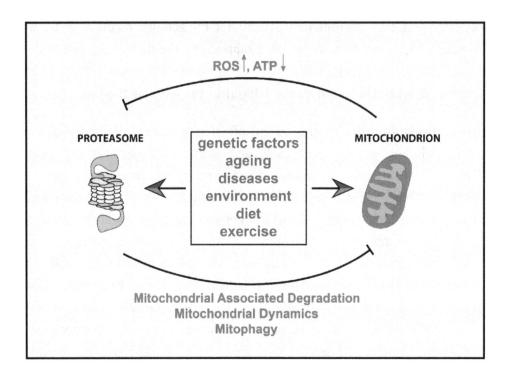

Figure 2. UPS and mitochondrial cross-talk. Several factors, including genes, environment, age, diseases, diet, and exercise can either positively or negatively affect UPS activity and mitochondrial function. Impairment of one of the two systems can then drive the malfunctioning of the other and result in a vicious cycle. A decrease in cellular ATP levels and an increase in ROS production can impair proteasomal function by affecting protein ubiquitination and proteasome assembly and stability, while a decrease in UPS activity could impair mitochondrial function by affecting mitochondrial dynamics, mitophagy, and the removal of damaged mitochondrial proteins.

ATP depletion is another mechanism through which mitochondrial dysfunction might affect proteasomal activity. ATP is required for both protein ubiquitination [87] and proteasome assembly and stability [88–90]. Intracellular ATP levels have been shown to regulate proteasomal activity both *in vitro* and in cultured cells [91], and manipulation of intracellular ATP levels by inhibition of complex I has been shown to decrease proteasomal activity in primary mesencephalic cell cultures, an effect which was counteracted by increasing the glucose concentration in the cellular medium [92].

6. The "Mitochondrion—Ubiquitin Proteasome System Axis" in Ageing and Age-Related Diseases

The UPS and mitochondria are two systems among several reportedly affected by ageing; an accumulation of mis-folded proteins and oxidative stress have been denoted as two features of the ageing process. A decline in UPS activity has been shown in yeast (*Saccharomyces cerevisiae*) [93], fly (*Drosophila melanogaster*) [94], rodents [95–97], and also in human-derived dermal fibroblasts [98]. Conversely, it has been shown that proteasome activation by genetic manipulation in different models can ameliorate the ageing process and also increase lifespan (reviewed in [99]). Several possibilities have been proposed to explain the UPS decline associated with ageing, including down-regulation and/or modification of proteasomal subunits, disassembly of the holoenzyme, an increase in substrates and aggregates that could clog the proteasome, and reduction in ATP levels, which could impair the overall process of protein ubiquitination and unfolding [100]. As mentioned, an increase in oxidative damage is a major contributor to the UPS decline, and with OXPHOS as the main source of ROS production, mitochondria have thus been suspected to play a central role in the ageing process. Based on this notion, Denham Harman proposed the "Free Radical Theory of Aging" (FRTA) in 1956, suggesting that ageing is driven by the accumulation of oxidative damage to cellular structures over time [101]. It has been proposed that accumulation of mtDNA mutations could be a possible cause of the mitochondrial dysfunction described in ageing, and in this regard data from different groups, including ours, have shown a cause-effect relationship between increased mtDNA mutational load and ageing phenotypes [102–110]. However, it has also been argued that the level of mtDNA mutations observed in normally aged tissues is much less than the threshold needed to cause respiratory chain dysfunction [111,112]. Thus, another possibility for the age-associated decline in mitochondrial function could be a loss in protein homeostasis due to the impairment of the UPS and/or autophagic systems.

As described, the UPS and mitochondria systems are tightly interdependent, and once a vicious cycle of dysfunction starts it is difficult to identify which one was the trigger (Figure 2). This is demonstrated in neurodegenerative diseases, such as Alzheimer's disease (AD) and Parkinson's disease (PD), with ageing consistently implicated as the major risk factor. In both diseases, it has been seemingly difficult to isolate UPS impairment from dysfunctional mitochondria, and *vice versa*, in order to understand the contribution of each system in disease onset and progression. PD is a neurodegenerative disorder that arises from the loss of dopaminergic neurons, mainly in substantia nigra, and is characterized by resting tremor, bradykinesia, and muscle rigidity. The discovery of Lewy bodies in neurons, aggregates containing α-synuclein, ubiquitinated proteins, and components of the UPS, strongly implicated the proteasome in the pathogenesis of the disease [113]. However, other studies have reported a compelling correlation between mitochondrial dysfunction and PD, and mouse models mimicking the disease have been generated by genetically impairing mitochondrial function in dopaminergic neurons [114] or by using toxins that affect mitochondria, such as 1-methyl-4-phenyl-1,2,3,6-tetrahydropyridine (MPTP) [115]. In all likelihood, PD will turn out to be several different diseases characterized by different etiologies, although only partially different phenotypes. AD patients exhibit gross brain atrophy, with both neuronal and synaptic loss, accumulation of amyloid plaques containing amyloid β peptides, and intracellular neurofibrillary tangles of phosphorylated Tau protein [116]. The involvement of the UPS in AD has been postulated based on studies demonstrating a decrease in proteasome activity associated with AD and the presence of ubiquitin and UPS components in the plaques [117]. As similarly shown with PD, another body of literature has focused on mitochondrial dysfunction as representing the major etiopathogenesis of AD [118]. Taking both perspectives into consideration, perhaps these two interconnected systems should be regarded as the "Mitochondrion-UPS Axis" when trying to understand and dissect the cellular dysfunction observed in ageing and age-related diseases. That is, UPS impairment and mitochondrial dysfunction could be two sides of the same coin in that either system cannot be separated from the other since they affect each other in a vicious cycle (Figure 2).

In order to explain the differences observed among individuals during ageing, we propose a model that takes into consideration the decline in both mitochondrial function and UPS activity over time. We speculate that the point of interception between the two systems might represent the age at which cellular dysfunction begins (Figure 3). While both systems decline with age in a dependent manner, the shape of each curve will vary slightly between individuals, due to the compounded effects of an individual's genetic background, environmental stressors (*i.e.*, toxins, smoking), diet, and exercise. Taking these factors into account, the age of cellular dysfunction onset for a given person could start decades earlier as compared to another, leading to the ageing heterogeneity of the human population.

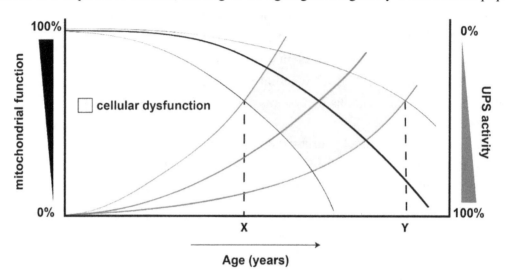

Figure 3. Hypothetical model to explain the heterogeneity of the ageing process among individuals taking into consideration changes in both UPS and mitochondrial function. A theoretical model to explain the idiosyncratic differences observed during ageing by taking into consideration the variation of both UPS activity and mitochondrial function over time. Both systems decline with age in a dependent manner, but the slope of the curve may vary between individuals, depending on factors such as genetics, environment, diet, and exercise, as depicted by the thin lines. The point of interception of the two curves hypothetically represents the age of onset of cellular dysfunction, defined as any point in time when cellular homeostasis is perturbed. Thus, two individuals, each following different extremities of mitochondrial dysfunction and UPS decline, might experience the onset of cellular dysfunction at different ages (X and Y), which could be decades apart from each other.

7. Conclusions and Future Prospects

The last century has witnessed a considerable increase of life expectancy due to better living conditions and medical advancements in the cure and prevention of many once fatal diseases. Several compounds, such as resveratrol, metformin, and rapamycin, have shown potential in improving overall health and lifespan in experimental organisms. Finding drugs to combat ageing might therefore not be just fantasy, but actually feasible [119,120]. However, the only currently known proven interventions shown to improve ageing phenotypes in humans are a hypocaloric diet and exercise [121,122]. Therefore, understanding the underlying molecular mechanism of the ageing process is the *condicio sine qua non* for developing any promising therapeutic intervention to slow the ageing process. In this regard, we suggest that dissecting the "Mitochondrion-UPS Axis" may help in the search for drugs to counteract ageing and age-related diseases.

Acknowledgments

The Swedish Research Council (537-2014-6856; JMR, K2012-62X-03185-42-4; LO), the Swedish Brain Foundation (Jaime M. Ross), Swedish Lundbeck Foundation (Jaime M. Ross), Swedish Brain Power (Jaime M. Ross, Lars Olson, Giuseppe Coppotelli), the Swedish Society for Medical Research (Giuseppe Coppotelli), the Foundation for Geriatric Diseases at Karolinska Institutet (Giuseppe Coppotelli), Karolinska Institutet Research Foundations (Giuseppe Coppotelli), Loo och Hans Ostermans Foundation for Medical Research (Giuseppe Coppotelli), ERC Advanced Investigator grant (322744; Lars Olson), and the Karolinska Distinguished Professor Award (Lars Olson).

Abbreviations

AD = Alzheimer's Disease; DUBs = Deubiquitinating enzymes; HECT = Homologous to the E6-AP Carboxyl Terminus; IMM = Inner Mitochondrial Membrane; IMS = Intermembrane Space; RC = Respiratory Chain; MAD = Mithochondrial Associated Degradation; OMM = Outer Mitochondrial Membrane; OXPHOS = Oxidative Phosphorylation; PD = Parkinson's Disease; RING = Really Interesting New Gene; ROS = Reactive Oxygen Species; Ub = Ubiquitin; UPS = Ubiquitin Proteasome System.

References

1. López-Otín, C.; Blasco, M.A.; Partridge, L.; Serrano, M.; Kroemer, G. The hallmarks of aging. *Cell* **2013**, *153*, 1194–1217.
2. Wang, X.; Wang, W.; Li, L.; Perry, G.; Lee, H.-G.; Zhu, X. Oxidative stress and mitochondrial dysfunction in Alzheimer's disease. *Biochim. Biophys. Acta* **2014**, *1842*, 1240–1247.
3. Morimoto, R.I. Proteotoxic stress and inducible chaperone networks in neurodegenerative disease and aging. *Genes Dev.* **2008**, *22*, 1427–1438.
4. Keller, J.N.; Hanni, K.B.; Markesbery, W.R. Possible involvement of proteasome inhibition in aging: Implications for oxidative stress. *Mech. Ageing Dev.* **2000**, *113*, 61–70.
5. Gautier, C.A.; Corti, O.; Brice, A. Mitochondrial dysfunctions in Parkinson's disease. *Rev. Neurol.* **2014**, *170*, 339–343
6. Büeler, H. Impaired mitochondrial dynamics and function in the pathogenesis of Parkinson's disease. *Exp. Neurol.* **2009**, *218*, 235–246.
7. Jung, T.; Catalgol, B.; Grune, T. The proteasomal system. *Mol. Asp. Med.* **2009**, *30*, 191–296.
8. Hershko, A.; Ciechanover, A. The ubiquitin system. *Annu. Rev. Biochem.* **1998**, *67*, 425–479.
9. Glickman, M.H.; Ciechanover, A. The ubiquitin-proteasome proteolytic pathway: Destruction for the sake of construction. *Physiol. Rev.* **2002**, *82*, 373–428.

10. Hochstrasser, M. Ubiquitin-dependent protein degradation. *Annu. Rev. Genet.* **1996**, *30*, 405–439.

11. Kim, A. A panoramic overview of mitochondria and mitochondrial redox biology. *Toxicol. Res.* **2014**, *30*, 221–234.

12. Mishra, P.; Chan, D.C. Mitochondrial dynamics and inheritance during cell division, development and disease. *Nat. Rev. Mol. Cell Biol.* **2014**, *15*, 634–646.

13. Green, D.R.; Galluzzi, L.; Kroemer, G. Cell biology. Metabolic control of cell death. *Science* **2014**, *345*, 1250256.

14. De Duve, C.; Pressman, B.C.; Gianetto, R.; Wattiaux, R.; Appelmans, F. Tissue fractionation studies. 6. Intracellular distribution patterns of enzymes in rat-liver tissue. *Biochem. J.* **1955**, *60*, 604–617.

15. Baraibar, M.A.; Friguet, B. Changes of the proteasomal system during the aging process. *Prog. Mol. Biol. Transl. Sci.* **2012**, *109*, 249–275.

16. Kaushik, S.; Cuervo, A.M. Chaperone-mediated autophagy: A unique way to enter the lysosome world. *Trends Cell Biol.* **2012**, *22*, 407–417.

17. Mizushima, N. Autophagy: Process and function. *Genes Dev.* **2007**, *21*, 2861–2873.

18. Ciechanover, A. Proteolysis: From the lysosome to ubiquitin and the proteasome. *Nat. Rev. Mol. Cell Biol.* **2005**, *6*, 79–87.

19. Pickart, C.M.; Eddins, M.J. Ubiquitin: Structures, functions, mechanisms. *Biochim. Biophys. Acta* **2004**, *1695*, 55–72.

20. Komander, D.; Rape, M. The ubiquitin code. *Annu. Rev. Biochem.* **2012**, *81*, 203–229.

21. Finley, D. Recognition and processing of ubiquitin-protein conjugates by the proteasome. *Annu. Rev. Biochem.* **2009**, *78*, 477–513.

22. Pelzer, C.; Kassner, I.; Matentzoglu, K.; Singh, R.K.; Wollscheid, H.P.; Scheffner, M.; Schmidtke, G.; Groettrup, M. UBE1L2, a novel E1 enzyme specific for ubiquitin. *J. Biol. Chem.* **2007**, *282*, 23010–23014.

23. Metzger, M.B.; Hristova, V.A.; Weissman, A.M. HECT and RING finger families of E3 ubiquitin ligases at a glance. *J. Cell Sci.* **2012**, *125*, 531–537.

24. Amerik, A.Y.; Hochstrasser, M. Mechanism and function of deubiquitinating enzymes. *Biochim. Biophys. Acta* **2004**, *1695*, 189–207.

25. Reyes-Turcu, F.E.; Ventii, K.H.; Wilkinson, K.D. Regulation and cellular roles of ubiquitin-specific deubiquitinating enzymes. *Annu. Rev. Biochem.* **2009**, *78*, 363–397.

26. Jung, T. and Grune, T. Structure of the proteasome. *Prog. Mol. Biol. Transl. Sci.* **2012**, *109*, 1–39.

27. Lander, G.C.; Estrin, E.; Matyskiela, M.E.; Bashore, C.; Nogales, E.; Martin, A. Complete subunit architecture of the proteasome regulatory particle. *Nature* **2012**, *482*, 186–191.

28. Van Nocker, S.; Sadis, S.; Rubin, D.M.; Glickman, M.; Fu, H.; Coux, O.; Wefes, I.; Finley, D.; Vierstra, R.D. The multiubiquitin-chain-binding protein Mcb1 is a component of the 26S proteasome in *Saccharomyces cerevisiae* and plays a nonessential, substrate-specific role in protein turnover. *Mol. Cell. Biol.* **1996**, *16*, 6020–6028.

29. Deveraux, Q.; Ustrell, V.; Pickart, C.; Rechsteiner, M. A 26 S protease subunit that binds ubiquitin conjugates. *J. Biol. Chem.* **1994**, *269*, 7059–7061.

30. Husnjak, K.; Elsasser, S.; Zhang, N.; Chen, X.; Randles, L.; Shi, Y.; Hofmann, K.; Walters, K.J.; Finley, D.; Dikic, I. Proteasome subunit Rpn13 is a novel ubiquitin receptor. *Nature* **2008**, *453*, 481–488.

31. Braun, B.C.; Glickman, M.; Kraft, R.; Dahlmann, B.; Kloetzel, P.M.; Finley, D.; Schmidt, M. The base of the proteasome regulatory particle exhibits chaperone-like activity. *Nat. Cell Biol.* **1999**, *1*, 221–226.

32. Liu, C.W.; Li, X.; Thompson, D.; Wooding, K.; Chang, T.; Tang, Z.; Yu, H.; Thomas, P.J.; DeMartino, G.N. ATP binding and ATP hydrolysis play distinct roles in the function of 26S proteasome. *Mol. Cell* **2006**, *24*, 39–50.

33. Verma, R.; Aravind, L.; Oania, R.; McDonald, W.H.; Yates, J.R.; Koonin, E.V.; Deshaies, R.J. Role of Rpn11 metalloprotease in deubiquitination and degradation by the 26S proteasome. *Science* **2002**, *298*, 611–615.

34. Müller, M.; Mentel, M.; van Hellemond, J.J.; Henze, K.; Woehle, C.; Gould, S.B.; Yu, R.Y.; van der Giezen, M.; Tielens, A.G.; Martin, W.F. Biochemistry and evolution of anaerobic energy metabolism in eukaryotes. *Microbiol. Mol. Biol. Rev.* **2012**, *76*, 444–495.

35. Rafelski, S.M. Mitochondrial network morphology: Building an integrative, geometrical view. *BMC Biol.* **2013**, doi:10.1186/1741-7007-11-71.

36. Dhingra, R.; Kirshenbaum, L.A. Regulation of mitochondrial dynamics and cell fate. *Circ. J.* **2014**, *78*, 803–810.

37. Van der Bliek, A.M.; Shen, Q.; Kawajiri, S. Mechanisms of mitochondrial fission and fusion. *Cold Spring Harb. Perspect. Biol.* **2013**, *5*, doi:10.1101/cshperspect.a011072.

38. Kuznetsov, A.V.; Hermann, M.; Saks, V.; Hengster, P.; Margreiter, R. The cell-type specificity of mitochondrial dynamics. *Int. J. Biochem. Cell Biol.* **2009**, *41*, 1928–1939.

39. Kuznetsov, A.V.; Margreiter, R. Heterogeneity of mitochondria and mitochondrial function within cells as another level of mitochondrial complexity. *Int. J. Mol. Sci.* **2009**, *10*, 1911–1929.

40. Pagliarini, D.J.; Calvo, S.E.; Chang, B.; Sheth, S.A.; Vafai, S.B.; Ong, S.E.; Walford, G.A.; Sugiana, C.; Boneh, A.; Chen, W.K. A mitochondrial protein compendium elucidates complex I disease biology. *Cell* **2008**, *134*, 112–123.

41. Chacinska, A.; Koehler, C.M.; Milenkovic, D.; Lithgow, T.; Pfanner, N. Importing mitochondrial proteins: Machineries and mechanisms. *Cell* **2009**, *138*, 628–644.

42. Baker, M.J.; Frazier, A.E.; Gulbis, J.M.; Ryan, M.T. Mitochondrial protein-import machinery: Correlating structure with function. *Trends Cell Biol.* **2007**, *17*, 456–464.

43. Baker, M.J.; Palmer, C.S.; Stojanovski, D. Mitochondrial protein quality control in health and disease. *Br. J. Pharmacol.* **2014**, *171*, 1870–1889.

44. Baker, M.J.; Tatsuta, T.; Langer, T. Quality control of mitochondrial proteostasis. *Cold Spring Harb. Perspect. Biol.* **2011**, *3*, doi:10.1101/cshperspect.a007559.

45. Voos, W.; Ward, L.A.; Truscott, K.N. The role of AAA+ proteases in mitochondrial protein biogenesis, homeostasis and activity control. *Subcell Biochem.* **2013**, *66*, 223–263.

46. Taylor, E.B.; Rutter, J. Mitochondrial quality control by the ubiquitin-proteasome system. *Biochem. Soc. Trans.* **2011**, *39*, 1509–1513.

47. Fritz, S.; Weinbach, N.; Westermann, B. Mdm30 is an F-box protein required for maintenance of fusion-competent mitochondria in yeast. *Mol. Biol. Cell* **2003**, *14*, 2303–2313.

48. Sickmann, A.; Reinders, J.; Wagner, Y.; Joppich, C.; Zahedi, R.; Meyer, H.E.; Schönfisch, B.; Perschil, I.; Chacinska, A.; Guiard, B. The proteome of *Saccharomyces cerevisiae* mitochondria. *Proc. Natl. Acad. Sci. USA* **2003**, *100*, 13207–13212.

49. Jeon, H.B.; Choi, E.S.; Yoon, J.H.; Hwang, J.H.; Chang, J.W.; Lee, E.K.; Choi, H.W.; Park, Z.Y.; Yoo, Y.J. A proteomics approach to identify the ubiquitinated proteins in mouse heart. *Biochem. Biophys. Res. Commun.* **2007**, *357*, 731–736.

50. Schubert, U.; Antón, L.C.; Gibbs, J.; Norbury, C.C.; Yewdell, J.W.; Bennink, J.R. Rapid degradation of a large fraction of newly synthesized proteins by proteasomes. *Nature* **2000**, *404*, 770–774.

51. Chatenay-Lapointe, M.; Shadel, G.S. Stressed-out mitochondria get MAD. *Cell Metab.* **2010**, *12*, 559–560.

52. Heo, J.-M.; Livnat-Levanon, N.; Taylor, E.B.; Jones, K.T.; Dephoure, N.; Ring, J.; Xie, J.; Brodsky, J.L.; Madeo, F.; Gygi, S.P. A stress-responsive system for mitochondrial protein degradation. *Mol. Cell* **2010**, *40*, 465–480.

53. Neutzner, A.; Youle, R.J.; Karbowski, M. Outer mitochondrial membrane protein degradation by the proteasome. *Novartis Found. Symp.* **2007**, *287*, 4–14.

54. Margineantu, D.H.; Emerson, C.B.; Diaz, D.; Hockenbery, D.M. Hsp90 inhibition decreases mitochondrial protein turnover. *PLoS ONE* **2007**, *2*, e1066.

55. Azzu, V.; Brand, M.D. Degradation of an intramitochondrial protein by the cytosolic proteasome. *J. Cell Sci.* **2010**, *123*, 578–585.

56. Clarke, K.J.; Adams, A.E.; Manzke, L.H.; Pearson, T.W.; Borchers, C.H.; Porter, R.K. A role for ubiquitinylation and the cytosolic proteasome in turnover of mitochondrial uncoupling protein 1 (UCP1). *Biochim. Biophys. Acta* **2012**, *1817*, 1759–1767.

57. Radke, S.; Chander, H.; Schäfer, P.; Meiss, G.; Krüger, R.; Schulz, J.B.; Germain, D. Mitochondrial protein quality control by the proteasome involves ubiquitination and the protease Omi. *J. Biol. Chem.* **2008**, *283*, 12681–12685.

58. Xu, S.; Peng, G.; Wang, Y.; Fang, S.; Karbowski, M. The AAA-ATPase p97 is essential for outer mitochondrial membrane protein turnover. *Mol. Biol. Cell.* **2011**, *22*, 291–300.

59. Braun, R.J.; Sommer, C.; Leibiger, C.; Gentier, R.J.G.; Dumit, V.I.; Paduch, K.; Eisenberg, T.; Habernig, L.; Trausinger, G.; Magnes, C. Accumulation of basic amino acids at mitochondria dictates the cytotoxicity of aberrant ubiquitin. *Cell Rep.* **2015**, doi:10.1016/j.celrep.2015.02.009.

60. Bartolome, F.; Wu, H.C.; Burchell, V.S.; Preza, E.; Wray, S.; Mahoney, C.J; Fox, N.C.; Calvo, A.; Canosa, A.; Moglia, C.; *et al.* Pathogenic *VCP* mutations induce mitochondrial uncoupling and reduced ATP levels. *Neuron* **2013**, *78*, 57–64.

61. Braun, R.J.; Zischka, H.; Madeo, F.; Eisenberg, T.; Wissing, S.; Büttner, S.; Engelhardt, S.M.; Büringer, D.; Ueffing, M. Crucial mitochondrial impairment upon CDC48 mutation in apoptotic yeast. *J. Biol. Chem.* **2006**, *281*, 25757–25767.

62. Kitada, T.; Asakawa, S.; Hattori, N.; Matsumine, H.; Yamamura, Y.; Minoshima, S.; Yokochi, M.; Mizuno, Y.; Shimizu, N. Mutations in the *parkin* gene cause autosomal recessive juvenile parkinsonism. *Nature* **1998**, *392*, 605–608.

63. Koyano, F.; Matsuda, N. Molecular mechanisms underlying PINK1 and Parkin catalyzed ubiquitylation of substrates on damaged mitochondria. *Biochim. Biophys. Acta* **2015**, doi:10.1016/j.bbamcr.2015.02.009.

64. Wenzel, D.M.; Lissounov, A.; Brzovic, P.S.; Klevit, R.E. UBCH7 reactivity profile reveals parkin and HHARI to be RING/HECT hybrids. *Nature* **2011**, *474*, 105–108.

65. Matsuda, N.; Sato, S.; Shiba, K.; Okatsu, K.; Saisho, K.; Gautier, C.A.; Sou, Y.S.; Saiki, S.; Kawajiri, S.; Sato, F.; Kimura, M.; *et al.* PINK1 stabilized by mitochondrial depolarization recruits Parkin to damaged mitochondria and activates latent Parkin for mitophagy. *J. Cell Biol.* **2010**, *189*, 211–221.

66. Kane, L.A.; Lazarou, M.; Fogel, A.I.; Li, Y.; Yamano, K.; Sarraf, S.A.; Banerjee, S.; Youle, R.J. PINK1 phosphorylates ubiquitin to activate Parkin E3 ubiquitin ligase activity. *J. Cell Biol.* **2014**, *205*, 143–153.

67. Koyano, F.; Okatsu, K.; Kosako, H.; Tamura, Y.; Go, E.; Kimura, M.; Kimura, Y.; Tsuchiya, H.; Yoshihara, H.; Hirokawa, T.; *et al.* Ubiquitin is phosphorylated by PINK1 to activate parkin. *Nature* **2014**, *510*, 162–166.

68. Kazlauskaite, A.; Kondapalli, C.; Gourlay, R.; Campbell, D.G.; Ritorto, M.S.; Hofmann, K.; Alessi, D.R.; Knebel, A.; Trost, M.; Muqit, M.M.K. Parkin is activated by PINK1-dependent phosphorylation of ubiquitin at Ser65. *Biochem. J.* **2014**, *460*, 127–139.

69. Geisler, S.; Holmström, K.M.; Skujat, D.; Fiesel, F.C.; Rothfuss, O.C.; Kahle, P.J.; Springer, W. PINK1/Parkin-mediated mitophagy is dependent on VDAC1 and p62/SQSTM1. *Nat. Cell Biol.* **2010**, *12*, 119–131.

70. Glauser, L.; Sonnay, S.; Stafa, K.; Moore, D.J. Parkin promotes the ubiquitination and degradation of the mitochondrial fusion factor mitofusin 1. *J. Neurochem.* **2011**, *118*, 636–645.

71. Narendra, D.; Tanaka, A.; Suen, D.-F.; Youle, R.J. Parkin is recruited selectively to impaired mitochondria and promotes their autophagy. *J. Cell Biol.* **2008**, *183*, 795–803.

72. Sarraf, S.A.; Raman, M.; Guarani-Pereira, V.; Sowa, M.E.; Huttlin, E.L.; Gygi, S.P.; Harper, J.W. Landscape of the PARKIN-dependent ubiquitylome in response to mitochondrial depolarization. *Nature* **2013**, *496*, 372–376.

73. Rana, A.; Rera, M.; Walker, D.W. Parkin overexpression during aging reduces proteotoxicity, alters mitochondrial dynamics, and extends lifespan. *Proc. Natl. Acad. Sci. USA* **2013**, *110*, 8638–8643.

74. Melrose, H.L.; Lincoln, S.J.; Tyndall, G.M.; Farrer, M.J. Parkinson's disease: A rethink of rodent models. *Exp. Brain Res.* **2006**, *173*, 196–204.

75. Sterky, F.H.; Lee, S.; Wibom, R.; Olson, L.; Larsson, N.G. Impaired mitochondrial transport and Parkin-independent degeneration of respiratory chain-deficient dopamine neurons *in vivo*. *Proc. Natl. Acad. Sci. USA* **2011**, *108*, 12937–12942.

76. Nagashima, S.; Tokuyama, T.; Yonashiro, R.; Inatome, R.; Yanagi, S. Roles of mitochondrial ubiquitin ligase MITOL/MARCH5 in mitochondrial dynamics and diseases. *J. Biochem.* **2014**, *155*, 273–279.

77. Karbowski, M.; Neutzner, A.; Youle, R.J. The mitochondrial E3 ubiquitin ligase MARCH5 is required for Drp1 dependent mitochondrial division. *J. Cell Biol.* **2007**, *178*, 71–84.

78. Yonashiro, R.; Ishido, S.; Kyo, S.; Fukuda, T.; Goto, E.; Matsuki, Y.; Ohmura-Hoshino, M.; Sada, K.; Hotta, H.; Yamamura, H.; *et al.* A novel mitochondrial ubiquitin ligase plays a critical role in mitochondrial dynamics. *EMBO J.* **2006**, *25*, 3618–3626.

79. Yonashiro, R.; Sugiura, A.; Miyachi, M.; Fukuda, T.; Matsushita, N.; Inatome, R.; Ogata, Y.; Suzuki, T.; Dohmae, N.; Yanagi, S. Mitochondrial ubiquitin ligase MITOL ubiquitinates mutant SOD1 and attenuates mutant SOD1-induced reactive oxygen species generation. *Mol. Biol. Cell* **2009**, *20*, 4524–4530.

80. Durcan, T.M.; Kontogiannea, M.; Thorarinsdottir, T.; Fallon, L.; Williams, A.J.; Djarmati, A.; Fantaneanu, T.; Paulson, H.L.; Fon, E.A. The Machado–Joseph disease-associated mutant form of ataxin-3 regulates parkin ubiquitination and stability. *Hum. Mol. Genet.* **2011**, *20*, 141–154.

81. Huang, Q.; Wang, H.; Perry, S.W.; Figueiredo-Pereira, M.E. Negative regulation of 26S proteasome stability via calpain-mediated cleavage of Rpn10 upon mitochondrial dysfunction in neurons. *J. Biol. Chem.* **2013**, *288*, 12161–12174.

82. Livnat-Levanon, N.; Kevei, É.; Kleifeld, O.; Krutauz, D.; Segref, A.; Rinaldi, T.; Erpapazoglou, Z.; Cohen, M.; Reis, N.; Hoppe, T.; *et al.* Reversible 26S proteasome disassembly upon mitochondrial stress. *Cell Rep.* **2014**, *7*, 1371–1380.

83. Segref, A.; Kevei, É.; Pokrzywa, W.; Schmeisser, K.; Mansfeld, J.; Livnat-Levanon, N.; Ensenauer, R.; Glickman, M.H.; Ristow, M.; Hoppe, T. Pathogenesis of human mitochondrial diseases is modulated by reduced activity of the ubiquitin/proteasome system. *Cell Metab.* **2014**, *19*, 642–652.

84. Grune, T.; Reinheckel, T.; Davies, K.J. Degradation of oxidized proteins in K562 human hematopoietic cells by proteasome. *J. Biol. Chem.* **1996**, *271*, 15504–15509.

85. Grune, T.; Merker, K.; Sandig, G.; Davies, K.J.A. Selective degradation of oxidatively modified protein substrates by the proteasome. *Biochem. Biophys. Res. Commun.* **2003**, *305*, 709–718.

86. Shringarpure, R.; Grune, T.; Mehlhase, J.; Davies, K.J.A. Ubiquitin conjugation is not required for the degradation of oxidized proteins by proteasome. *J. Biol. Chem.* **2003**, *278*, 311–318.

87. Hershko, A.; Heller, H.; Elias, S.; Ciechanover, A. Components of ubiquitin-protein ligase system. Resolution, affinity purification, and role in protein breakdown. *J. Biol. Chem.* **1983**, *258*, 8206–8214.

88. Eytan, E.; Ganoth, D.; Armon, T.; Hershko, A. ATP-dependent incorporation of 20S protease into the 26S complex that degrades proteins conjugated to ubiquitin. *Proc. Natl. Acad. Sci. USA* **1989**, *86*, 7751–7755.

89. Dahlmann, B.; Kuehn, L.; Reinauer, H. Studies on the activation by ATP of the 26 S proteasome complex from rat skeletal muscle. *Biochem. J.* **1995**, *309*, 195–202.

90. Kleijnen, M.F.; Roelofs, J.; Park, S.; Hathaway, N.A.; Glickman, M.; King, R.W.; Finley, D. Stability of the proteasome can be regulated allosterically through engagement of its proteolytic active sites. *Nat. Struct. Mol. Biol.* **2007**, *14*, 1180–1188.

91. Huang, H.; Zhang, X.; Li, S.; Liu, N.; Lian, W.; McDowell, E.; Zhou, P.; Zhao, C.; Guo, H.; Zhang, C.; *et al.* Physiological levels of ATP negatively regulate proteasome function. *Cell Res.* **2010**, *20*, 1372–1385.

92. Höglinger, G.U.; Carrard, G.; Michel, P.P.; Medja, F.; Lombès, A.; Ruberg, M.; Friguet, B.; Hirsch, E.C. Dysfunction of mitochondrial complex I and the proteasome: Interactions between two biochemical deficits in a cellular model of Parkinson's disease. *J. Neurochem.* **2003**, *86*, 1297–1307.

93. Chen, Q.; Thorpe, J.; Ding, Q.; El-Amouri, I.S.; Keller, J.N. Proteasome synthesis and assembly are required for survival during stationary phase. *Free Radic. Biol. Med.* **2004**, *37*, 859–868.

94. Vernace, V.A.; Arnaud, L.; Schmidt-Glenewinkel, T.; Figueiredo-Pereira, M.E. Aging perturbs 26S proteasome assembly in *Drosophila melanogaster*. *FASEB J.* **2007**, *21*, 2672–2682.

95. Keller, J.N.; Huang, F.F.; Markesbery, W.R. Decreased levels of proteasome activity and proteasome expression in aging spinal cord. *Neuroscience* **2000**, *98*, 149–156.

96. Dasuri, K.; Zhang, L.; Ebenezer, P.; Liu, Y.; Fernandez-Kim, S.O.; Keller, J.N. Aging and dietary restriction alter proteasome biogenesis and composition in the brain and liver. *Mech. Ageing Dev.* **2009**, *130*, 777–783.

97. Ferrington, D.A.; Husom, A.D.; Thompson, L.V. Altered proteasome structure, function, and oxidation in aged muscle. *FASEB J.* **2005**, *19*, 644–646.

98. Hwang, J.S.; Hwang, J.S.; Chang, I.; Kim, S. Age-associated decrease in proteasome content and activities in human dermal fibroblasts: Restoration of normal level of proteasome subunits reduces aging markers in fibroblasts from elderly persons. *J. Gerontol. A Biol. Sci. Med. Sci.* **2007**, *62*, 490–499.

99. Chondrogianni, N.; Voutetakis, K.; Kapetanou, M.; Delitsikou, V.; Papaevgeniou, N.; Sakellari, M.; Lefaki, M.; Filippopoulou, K.; Gonos, E.S. Proteasome activation: An innovative promising approach for delaying aging and retarding age-related diseases. *Ageing Res. Rev.* **2015**, *23*, 37–55.

100. Vernace, V.A.; Schmidt-Glenewinkel, T.; Figueiredo-Pereira, M.E. Aging and regulated protein degradation: Who has the UPPer hand? *Aging Cell.* **2007**, *6*, 599–606.

101. Harman, D. Aging: A theory based on free radical and radiation chemistry. *J. Gerontol.* **1956**, *11*, 298–300.

102. Schwarze, S.R.; Lee, C.M.; Chung, S.S.; Roecker, E.B.; Weindruch, R.; Aiken, J.M. High levels of mitochondrial DNA deletions in skeletal muscle of old rhesus monkeys. *Mech. Ageing Dev.* **1995**, *83*, 91–101.

103. Khaidakov, M.; Heflich, R.H.; Manjanatha, M.G.; Myers, M.B.; Aidoo, A. Accumulation of point mutations in mitochondrial DNA of aging mice. *Mutat. Res.* **2003**, *526*, 1–7.

104. Corral-Debrinski, M.; Horton, T.; Lott, M.T.; Shoffner, J.M.; Beal, M.F.; Wallace, D.C. Mitochondrial DNA deletions in human brain: Regional variability and increase with advanced age. *Nat. Genet.* **1992**, *2*, 324–329.

105. Soong, N.W.; Hinton, D.R.; Cortopassi, G.; Arnheim, N. Mosaicism for a specific somatic mitochondrial DNA mutation in adult human brain. *Nat. Genet.* **1992**, *2*, 318–323.

106. Ross, J.M.; Stewart, J.B.; Hagström, E.; Brené, S.; Mourier, A.; Coppotelli, G.; Freyer, C.; Lagouge, M.; Hoffer, B.J.; Olson, L.; *et al.* Germline mitochondrial DNA mutations aggravate ageing and can impair brain development. *Nature* **2013**, *501*, 412–415.

107. Ross, J.M.; Öberg, J.; Brené, S.; Coppotelli, G.; Terzioglu, M.; Pernold, K.; Goiny, M.; Sitnikov, R.; Kehr, J.; Trifunovic, A.; *et al.* High brain lactate is a hallmark of aging and caused by a shift in the lactate dehydrogenase A/B ratio. *Proc. Natl. Acad. Sci. USA* **2010**, *107*, 20087–20092.

108. Ross, J.M.; Coppotelli, G.; Hoffer, B.J.; Olson, L. Maternally transmitted mitochondrial DNA mutations can reduce lifespan. *Sci. Rep.* **2014**, doi:10.1038/srep06569.

109. Trifunovic, A.; Wredenberg, A.; Falkenberg, M.; Spelbrink, J.N.; Rovio, A.T.; Bruder, C.E.; Bohlooly, Y.M.; Gidlöf, S.; Oldfors, A.; Wibom, R.; *et al.* Premature ageing in mice expressing defective mitochondrial DNA polymerase. *Nature* **2004**, *429*, 417–423.

110. Kujoth, G.C.; Hiona, A.; Pugh, T.D.; Someya, S.; Panzer, K.; Wohlgemuth, S.E.; Hofer, T.; Seo, A.Y.; Sullivan, R.; Jobling, W.A.; *et al.* Mitochondrial DNA mutations, oxidative stress, and apoptosis in mammalian aging. *Science* **2005**, *309*, 481–484.

111. Larsson, N.G.; Oldfors, A. Mitochondrial myopathies. *Acta Physiol. Scand.* **2001**, *171*, 385–393.

112. Cottrell, D.A.; Turnbull, D.M. Mitochondria and ageing. *Curr. Opin. Clin. Nutr. Metab. Care* **2000**, *3*, 473–478.

113. Cook, C.; Petrucelli, L. A critical evaluation of the ubiquitin-proteasome system in Parkinson's disease. *Biochim. Biophys. Acta* **2009**, *1792*, 664–675.

114. Ekstrand, M.I.; Terzioglu, M.; Galter, D.; Zhu, S.; Hofstetter, C.; Lindqvist, E.; Thams, S.; Bergstrand, A.; Hansson, F.S.; Trifunovic, A.; *et al.* Progressive parkinsonism in mice with respiratory-chain-deficient dopamine neurons. *Proc. Natl. Acad. Sci. USA* **2007**, *104*, 1325–1330.

115. Schmidt, N.; Ferger, B. Neurochemical findings in the MPTP model of Parkinson's disease. *J. Neural. Transm.* **2001**, *108*, 1263–1282.

116. Harrington, C.R. The molecular pathology of Alzheimer's disease. *Neuroimaging Clin. N. Am.* **2012**, *22*, 11–22.

117. Riederer, B.M.; Leuba, G.; Vernay, A.; Riederer, I.M. The role of the ubiquitin proteasome system in Alzheimer's disease. *Exp. Biol. Med.* **2011**, *236*, 268–276.

118. Friedland-Leuner, K.; Stockburger, C.; Denzer, I.; Eckert, G.P.; Müller, W.E. Mitochondrial dysfunction: Cause and consequence of Alzheimer's disease. *Prog. Mol. Biol. Transl. Sci.* **2014**, *127*, 183–210.

119. Argyropoulou, A.; Aligiannis, N.; Trougakos, I.P.; Skaltsounis, A.L. Natural compounds with anti-ageing activity. *Nat. Prod. Rep.* **2013**, *30*, 1412–1437.

120. De Cabo, R.; Carmona-Gutierrez, D.; Bernier, M.; Hall, M.N.; Madeo, F. The search for antiaging interventions: From elixirs to fasting regimens. *Cell* **2014**, *157*, 1515–1526.

121. Mizushima, S.; Moriguchi, E.H.; Ishikawa, P.; Hekman, P.; Nara, Y.; Mimura, G.; Moriguchi, Y.; Yamori, Y. Fish intake and cardiovascular risk among middle-aged Japanese in Japan and Brazil. *J. Cardiovasc. Risk* **1997**, *4*, 191–199.

122. Huffman, K.M.; Slentz, C.A.; Bateman, L.A.; Thompson, D.; Muehlbauer, M.J.; Bain, J.R.; Stevens, R.D.; Wenner, B.R.; Kraus, V.B.; Newgard, C.B.; *et al.* Exercise-induced changes in metabolic intermediates, hormones, and inflammatory markers associated with improvements in insulin sensitivity. *Diabetes Care* **2011**, *34*, 174–176.

4

The Role of Mitochondrial DNA in Mediating Alveolar Epithelial Cell Apoptosis and Pulmonary Fibrosis

Seok-Jo Kim [1,2], Paul Cheresh [1,2], Renea P. Jablonski [1,2], David B. Williams [1,2] and David W. Kamp [1,2,*]

[1] Department of Medicine, Division of Pulmonary and Critical Care Medicine, Jesse Brown VA Medical Center, Chicago, IL 60612, USA; E-Mails: seokjo.kim@northwestern.edu (S.-J.K.); p-cheresh@northwestern.edu (P.C.); renea.jablonski@northwestern.edu (R.P.J.); D-Williams@northwestern.edu (D.B.W.)

[2] Division of Pulmonary & Critical Care Medicine, Northwestern University Feinberg School of Medicine, Chicago, IL 60611, USA

* Authors to whom correspondence should be addressed; E-Mail: d-kamp@northwestern.edu

Academic Editors: Jaime M. Ross and Giuseppe Coppotelli

Abstract: Convincing evidence has emerged demonstrating that impairment of mitochondrial function is critically important in regulating alveolar epithelial cell (AEC) programmed cell death (apoptosis) that may contribute to aging-related lung diseases, such as idiopathic pulmonary fibrosis (IPF) and asbestosis (pulmonary fibrosis following asbestos exposure). The mammalian mitochondrial DNA (mtDNA) encodes for 13 proteins, including several essential for oxidative phosphorylation. We review the evidence implicating that oxidative stress-induced mtDNA damage promotes AEC apoptosis and pulmonary fibrosis. We focus on the emerging role for AEC mtDNA damage repair by 8-oxoguanine DNA glycosylase (OGG1) and mitochondrial aconitase (ACO-2) in maintaining mtDNA integrity which is important in preventing AEC apoptosis and asbestos-induced pulmonary fibrosis in a murine model. We then review recent studies linking the sirtuin (SIRT) family members, especially SIRT3, to mitochondrial integrity and mtDNA damage repair and aging. We present a conceptual model of how SIRTs modulate reactive oxygen species (ROS)-driven mitochondrial metabolism that may be important for their tumor suppressor function. The emerging insights into the pathobiology underlying AEC mtDNA damage and apoptosis is suggesting novel therapeutic targets that may prove useful for the management of age-related diseases, including pulmonary fibrosis and lung cancer.

Keywords: mitochondrial DNA damage; oxidative stress; Sirtuin 3; alveolar epithelial cell; pulmonary fibrosis

---

1. Introduction

Pulmonary fibrosis is characterized by an over abundant accumulation of extracellular matrix (ECM) collagen deposition in the distal lung interstitial tissue in association with an injured overlying epithelium and activated myofibroblasts. Idiopathic pulmonary fibrosis (IPF) is the most common variety of lung fibrosis and carries a sobering mortality approaching 50% at 3–4 years [1]. Although many of the cellular and molecular mechanisms underlying the pathophysiology of lung fibrosis have emerged from numerous studies over the past several decades, the precise pathways involved, their regulation, and the role of crosstalk between cells are not fully understood. With the exception of two FDA-approved drug therapies (pirfenidone and nintenanib) emerging in the fall of 2014, there are no effective therapies for patients with IPF. Furthermore, these two drugs primarily slow disease progression rather than improve lung function or symptoms. A better understanding of the pathobiology of pulmonary fibrosis is critically important in the design of more useful therapies.

As will be reviewed herein, the extent of alveolar epithelial cell (AEC) injury, repair, and aging are emerging as critical determinants underlying pulmonary fibrosis. The purpose of this review is to highlight our current understanding of the causal role of AEC mitochondrial DNA (mtDNA) damage following oxidative stress in promoting AEC apoptosis and pulmonary fibrosis. Although oxidative mtDNA damage in other cell types (*i.e.*, vascular endothelial cells, macrophages, fibroblasts, *etc.*) are likely important, we concentrate on the lung epithelium given its prominent role in the pathophysiology of lung fibrosis. In particular, we focus on asbestosis (pulmonary fibrosis arising following asbestos exposure) as it shares radiographic and pathologic features with IPF though IPF is more common and carries a worse prognosis. Our group is using the asbestos paradigm to better understand the pathophysiologic mechanisms underlying pulmonary fibrosis. We begin with a brief overview of the evidence implicating that oxidative stress induces mtDNA damage and thereby promotes AEC apoptosis and pulmonary fibrosis. We explore the evidence that mitochondrial-derived reactive oxygen species (ROS) trigger an AEC mtDNA damage response and apoptosis that can promote lung fibrosis and other degenerative lung diseases (*i.e.*, lung cancer and chronic obstructive pulmonary disease [COPD]). We discuss the emerging role for AEC mtDNA damage repair by 8-oxoguanine DNA glycosylase (OGG1) and mitochondrial aconitase (ACO-2) in maintaining mtDNA integrity, which is important in preventing AEC apoptosis and asbestos-induced pulmonary fibrosis. We review the emerging evidence on the important crosstalk between mitochondrial ROS production, mtDNA damage, p53 activation, OGG1, and ACO-2 acting as a mitochondrial redox-sensor involved in mtDNA maintenance in animal models of lung fibrosis. We summarize recent studies linking the sirtuin (SIRT) family members, especially SIRT3, to mitochondrial integrity and mtDNA damage repair and aging. SIRT3 is considered the 'guardian of the mitochondria' because it is the major mitochondrial deactylase controlling mitochondrial metabolism playing important roles in mtDNA integrity and the prevention of aging. Finally, we present a conceptual model of how SIRTs modulate ROS-driven mitochondrial metabolism that may be important for cell survival as well as their tumor suppressor function. A general hypothetical model linking mtDNA damage and mitochondrial dysfunction to diverse degenerative diseases, including pulmonary fibrosis, aging, and tumorigenesis is shown in Figure 1. Specifically, herein we focus on a proposed model of AEC mtDNA damage in mediating AEC-intrinsic apoptosis and pulmonary fibrosis as illustrated in Figure 2. Collectively, these studies are revealing novel insights into the pathobiology underlying AEC mtDNA damage and apoptosis that should provide the rationale for developing novel therapeutic targets for managing age-related diseases such as pulmonary fibrosis, COPD, and lung cancer.

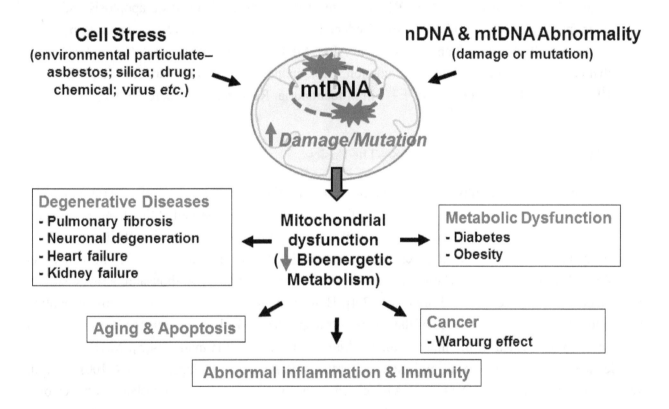

Figure 1. Hypothetical model whereby mtDNA damage induces diverse degenerative diseases. MtDNA damage and mutation can be induced by cell stress from environmental particulates and/or DNA abnormality. MtDNA damage/mutation cause mitochondrial dysfunction reducing bioenergeneric metabolism that can promote degenerative diseases, metabolic dysfunction, aging, apoptosis and cancer. Red-up arrow, increase; red-down arrow, decrease.

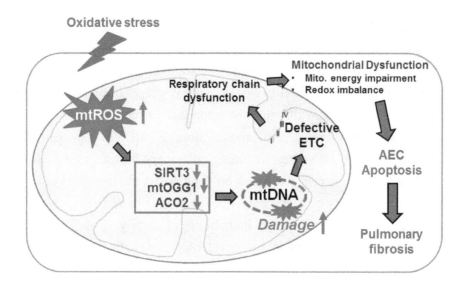

Figure 2. Proposed model of mtDNA damage in mediating AEC intrinsic apoptosis and pulmonary fibrosis. Oxidative stress-induced mtROS induces mtDNA damage by decreasing SIRT3, ACo-2 and mtOGG1 in AEC. MtDNA damage causes a defective ETC that can promote mitochondrial dysfunction, AEC apoptosis, and pulmonary fibrosis. I, II, III, IV, four different complex of ETC in mitochondria. Red-up arrow, increase; red-down arrow, decrease.

2. The Mitochondria, mtDNA, and ROS—The Basics

Mitochondria are maternally inherited and have an essential cellular function of generating energy in the form of ATP via respiration, hence are the "powerhouse" of the cell. Mitochondria also are critically important in regulating complex survival signals that determine whether cells live or die and are closely involved in additional functions, such as cellular differentiation, growth, and cell cycle control [2]. The number of mitochondria in a cell ranges from one to several thousand, a range largely determined by the tissue type and organism [3,4]. Human mtDNA is composed of 16,569 nucleotide bases and encodes 13 polypeptides of the electron transport chain (ETC), 22 transfer RNAs, and two ribosomal RNAs located in the inner mitochondrial membrane (IMM) matrix [4,5]. MtDNA, which encodes approximately 3% of all mitochondrial proteins, is present in multiple copies (~100) per cell, whereas nearly 1200 nuclear DNA (nDNA)-encoded mitochondrial proteins are translated in the cytosol and imported into the mitochondria [3–5]. Interestingly, the extent of mtDNA alterations that occurs during development affects the presence and emergence of mtDNA genetic variations and mutations primarily in a region termed the D-loop [6,7]. This D-loop on the mtDNA forms the basis of forensic medicine in human identification and has been a useful tool in molecular anthropological studies on human origins [7]. Some proteins encoded by nDNA have been shown to be essential for maintaining mtDNA integrity including OGG1, ACO-2, mitochondrial transcription factor A (Tfam), and others [8–13]. However, the mitochondrial proteins involved in mtDNA repair (mostly base excision repair [BER]) are all nuclear encoded and highly dependent on the nDNA repair machinery systems [14,15]. Notably, compared to nDNA, mtDNA is ~50-fold more sensitive to oxidative damage, in part due to its proximity to the ETC and ROS production, lack of a histone protective shield overlying the mtDNA, and relatively limited DNA repair mechanisms [12,13,16,17]. As compared to nDNA, oxidative stress-induced mtDNA damage has a mutation rate that is 10-fold greater [18–23]. Not surprisingly, mtDNA damage and subsequent mutations can lead to mitochondrial dysfunction, including the collapse in the mitochondrial membrane potential ($\Delta\Psi_m$) and release of pro-apoptogenic agents which drives disease formation, aging, and tumorigenesis (Figure 1) [12,19].

ROS, such as hydroxyl radicals (•HO), superoxide anions ($O_2^{•-}$), hydrogen peroxide (H_2O_2), and others are primarily generated under physiologic conditions from the mitochondrial ETC but also from other intracellular sources [12,18,24–29]. Although low levels of ROS are important for promoting cell survival signaling pathways and antioxidant defenses, higher ROS levels, as occurs in the setting of disease or aging, cause oxidative damage to biomolecules, such as DNA, protein, and lipids. Oxidative DNA damage can result in apoptosis and senescence, tumorigenesis, and degenerative diseases ([7,12,18,24–26,28], Figure 1). Furthermore, mtDNA variants within cells can affect both energy and non-energy pathways (complement, inflammatory, and apoptotic) supporting a paradigm shift in thinking about the role of mitochondria beyond simply energy production [7,12,30].

Biological tissues, especially the lungs, are exposed to both extrinsic sources of ROS (e.g., tobacco, asbestos, silica, radiation, bleomycin, and other drugs) and intrinsic sources (such as those from inflammatory, mesenchymal, epithelial, and endothelial cells) primarily via the mitochondrial ETC as well as numerous enzyme systems including Nicotinamide adenine dinucleotide phosphate (NADPH) oxidases (NOXs), xanthine oxidase, and nitric oxide synthase (NOS) [12,19,31]. Intracellular ROS can also be generated from redox-active ferrous (Fe^{2+}) iron within or on the surface of asbestos fibers via the Haber-Weiss reaction [31,32], resulting in the accumulation of •HO and other free radicals. As reviewed in detail elsewhere, several lines of evidence demonstrate that ROS play a role in pulmonary fibrotic disease: (1) oxidized lipids and proteins have been identified from the exhaled air, BAL fluid, and lung tissue of patients with fibrotic lung disease [33,34]; and (2) Bleomycin-induced pulmonary fibrosis (the most common animal fibrosis model) is associated with increased levels of ROS, oxidized proteins, DNA, and lipids [35,36]; (3) Increased oxidative DNA damage is seen in IPF, silicosis, and asbestosis patients, as well in experimental animal models of silicosis or asbestos-induced lung fibrosis [37]; (4) Antioxidants and iron chelators can attenuate fibrosis induced by bleomycin or asbestos in rodent models [35,38]. Additionally, there is some evidence implying that mitochondria-generated ROS of lung parenchymal cells mediate pulmonary fibrosis [36]. Exogenous toxins, such as asbestos fibers, can also induce mitochondrial ROS in lung epithelial cells and macrophages; both of which are important target cells implicated in pulmonary fibrosis (see for reviews: [31,35,37]). However, more work is needed to determine the precise molecular mechanisms involved as well as any cross-talk between cell types. A key role of alveolar macrophage (AM) mitochondrial ROS in mediating asbestosis has been suggested in the studies by Carter and colleagues [39–42]. These investigators showed that mitochondrial Rac-1 levels are elevated in AM from patients with asbestosis, that Rac-1 augments asbestos-induced AM H_2O_2 production, and that ROS production is reduced by knockdown of the iron-sulfur complex III in the mitochondrial ETC. These data implicate H_2O_2 production via electron transfer from Rac-1 to complex III may activate cellular injury pathways that promote asbestosis.

Although the precise role of H_2O_2-induced AEC mtDNA damage in mediating pulmonary fibrosis is unclear, a possible causal role for H_2O_2 in promoting lung fibrosis is supported by several lines of evidence that we recently reviewed in detail elsewhere [35], and briefly summarize herein; some of the key points are: (1) catalase, a H_2O_2 scavenger, blocks H_2O_2-induced human IPF fibroblast activation [34];

and prevents asbestos-induced fibrosis in rats [43,44]; (2) glutathione (GSH), an antioxidant, is diminished in IPF lungs and epithelial lining fluid [34,45,46]; and (3) although n-acetyl cysteine (NAC), a GSH precursor, attenuates bleomycin-induced fibrosis in rodents and increases lung GSH levels, NAC administration to patients with IPF was recently proven no better than placebo [47,48]. Similar to H_2O_2, considerable evidence reviewed elsewhere, implicates NOXs, especially NOX1, 2, and 4 isoforms, in the pathogenesis of pulmonary fibrosis, including AEC apoptosis and apoptosis-resistant myofibroblasts [49–53].

3. AEC Apoptosis and Lung Fibrosis—Role of the Mitochondria

3.1. AEC Aging, Apoptosis and Pulmonary Fibrosis

Accumulating evidence firmly implicate that "exaggerated" aging lung has a crucial role in the pathogenesis of lung fibrosis, although the detailed molecular mechanisms involved are not fully established (see for reviews: [1,54]). The nine proposed pivotal hallmarks mediating the "aging phenotype" include: genomic instability, telomere shortening, epigenetic alterations, deficient proteostasis, dysregulated nutrient sensing, mitochondrial dysfunction, cellular senescence/apoptosis, stem cell depletion, and distorted intercellular communication [55]. However, many of the nine aging pathways are implicated in humans with IPF, including AEC DNA damage, activation of epigenetic signaling, shortened alveolar type II (AT2—the distal lung epithelial stem cell) cell telomeres, AEC mitochondria-mediated (intrinsic) apoptosis, and activated endoplasmic reticulum (ER) stress response in apoptotic AECs (see for reviews: [1,37,54,56–60]). Herein we focus on mtDNA damage since it is an early event in oxidant-exposed cells that may contribute to the inflammatory, fibrogenic and malignant potential of asbestos [37,57,61,62]. Notably, genome-wide association studies (GWAS) have established an important role for aberrant DNA repair pathways in patients with IPF [55,63–65]. As reviewed in detail elsewhere [7,66], mutations in maternally-inherited mtDNA encoding for key genes of mitochondrial energy-generating oxidative phosphorylation, rather than Mendelian nuclear genetic principles, better accounts for the complex clinical-pathological features of many common degenerative and metabolic disease whose tissue stem cells are bioenergetically abnormal (Figure 1).

In contrast to catastrophic lytic/necrotic cell death that can trigger an inflammatory response, apoptosis is a regulated, ATP-dependent process of cell death that results in the elimination of cells with extensive DNA damage without eliciting an inflammatory response. Apoptotic cellular responses occur by two mechanisms: (1) the extrinsic (death receptor) pathway and (2) the intrinsic (mitochondria-regulated) pathway. Others [19,67] as well as ourselves [35,37] have extensively reviewed these pathways recently we, therefore, confine our comments to some of the more recent updates centered on mitochondrial dysfunction and mtDNA damage in driving AEC apoptosis.

Considerable evidence reviewed elsewhere convincingly demonstrates that AEC apoptosis is one of the key pathophysiologic events hindering normal lung repair and thus promoting pulmonary fibrosis [1,35,37,52,56–59,68–71]. Briefly summarizing some of the key findings includes the following: (1) patients with IPF and animal models of asbestos- and silica-induced pulmonary fibrosis show significant lung epithelial cell injury, ER stress and apoptosis; (2) fibrogenic dusts, such as asbestos and silica, can induce both lytic and apoptotic AEC death in part by generating ROS derived from the mitochondria or NOXs; (3) DNA damage, which is a strong activator of intrinsic apoptosis, occurs in the AEC of human patients with IPF and murine models of asbestos-induced lung fibrosis and can activate p53, an important DNA damage response molecule; (4) protein S-glutathionylation, in part through effects occurring in the ER, mediates redox-based alterations in the FAS death receptor important for triggering extrinsic lung epithelial cell apoptosis and pulmonary fibrosis; and (5) blocking $\alpha v \beta 6$ integrin release from injured lung epithelial cells, prevents latent TGF-β activation and pulmonary fibrosis following radiation or bleomycin exposure.

Perhaps the most convincing evidence implicating AEC apoptosis in the pathophysiology of pulmonary fibrosis is that genetic approaches targeting apoptosis of Alveolar epithelial type 2 cell (AT2 cells) in mice and humans demonstrate an important role for AECs (see for reviews: [56,58]). A primary requirement for AEC death and inadequate epithelial cell repair in causing pulmonary fibrosis as first pointed out by Haschek and Witschi 35 years ago has now been elegantly verified by various transgenic murine models of pulmonary fibrosis and genetic mutations in 10 different surfactant protein C (SPC) BRICHOS domain mutations that are only evident in AT2 cells in humans with interstitial pulmonary fibrosis [56]. A clear genetic predisposition to developing IPF is evident in 5%–20% of patients [1,56,58,59,63–65]. Notably, many mutations associated with the development of pulmonary fibrosis are only expressed in epithelial cells (*i.e.*, surfactant C and A2 genes, MUC5b), while others are more ubiquitously expressed. Although a detailed discussion of these mutations is beyond the scope of this article, SPC mutations can induce AEC ER stress response that promotes AEC apoptosis and pulmonary fibrosis [59]. Among the most common gene mutations seen in patients with IPF and familial pulmonary fibrosis involve telomerase (TERT and TERTC). Unlike surfactant mutations, telomerase mutations are ubiquitously expressed in cells, especially in stem cells [72]. Shortened telomeres, which are associated with aging-related diseases due to oxidative stress, are evident in the majority of AT2 cells (the distal lung epithelial stem cells) in patients with lung fibrosis [72,73]. One study showed that AT2 cells from 97% of 62 IPF patients (both sporadic and familial) had shortened telomeres [73]. Although mitochondrial dysfunction and ROS production appear important in driving telomerase-dependent cell senescence, the role of mtDNA damage is uncertain [74]. The finding that AEC telomerase shortening, alone, does not trigger lung fibrosis, nor augment bleomycin-induced lung fibrosis in mice, strongly implicates other genetic and/or environmental factors are likely crucial [75].

3.2. Mitochondria-Regulated AEC Apoptosis

The intrinsic apoptotic death pathway is activated by various fibrotic stimuli (*i.e.*, ROS, DNA damage, asbestos, *etc.*) that stimulate pro-apoptotic Bcl-2 family members action at the mitochondria that results in increased permeability of the outer mitochondrial membrane, reduced $\Delta \Psi_m$, and the release of numerous apoptotic proteins (*i.e.*, cytochrome c, *etc.*) that subsequently activate pro-apoptotic caspase-9 and caspase-3 (see for reviews: [19,35,37,58,67,68]). Notably, a crucial role for mtDNA damage in driving intrinsic apoptosis was established in cell-sorting studies demonstrating that persistent mtDNA damage results in the collapse in the $\Delta \Psi_m$ and intrinsic apoptosis [76]. Bleomycin-induced fibrosis in mice is blocked in the pro-apoptotic Bid deficient mice [77]. Bid is activated by the death receptor pathway and triggers intrinsic apoptosis by blocking anti-apoptotic Bcl-2 molecules and thereby enabling Bax/Bak-mediated apoptosis [77]. However, additional studies are warranted to better understand how Bcl-2 family members modulate mtDNA integrity to impact AEC survival and prevent lung fibrosis. More recently, two groups have established that PTEN-induced putative kinase 1 (PINK1) deficiency impairs AEC mitochondrial function in patients with IPF and PINK1-deficient mice have increased AEC intrinsic apoptosis and lung fibrosis following viral-induced ER stress or bleomycin exposure [78,79]. Interestingly, the pro-fibrotic cytokine TGF-β may be protective to lung epithelial by promoting PINK1 expression and attenuating AEC apoptosis that drives lung fibrosis [79]. Collectively, these studies firmly support an important role of AEC mitochondria-regulated apoptosis in the pathophysiology of pulmonary fibrosis. Additional studies are required to further characterize the precise molecular mechanisms involved, the role of mtDNA damage, and crosstalk between AEC and macrophages. Furthermore, the translational significance of any identified targets in animals exposed to fibrogenic agents will need to be investigated in humans with IPF.

Others as well as our group have been using the asbestos paradigm to better inform our understanding of how oxidative stress resulting from fiber exposure promotes lung epithelial cell intrinsic apoptosis important in the development of pulmonary fibrosis. As we have extensively reviewed these studies from our group elsewhere [35,37], we summarize herein only some of the salient supporting findings including: (1) asbestos fibers are internalized by AECs soon after exposure, resulting in the production of iron-derived ROS, mtDNA damage, and intrinsic apoptosis as evidenced by decreased $\Delta\Psi_m$, mitochondrial cytochrome c release into the cytosol, and activation of caspase-9 and 3 (but not caspase-8); (2) these deleterious actions by asbestos on AECs are blocked by phytic acid (an iron chelator), benzoic acid (a free-radical scavenger), and overexpression of Bcl-XL; and (3) an important role for mitochondrial ROS is suggested by the findings that asbestos-induced AEC intrinsic apoptosis and p53 activation are blocked in cells unable to produce mitochondrial ROS and that asbestos preferentially induces mitochondrial ROS production as assessed using a highly sensitive rho-GFP probes targeted to the mitochondria or cytosol. Furthermore, as reviewed below (see Section 3.3), we find a direct relationship between asbestos-induced mtDNA damage and intrinsic AEC apoptosis. Mossman and colleagues showed that activated protein kinase delta (PKCδ) migrates to the mitochondria of lung epithelial cells in vitro and in vivo following asbestos exposure and is crucial for promoting asbestos-induced mitochondria-regulated apoptosis and fibrosis via mechanisms dependent upon pro-apoptotic Bim activation [80,81]. Taken together, mitochondrial ROS production and PKCδ activation following asbestos exposure appear important for inducing p53 activation and intrinsic lung epithelial cell apoptosis. However, the role of mtDNA integrity in modulating p53 and PKCδ activation requires additional study.

3.3. mtDNA Damage and Repair—Role in Cancer and Lung Fibrosis

Prompt repair of damaged mtDNA is important given the accumulating evidence convincingly showing that mtDNA damage and mutations are linked to various pathologic conditions, including lung fibrosis (see for reviews: [7,12,18,19,82]). MtDNA mutations accumulate in tissues with aging in part via disruptions in mitochondrial quality control pathways. MtDNA deletions that occur early in development can become widely disseminated throughout the body and cause spontaneous mitochondrial dysfunction [7]. Further, mtDNA deletions [83] and mutations [84] can arise in cells of various tissues throughout life and their accumulation modulates aging and longevity [7,84]. These findings suggest that the accumulation of mtDNA mutations arising from mtDNA damage caused by aging, environmental exposure, and other forms of oxidative stress support the "mitochondrial theory of aging" that may be crucial in depleting the longevity of important stem cells (*i.e.*, AT2 cells in the distal lung) and promoting the pathobiology of degenerative diseases and tumorigenesis [3,7,12].

Cancer is characterized by altered energy metabolism (Warburg effect) arising from mtDNA mutations and changes in mtDNA copy number [85,86]. Of 41 human lung, bladder, and head and neck tumors examined, mutated mtDNA occurred 19–220 times more frequently than nDNA [87]. The importance of mtDNA mutations in lung cancer is supported by the observation that over 40% of patients with lung cancer demonstrate mutations in their mtDNA [88]. MtDNA mutations can compromise ETC function and contribute to altered metabolism driving accelerated aerobic glycolysis in the setting of metastatic progression [89]. Additionally, severe mtDNA damage promotes mitochondrial genome deletion [90]. Tumor cells lacking mtDNA can acquire mtDNA of host origin, resulting in sequential recovery of respiration from primary to metastatic tumor cells [91]. There is also evidence that mtDNA mutations can preferentially accumulate in non-small cell lung cancer (NSCLC) tissues as compared to matched blood samples [88]. Taken together, these studies demonstrate that mtDNA damage and mutations occur in malignant cells, including lung cancers, and that preservation of mtDNA integrity may be an innovative preventative therapeutic target.

Base excision repair (BER), which is the major mtDNA repair mechanism, has been reviewed in detail elsewhere [18]. All mtDNA repair proteins are nuclear-encoded and imported into mitochondria. 8OHdG, the most common of ~50 DNA base changes that occur with oxidative stress, is highly mutagenic in replicating cells by causing G:C→A:T transversions that can contribute to tumorigenesis and aging [12,18]. Mutations in the hOGG1 gene occur in patients with lung cancer and other malignancies [92]. OGG1 is over three-fold more active in the mitochondria as compared to the nucleus and *Ogg1*$^{-/-}$ mice have a 20-fold increase in liver mitochondrial 8OHdG levels [18,92]. Mitochondria-targeted OGG1 (mt-OGG1) over-expression prevents mitochondria-regulated apoptosis caused by oxidative stress, including AEC apoptosis following asbestos exposure [8,9,12,13,62,93,94]. OGG1 has two isoforms (α and β), yet curiously the βOGG1 isoform has negligible DNA repair activity despite being in 50-fold excess as compared to the αOGG1 isoform in the mitochondria [95]. This suggests that βOGG1 isoform plays a role in mitigating mitochondrial oxidative stress independent of its BER activity. We recently showed that overexpression of mt-OGG1 or mt-OGG1 mutants incapable of DNA repair promote AEC survival despite high levels of asbestos-induced mitochondrial ROS stress [9]. Although one mechanism by which mt-OGG1 preserves mitochondrial function is by increasing mtDNA repair, we identified a novel function of OGG1 in chaperoning mitochondrial aconitase (ACO-2) from oxidative degradation and, thereby, preserving mtDNA integrity [9]. ACO-2, a mitochondrial tricarboxylic acid cycle (TCA) enzyme, is a sensitive marker of oxidative stress and, notably, preserves mtDNA in yeast independent of ACO-2 activity [96,97]. We also reported that oxidative stress (asbestos or H_2O_2) preferentially induces mtDNA than nuclear DNA damage in AEC both *in vitro* as well as *in vivo* and that OGG1 preservation of ACO-2 is crucial for preventing asbestos-induced AEC mtDNA damage, intrinsic apoptosis, and pulmonary fibrosis [8,98]. Additional support for a protective role of ACO-2 is that ACO-2 inactivation has been linked to decreased lifespan in yeast and progressive neurodegenerative diseases in humans [99]. Thus, ACO-2 appears to have a dual function in the TCA cycle for mitochondrial bioenergy production as well as for preserving mtDNA. The precise molecular mechanisms by which mt-OGG1 and ACO-2 interact to preserve AEC mtDNA integrity are not fully understood. Furthermore, additional studies are necessary to assess the translational significance of AEC OGG1 and ACO-2 in preserving mtDNA integrity and preventing pulmonary fibrosis.

3.4. Animals Models of Pulmonary Fibrosis—Role of Mitochondrial ROS, mtDNA Damage, and Mitochondrial Dysfunction

Accumulating evidence reviewed above strongly implicates mitochondrial ROS production, mtDNA damage, and mitochondrial dysfunction (in part due to PINK1 deficiency) in the pathophysiology of AEC apoptosis and pulmonary fibrosis. Herein we review some of the other more recent animal lung fibrosis models that have better informed our understanding of the field. Gadzhar *et al.* [36] examined adult Wistar rat lungs at various time points after a single intratracheal dose of bleomycin and observed lung fibrosis, as measured by Ashcroft scores, collagen, and TGF-β levels at day 14. Evidence of ROS, as assessed by malondialdehyde (MDA) production, was noted as early as 24 h after bleomycin treatment and continued to increase over 14 days. By day seven, mtDNA deletions were significantly elevated and disruption of the mitochondrial architecture as assessed by electron microscopy was noted in lung tissue. Notably, these mitochondrial abnormalities resulted in dysfunction of ETC subunits encoded by mtDNA, but not nDNA, and mtDNA deletions and mtDNA-encoded ETC dysfunction were directly associated with pulmonary TGF-β levels that were predictive of developing lung fibrosis in a multivariate model.

As pulmonary fibrosis is a disease of aging, Hecker *et al.* [53] compared the capacity of young (two months) and aged (18 months) mice to repair bleomycin-induced lung injury and fibrosis. Although the severity of lung fibrosis in each group was similar at three weeks following bleomycin exposure, the aged mice were unable to resolve fibrotic lung injury at two months whereas young mice were largely free of fibrotic injury. Persistent lung fibrosis in the aged mice was characterized by the accumulation of senescent and apoptosis-resistant myofibroblasts, as well as sustained alterations in redox balance resulting from the elevated expression of NOX4 and an impaired capacity to induce the nuclear factor erythroid 2-related factor 2 (Nrf2)-mediated antioxidant response. Human IPF lung tissues also exhibited the imbalance between NOX4 and Nrf2, as well as NOX4 mediated senescence and apoptosis resistance in IPF fibroblasts. Genetic and pharmacological inhibition of NOX4 (with NOX4 siRNA and GKT137831) in older mice with established fibrosis attenuated the senescent and apoptosis-resistant myofibroblast phenotype and led to a reversal of persistent fibrosis. These findings implicating Nrf2 are in accord with prior studies showing that Nrf2 knockout mice are more sensitive to bleomycin and paraquat-induced lung injury than their wild-type counterparts, that primary lung fibroblasts isolated from IPF patients, as compared to healthy controls, have decreased Nrf2 expression and a myofibroblast (pro-fibrotic) differentiated phenotype, and that treatment with sulfaphane, an Nrf2 activator, increases antioxidant levels that results in decreased ROS levels, myofibroblastic de-differentiation, and TGF-β profibrotic effects. Although the role of the NOX4/Nrf2 pathway in AEC and mtDNA damage is unknown, these studies firmly suggest that the restoration of NOX4-Nrf2 redox imbalance in myofibroblasts may be an important therapeutic target.

Our group recently reported that mice globally deficient in $Ogg1^{-/-}$ are more prone to pulmonary fibrosis following asbestos exposure than their wild-type counterparts due in part to increased AEC mtDNA damage and apoptosis [98]. Interestingly, compared to AT2 cells isolated from WT mice, AT2 cells from $Ogg1^{-/-}$ mice have increased mtDNA damage, reduced ACO-2 expression, and increased p53 expression at baseline and these changes were augmented following crocidolite asbestos exposure for three weeks. Collectively, these data support a key role for AEC OGG1 and ACO-2 in the maintenance of mtDNA necessary for preventing AEC apoptosis and pulmonary fibrosis. These findings implicating AEC mtDNA damage signaling in mediating pulmonary fibrosis parallels work by other groups implicating mtDNA damage in the pathophysiology of diverse conditions, such as atherosclerosis, cardiac fibrosis/heart failure, diaphragmatic dysfunction from mechanical ventilation, and cancer [100–106]. Interestingly, mitochondria-targeted OGG1 diminishes ventilator-induced lung injury in mice by reducing the levels of mtDNA damage in the lungs [107]. Accumulating evidences also support an important association between p53, OGG1, and ACO-2, including (1) p53 regulates $OGG1$ gene transcription in colon and renal epithelial cells [93]; (2) p53 deficient cells have reduced OGG1 protein expression and activity [93]; (3) p53 can reduce Aco-2 gene expression [108]; (4) p53 activation is required for oxidant-induced apoptosis in $OGG1$-deficient human fibroblasts [93]; and (5) p53 sensitizes HepG2 cells to oxidative stress by reducing mtDNA [109]. Collectively, these data support a key role for p53 in modulating AEC mtDNA damage in the pro-fibrotic lung response following asbestos exposure that also has important implications for our understanding of the malignant potential of asbestos fibers. However, the precise molecular mechanisms by which OGG1, ACO-2, and p53 coordinately regulate mtDNA integrity in AEC as well as the translational significance of these findings in humans await further study.

A number of animal models of pulmonary fibrosis beyond the scope of this review have implicated excess plasminogen activator inhibitor (PAI-1) in augmenting AEC apoptosis. Shetty and colleagues have recently published a number of elegant studies showing an important dichotomous role of PAI-1 in promoting AEC apoptosis but reducing fibroblast proliferation and collagen production in the pathobiology of lung fibrosis [110–112]. Similar to older studies, these investigators showed that lung injury and pulmonary fibrosis are more evident in mice deficient in urokinase-type plasminogen activator (uPA), whereas mice deficient in PAI-1 are protected. To explore whether changes in AT2 cell uPA and PAI-1 contribute to epithelial-mesenchymal transition (EMT), AT2 cells from patients with IPF and COPD, and mice with bleomycin-, transforming growth factor β-, or passive cigarette smoke-induced lung injury all had reduced expression of E-cadherin and zona occludens-1, whereas collagen-I and α-smooth muscle actin (markers of EMT) were increased along with a parallel increase in PAI-1 and reduced uPA expression [110]. These studies suggest that induction of PAI-1 and inhibition of uPA during fibrotic lung injury promotes EMT in AT2 cells. These same investigators showed that fibroblasts isolated from human IPF lungs and from mice with bleomycin-induced lung fibrosis had an increased rate of proliferation compared with normal lung fibroblasts [111]. Basal expression of plasminogen activator inhibitor-1 (PAI-1) in human and murine fibroblasts was reduced, whereas collagen-I and α-smooth muscle actin were markedly elevated. In contrast, AT2 cells surrounding the fibrotic foci, as well as those isolated from IPF lungs, showed increased caspase-3 and PAI-1 activation with a parallel reduction in uPA expression. PAI-1 depletion and enforced expression studies in cultured fibroblast confirmed the inverse relationship between PAI-1 activation and collagen production. The authors suggested that depletion of PAI-1 in fibroblasts promotes an activated collagen producing cell that is resistant to senescence/apoptosis whereas activated PAI-1 augments AT2 cell apoptosis important for the propagation of lung fibrosis. Using a silica-induced model of lung fibrosis, these investigators showed p53-mediated changes in the uPA system promote lung fibrosis in part by reducing caveolin-1 scaffolding domain peptide (CSP), which is necessary for inhibiting p53 expression and silica-induced lung injury [112]. Notably, as compared to untreated WT mice, silica-exposed WT mice treated with CSP inhibited PAI-1, augmented uPA expression and prevented AEC apoptosis by suppressing p53. The authors suggested that silica-induced lung fibrosis is driven by important crosstalk between the p53-uPA fibrinolytic system in AT2 cells and provide support for a novel pharmacologic target (*i.e.*, CSP), in modulating this pathway. In contrast, another group working with murine fibroblasts recently showed that increased PAI-1 may drive age-related and bleomycin-induced pulmonary fibrosis at least in part by blocking fibroblast apoptosis [113]. Additional studies are required to better understand how precisely PAI-1 affects AEC and fibroblast mtDNA damage response, mitochondrial function and apoptosis as well as how this impacts lung fibrosis.

Mitochondrial ROS and mtDNA can also trigger NACHT, LRR, and PYD domains-containing protein 3 (NALP3) inflammasome signaling important in driving lung fibrosis following asbestos or silica exposure [37,57,114,115]. The mtDNA released into the circulation can act as a sentinel molecule triggering a DNA damage-associated molecular pattern (DAMP) that activates innate immune responses, especially toll like receptor (TLR)-9 signaling, leading to change a phenotype in lung fibroblasts and tissue injury, including lung fibrosis [12,116]. Gu and associates recently showed that intratracheal instillation of mtDNA into murine lungs triggers infiltration of inflammatory cells and production of inflammatory cytokines (*i.e.*, IL-1β, IL-6, and TNF-β) and that these effects were blocked when the lungs were pretreated with TLR-9 siRNA [117]. This suggests that the mtDNA DAMPs can activate innate immune signaling in the lungs via the TLR-9 pathway. Interestingly, Kuck and colleagues showed that mitochondria-targeted OGG1 protein infusion mitigates mtDNA DAMP formation and TLR-9-dependent vascular injury induced by intratracheally-instilled bacteria [118]. Using mice lacking vimentin, a type III intermediate filament, Dos Santos and colleagues demonstrated an important role for vimentin in regulating NLRP3 inflammasome signaling that promotes acute lung injury, IL-1β expression, alveolar epithelial barrier permeability, and lung fibrosis following exposure to lipopolysaccharide (LPS), crocidolite asbestos, and bleomycin [119]. Notably, a direct interaction between vimentin and NLRP3 was demonstrated as well as an important role for macrophages based upon the finding that bone marrow chimeric mice lacking vimentin have decreased lung fibrosis as well as levels of caspase-1 and IL-1β. Collectively, these recent studies provide insight into the role of mtDNA and vimentin in regulating the NLRP3 inflammasome signaling important in promoting lung inflammation and fibrosis.

4. The Role of Sirtuins in Mitochondrial Integrity, mtDNA Damage Repair, and Aging

4.1. Overview of the Sirtuin (SIRT) Family Members

The yeast silent information regulator protein (SIR2) is a highly-conserved protein that has been linked to increased longevity via maintenance of genomic stability in a variety of organisms, including

Drosophila melanogaster and *Caenorhabditis elegans* [120–122]. The homologous mammalian sirtuin family (SIRTs) consists of seven identified members to date, which are localized to the nucleus (SIRT1, SIRT6, SIRT7), cytoplasm (SIRT2), and mitochondria (SIRT3-5), respectively. All sirtuins contain a conserved core domain with NAD^+ binding activity, while most sirtuins catalyze NAD^+-dependent deacetylation of lysine residues though SIRT4 is known to have ADP-ribosyltransferase activity and SIRT5 both desuccinylase and demalonyase activity. Members of the sirtuin family play a role in maintenance of genomic stability at multiple levels by participating in DNA repair, altering chromatin structure and function via histone deacetylation [120], and via adaptation of cellular metabolic flow and energy demand [121]. As such, sirtuins have been considered by many to be the guardians of the genome [122].

4.2. The Role of SIRTs and Mitochondria; Normal and General Diseases

Changes in mitochondrial number and function are implicated in the pathogenesis of aging and many of its associated diseases, such as Parkinson's disease, presbycusis, diabetes and the metabolic syndrome, malignancy, and fibrosis. Though changes in mitochondria have been linked to many disease processes, the underlying detailed molecular mechanisms have yet to be fully elucidated as noted above. Major changes in the mitochondria occur with aging, including an increase in the $\Delta\psi_m$ with subsequent increases in ROS production and oxidative damage to mtDNA and other cellular macromolecules. Maintenance of intracellular redox balance is critical to cellular homeostasis and survival. Certain mtDNA haplogroups are associated with an increase in ROS production; these may be associated with a protective effect in early life due to protection against infection, though with age may in fact be maladaptive due to the presence of chronic oxidative stress [7].

Crosstalk between the mitochondria and nucleus has emerged as a potentially powerful regulator underlying age-related diseases. Using a mitochondrial cybrid model of age-related macular degeneration, Kenney *et al.* [30] showed varying bioenergetic profiles among mtDNA haplogroups and went further to demonstrate different gene expression profiles for both mitochondrial-encoded genes involved in cellular respiration and nuclear-encoded genes involved in inflammation and the alternative complement and apoptosis pathways. Based on their findings, they propose a constant interaction between the mitochondrial and nuclear DNA whereby the mtDNA haplotype sets a baseline bioenergetics profile for the cell which interacts with environmental factors to contribute to oxidative stress, mitochondrial dysfunction, cell death and disease. As extensively reviewed in detail elsewhere [18,123], considerable evidence demonstrate that preservation of the mitochondrial genome by various mechanisms beyond the scope of this review is critical for ensuring a functional mitochondria and, thereby, contributing to nuclear DNA stability and cell survival.

As emerging evidence reviewed above implicates the mitochondria as the sentinel organelle governing the cell's cytotoxic response to oxidative stress in the lung, important questions emerge about how the redox balance in the mitochondria is maintained [12]. A crucial role of the mitochondria is to balance energy generation via oxidative phosphorylation with cellular nutrient supply; failure to do so may result in damaging levels or ROS, with resultant mtDNA damage and decreased mitochondrial biogenesis, or decreased cellular availability of ATP. SIRT3 has emerged as a key regulator in cellular ROS balance due to its role modulating mitochondrial homeostasis via deacetylation of multiple mediators of energy metabolism and cellular ROS, including members of the ETC, TCA cycle, and mitochondrial enzymes which detoxify ROS. As such, SIRT3 is considered the "gatekeeper" of mitochondrial integrity [124]. Figure 3 highlights some of the key mitochondrial SIRT3 proteins whose functions are post-translationally regulated by acetylation. Given the hypothesized relation between chronic oxidative stress, SIRTs, and aging [122,124], it is interesting that SIRT3 is the only sirtuin that has been closely associated with longevity in humans based upon the presence of a variable nucleotide tandem repeat (VNTR) enhancer within the SIRT3 gene that is associated with increased survival in the elderly [125].

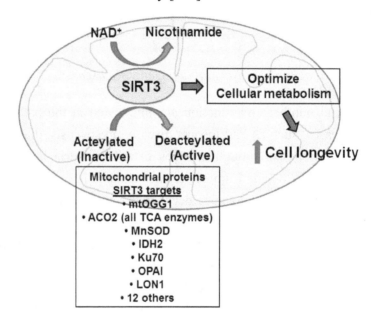

Figure 3. SIRT3 mitochondrial protein deactylation targets modulate cell metabolism and longevity. Red-up arrow, increase.

4.3. The Role of SIRT3 in mtDNA Damage, Aging and Diseases Including Lung

As reviewed briefly above, repair of mtDNA damage following oxidative injury is a complex process that remains incompletely understood. Emerging evidence suggest an important role for SIRT3 in mtDNA repair. SIRT3 deaceylates and activates many mitochondrial proteins involved in energy metabolism (including all the enzymes involved in the TCA cycle such as ACO-2, isocitrate dehydrogenase 2 [IDH2], *etc.*), ETC members, antioxidant defenses, and mtDNA repair (OGG1) [121,124,126]. Murine SIRT3 depletion studies have shown that SIRT3 is necessary for cellular resistance against genotoxic and oxidative stress by preserving mitochondrial function and genomic stability. SIRT3 deficiency promotes intrinsic apoptosis by several mechanisms identified to date, including (1) augmenting mitochondrial ROS production due to acetylation and inactivation of manganese superoxide dismutase (MnSOD) and IDH2 [124,127]; (2) increasing cyclophilin D activity and down-stream mitochondrial permeability transition (MPT) [128,129]; (3) promoting Bax-mediated apoptosis by acetylating Ku70 [129]; and (4) attenuating p53-mediated growth arrest [130,131]. Notably, a recent study using glioma and renal epithelial tumor cells showed that mitochondrial OGG1 is a direct SIRT3 deacetylation target and that SIRT3 deficiency reduces the oxygen consumption rate (OCR) and 8OHdG mtDNA BER that increases mtDNA damage and intrinsic apoptosis [126]. Further, mtDNA mutations/deletions can reduce SIRT3 expression [132,133]. Although unclear in AT2 cells, loss of SIRT3 in keratinocytes augments ROS levels, reduces NAD^+ levels, and promotes epidermal terminal differentiation [134]. These findings suggest SIRT3 may play an important role in maintaining AT2 cell mtDNA and cell survival in the setting of oxidative stress.

A decade ago, a novel function of ACO-2 was discovered, whereby this TCA cycle enzyme was also found to associate with mtDNA nucleoids and stabilize mtDNA in the setting of mtDNA instability [98]. ACO-2 activity is sensitive to the redox state of the cell, suggesting that in the setting of oxidative stress ACO-2 can be relocated from the TCA cycle to the nucleosome to aid in stabilization of the mtDNA with subsequent removal of oxidized Aco-2 by Lon protease [135]. As noted earlier, in an asbestos-induced model of pulmonary fibrosis, oxidant-induced mtDNA damage was blocked by overexpression of ACO-2, a mitochondria-targeted OGG1, and an OGG1 mutant incapable of DNA repair that chaperones ACO-2 [8,9]. The precise mechanism of mtDNA protection by mutant mt-OGG1 comparable to WT mt-OGG1 is not established but may involve blockade of oxidative modification sites on ACO-2, which are necessary for subsequent degradation by the Lon protease. Support for this possibility is that MG132, an inhibitor of Lon protease activity, prevents oxidant-induced reductions in ACO-2 activity in AECs [9]. Another possibility is via effects of SIRT3 on Lon protease since both proteins co-precipitate in breast cancer cells exposed to oxidative and hypoxic stress and SIRT3 silencing results in hyperacetylation and inactivation of Lon [136]. As activity of Lon can favor the transition from aerobic respiration to anaerobic glycolysis, regulate proteins of the TCA cycle and degrade proteins following oxidative damage, these findings suggest a unique coupling between Lon, SIRT3, OGG1, ACO-2, mtDNA repair and the metabolic state of the cell.

Chronic oxidative stress with resultant depletion of SIRT3 and perturbations in mitochondrial function and biogenesis has been increasingly identified as a vital element in the pathogenesis of age-related diseases. *Sirt3*-deficient *(Sirt3$^{-/-}$)*mice have no obvious phenotype but are susceptible to age-linked diseases including metabolic syndrome, cancer, cardiac hypertrophy-fibrosis/CHF, hearing loss, acute renal injury, neurodegeneration, and radiation-induced fibrosis [124,137–143]. Notably, *Sirt3$^{-/-}$* mice exposed to irradiation have reduced liver ACO-2 activity and increased mitochondrial p53 expression [140]. Aged mouse hematopoietic stem cells (mHSCs) have a diminished capacity to respond to oxidative injury induced by H_2O_2 resulting in decreased cell survival and increased apoptosis [144]. SIRT3 expression is reduced in aged mHSCs and SIRT3 overexpression in turn restored the proliferative ability of these cells. Whether SIRT3 affords similar changes in AT2 cells, the stem cell of the distal alveolar epithelium, is unknown. Interestingly, Huang *et al.* [145] showed that rat bone marrow mesenchymal stem cells can differentiate into AT2 cells and alleviate bleomycin-induced lung fibrosis when injected at the same time as bleomycin exposure. In skeletal muscle, aging is associated with oxidative damage to cellular macromolecules; exercise training has been associated with an increase in SIRT3 expression, in both young and old subjects, as well as reduced acetylation of IDH-2, a SIRT3 deacetylase target involved in cellular ROS detoxification [146]. In a murine model of acute kidney injury (AKI), cisplatin-induced oxidative injury decreased renal SIRT3 expression and increased mitochondrial fragmentation [141]. *Sirt3$^{-/-}$* mice were more susceptible to cisplatin-induced AKI as compared to their wild-type counterparts and treatment with antioxidants restored SIRT3 expression and activity and protected against renal dysfunction in the wild-type mice but not in $Sirt3^{-/-}$ animals. In an *in vitro* cortical neuron model of oxidative stress, overexpression of SIRT3 increases mtDNA and mitochondrial biogenesis that has pro-survival effects [147]. In a rodent model of pre-diabetes, oxidative stress induced by a high-fat diet was associated with disruption of the SIRT3/PGC-1α axis with impairment in mitochondrial bioenergetics and decreased testicular mtDNA and adenylate energy charge [148]. A potential role of targeting SIRT3 in diabetes was supported by a recent study showing that overexpression of SIRT3 can mitigate palmitate-mediated pancreatic β cell dysfunction [149].

Murine models of SIRT3 deficiency confirm its protective role in multiple models of age-associated diseases related to oxidative stress. Lysine deacetylation has emerged as a key post-translational protein modification employed to activate mitochondrial signaling [150,151]. Mice deficient in SIRT3 exhibit striking increases in global protein acetylation; effects that were notably not seen in SIRT4- and SIRT5-deficient mice, suggesting that SIRT3 serves as the key mitochondrial deacetylase [152]. In a model of cardiac fibrosis, $Sirt3^{-/-}$ mice develop severe interstitial cardiac fibrosis and hypertrophy following application of a hypertrophic stimulus, whereas mice engineered to overexpress SIRT3 maintain normal cardiac structure and function [137]. These investigators showed that the mechanism of SIRT3 protection was by activation of the FOXO3a-dependent antioxidant genes catalase and MnSOD which reduced cellular ROS [137]. Another group recently showed that $Sirt3^{-/-}$ mice developed age-related cardiac dysfunction likely due to increased acetylation of various mitochondrial energy producing proteins resulting in myocardial energy depletion [153]. SIRT3 also seems important in pulmonary arterial hypertension (PAH) since pulmonary artery smooth muscle cells (PASMC) from patients with PAH display down-regulation of SIRT3; $Sirt3^{-/-}$ mice spontaneously develop PAH and SIRT3 restoration in a rodent model and $Sirt3^{-/-}$ mice PASMC attenuates the disease phenotype [154]. In a murine model of presbycusis, which is postulated to be due to chronic oxidative stress, decreased SIRT3 expression in the central auditory cortex was noted with concurrent increases in ROS, mtDNA damage, and SOD2 acetylation [155]. Taken together, these data strongly support the protective role of SIRT3 against oxidative stress in a variety of cell types and murine models of various degenerative diseases. Additional studies are necessary to better define the role of mtDNA integrity in mediating the beneficial effects of SIRT3 as well as the translational significance in humans, including pulmonary fibrosis.

4.4. Therapeutic Approach: Resveratrol/Viniferin/Honokiol

The first techniques used to enhance sirtuin expression involved caloric restriction due to the putative link between SIRT3 deacetylase activity and the metabolic state of the cell [124]. The role of SIRT3 in modulating mitochondrial energy metabolism will be discussed in detail the final section below. Exercise training has been associated with increased SIRT3 expression and recently has been linked to a decrease in mitochondrial protein acetylation, increased ACO-2 and MnSOD activity, and improved mitochondrial biogenesis in a cardiac model of doxorubicin-induced oxidative injury [156].

Recently, small molecule sirtuin inducers have been under investigation. Resveratrol (RSV), a naturally occurring polyphenol, extends the lifespan of diverse model organisms in a Sir2 (a silent information regulator)-dependent fashion [157]. RSV induces both SIRT1 and SIRT3 expression via stimulation of NADH dehydrogenases and mitochondrial complex I resulting in increases in the mitochondrial NAD^+/NADH ratio [158]. Treatment with RSV has been shown to abrogate hyperoxia-mediated acute liver injury [158], airway remodeling and hyperreactivity in a model of allergic asthma [159], insulin resistance [160], and pulmonary fibrosis in a bleomycin mouse model [161]. Activation of SIRT3 via RSV in a murine model of cardiac fibrosis attenuated collagen deposition and cardiac hypertrophy via regulation of the TGF-β/Smad pathway; SIRT3 is required for the cardio-protective effects revealing a potential link between mitigation of oxidative stress and the signaling pathways responsible for fibrosis [142]. Viniferin, a natural dehydrodimer of RSV, may have increased antioxidant potential compared to RSV and has been shown to protect vascular endothelial cells from oxidative stress by suppressing intracellular ROS production [162]. Further, SIRT3 was shown to mediate the neuroprotective effect of viniferin in models of Huntington disease via an increase in the number of mtDNA copies, attenuation of the loss of mitochondrial membrane potential, and enhanced activity of MnSOD [163]. Pillai and colleagues showed that honokiol, a natural occurring compound from the bark of magnolia trees with anti-inflammatory, anti-oxidative, anti-tumor, and neuroprotective properties, reverses murine cardiac hypertrophy and fibrosis by a SIRT3-dependent mechanism [164]. Although it is unknown whether these small molecule sirtuin inducers are protective to AEC mtDNA and cell survival following exposure to oxidative stress, they represent an exciting therapeutic strategy for future studies addressing age-related diseases attributed to chronic oxidative stress, such as pulmonary fibrosis.

5. MtDNA and Metabolism in Mitochondria

5.1. Mitochondrial Metabolism—The Basics

As noted earlier, the mitochondria, long championed as the "powerhouse of the cell", are now well-recognized as being critically important in overall cellular health, intracellular signaling, and disease pathobiology [12]. However, that does not diminish the importance of the organelle's ATP-producing function, as mitochondrial metabolism is the main mechanism by which a cell synthesizes ATP. Mitochondrial metabolism is governed primarily by one aspect: the presence of oxygen. Under normal conditions, in the presence of oxygen, mitochondria utilize both oxygen and electrochemical gradients for the production of ATP via the ETC, known as oxidative phosphorylation (OXPHOS), and the TCA (or Krebs) cycle, while in the absence of oxygen the mitochondria rely on glycolysis and fatty acid oxidation for ATP production. Glycolysis produces pyruvate as an end product, which is then used by the TCA to produce the reducing equivalents (e.g., NADH and $FADH_2$) necessary for the ETC to convert ADP to ATP. Fatty acid oxidation, which occurs in the mitochondrial matrix, breaks fatty acids down from triacytlglycerols by β-oxidation and forms both acetyl-CoA (which is converted to citrate in the TCA cycle) and ATP [165]. The interaction between cytosolic liquid triacytlglycerol droplets and mitochondria in fatty acid oxidation must maintain a fine balance, as lipids can either inhibit or uncouple OXPHOS [166]. These anaerobic cycles produce less ATP per cycle, but can be much faster making them indispensable for cells that are not always under "ideal" conditions (i.e., oxidative stress). Cells typically utilize these anaerobic pathways under low-oxygen conditions or when the cell requires energy faster than can be produced by O_2-dependent means.

However, mitochondrial damage, be it due to mtDNA damage, ROS, or ETC complex inhibition, can lead the cell to favor these alternate ATP producing pathways. The Warburg effect, or aerobic glycolysis, is where the cell favors the glycolytic pathway over the ETC even in the presence of O_2, a phenomenon nearly synonymous with a cancerous phenotype as it can rapidly produce copious amounts of ATP, which are useful for the rapid growth of cancer cells [167]. However, excessive glycolysis, beyond that which is utilized by cancerous cells, can promote cell stasis, excessive mtDNA damage, and cytotoxicity [168].

5.2. Role of Mitochondria-Derived ROS, mtDNA Damage, and Mitochondrial Metabolism

ROS, especially $O_2^{\bullet-}$, is a natural byproduct of the ETC due to inefficiencies in electron transfer between the four complexes (I, II, III, and IV). ROS are not inherently detrimental, but increased mitochondrial metabolism or damage within the OXPHOS pathway (i.e., buildup of acetylated metabolic intermediates, ETC complex damage) increases cellular ROS, and, as detailed above, can cause mtDNA damage and harm components of the ETC, which further promotes ROS production. NAD^+, a natural byproduct of metabolism, is produced when NADH is reduced by electrons from the ETC; with an impaired ETC, cells instead use glycolytic pathways or fatty acid oxidation and, as such, metabolic reducing equivalents (i.e., NADH) build up in the mitochondria, reducing NAD^+ formation and down-stream NAD^+-dependent processes (e.g., SIRT3 deacetylation—see below) [165]. Decreased NAD^+ levels promote OXPHOS dysfunction leading to metabolic failure in cells, which is a common phenotype in the aged [169]. However, strategies to augment NAD^+ levels can prevent apoptosis-induced complex I inhibition, the depletion of intracellular ATP, and preserve mtDNA integrity, possibly by preventing an increase in BAX expression (6). Additionally, ACO-2, a TCA cycle intermediary metabolite, can stabilize the mtDNA and, thereby, linking mtDNA integrity with metabolic efficiency [135]. However, the mechanism by which ACO-2 toggles between these two ACO-2 functions is not well understood. Notably, mutations in *ACO-2* gene can cause syndromic optic neuropathy with encephalopathy and cerebellar atrophy in humans [170].

Disruption of mitochondrial dynamics is an early event in ROS-induced intrinsic apoptotic cell death. Excessive ROS production can induce ER Ca^{2+} release, reduce the cell's abilty to produce autophagosomes, and contribute to degenerative diseases via effects on mtDNA [12,171]. OXPHOS dysregulation arising from mtDNA mutations/damage results in an increase in the invasive cell phenotype via effects on matrix metalloproteinase (MMP) family members. It also mimics lack-of-oxygen by causing increased lactate production and acidification of the extracellular environment, and can act parallel to (and independent of) hypoxia inducible factor (HIF)-1α activation to increase angiogenesis and glucose uptake [172]. Inflammatory signaling typically increases oxygen consumption (OCR), ROS production, and $\Delta\psi_m$, but does not significantly affect spare respiratory capacity (SCR—the difference between a cell's maximal, uncoupled respiration, and its normal, basal respiration) when normalized to mitochondria content [173]. With progressive cellular stress, mitochondrial rupture and release of mtDNA can occur, which can lead to TLR-9/NLRP3 inflammasome activation and a vicious inflammatory cycle [115,117].

Mitophagy is the cellular mechanism in place to discard damaged and ineffective mitochondria with extensive mtDNA damage [3,174]. Healthy mitochondria can fuse, and such fusion acts as a buffer against mitophagy, ensuring that, optimally, fully-functional mitochondria will be spared, while those mitochondria that cannot fuse will be more easily mitophagized [3,174]. Full mitochondrial fusion can also allow for mtDNA and nucleoid transfer, thereby diminishing/alleviating mtDNA damage. However, fusion can still occur in mitochondria with extensive mtDNA damage if initiated by a healthy mitochondrion, which can revive the metabolic functioning of the damaged mitochondrion. Metabolically inefficient mitochondria that overexpress mitofusion genes can escape mitophagy [174]. Some inherited mitochondrial haplotypes display significant differences in ATP and ROS production and ETC complex expression; those that exhibit relatively lower productions of ATP and ROS appear to be more inclined toward dysfunction and resultant disease independent of nuclear DNA mutations [30]. As reviewed in detail elsewhere [7], there has been extensive study of mitochondrial lineage and how the inheritance of mitochondrial mutations can affect disease progression and severity. Notably, altered proteins resulting from damaged nDNA can allow mtDNA damage to accumulate [7,12]. For example, PINK1 and PARK2 mutations prevent the proper functioning of autophagosomes thereby preventing damaged mitochondria from being destroyed, leading to even greater mtDNA damage.

Although the role of mitochondrial metabolic pathways in regulating AEC function and maintaining mtDNA integrity are not well established, there is some information in other cell types. For example, in Huntington's disease there are increased numbers of large, unhealthy mitochondria with decreased $\Delta\psi_m$, PGC-1α, ATP production, ETC function, ADP-uptake, glucose metabolism, and SRC [175]. PGC-1α, a regulator of both metabolism and mitochondrial biogenesis, is upregulated by RIP1 (receptor-interacting protein 1); a decrease in RIP1 leads to an increase of dsDNA breakage and oxidative glycolysis, a reduction in the NAD^+ pools, and suppression of cell proliferation [168]. RIP1 maintains cancer cell glycolytic metabolism such that enhanced cell proliferation can occur, but its loss results in excessive glycolysis and p53-mediated cell stasis. Hyperglycemic damage in diabetic heart cells can cause alterations to mtDNA as a result of alterations in the supply of metabolic substrates (*i.e.*, $NAD(P)^+/NAD(P)H$, GSH/GSSG, and $TrxSH_2/TrxSS$) that can affect mitochondrial health [166]. Using a diabetic heart mouse model, these same investigators showed that cardiac muscle contraction and Ca^{2+} signaling are reduced largely because of alterations in complex I resulting from mitochondrial metabolic damage. Impaired pulmonary artery endothelial cell regeneration is linked to mitochondrial DNA deletion, and hypoxia-reoxygenation reduces p53, PGC-1α, ATP, $\Delta\psi_m$, caspase-induced apoptosis, the levels of mitofusin 1 and 2, and mitophagy [176]. Hypoxic conditions also render significant damage to mtDNA, through increased complex III $O_2^{\bullet-}$ production [12]. Lung fibrosis in bleomycin-treated rats is associated with significant mtDNA damage, dysfunction of mtDNA-encoded ETC subunits, and increased ROS production and TGFβ levels [36]. Although the primary cell type mediating these effects was not identified, future studies focusing on mitochondrial metabolism in AECs will be of considerable interest. We reason that AEC mtDNA damage that accumulates over time can promote "aged" AT2 cells that are more prone to triggering pulmonary fibrosis following an environmental or oxidative stress insult.

5.3. Role of Sirtuins and Energy Metabolism in Mitochondria

Convincing evidences implicate SIRT-induced mitochondrial dysfunction in aging as well as diseases associated with aging (*i.e.*, cancer, neurodegeneration, CHF, and metabolic syndrome/diabetes) and will likely prove important in the pathophysiology of lung disease, such as IPF, asbestosis, and lung cancer [177–179]. The paradigm that is emerging by which SIRT3 affects cell metabolism and longevity is illustrated in Figure 3. As noted above (see Section 4), SIRT3 deaceylates and activates numerous mitochondrial proteins involved in diverse functions involving mitochondrial energy metabolism (including all the enzymes involved in the TCA cycle such as ACO-2, *etc.*), ETC members, antioxidant defenses, and mtDNA repair. Global loss of the *Sirt3* gene augments mitochondrial ROS levels, reduces OCR, NAD^+ levels, and ATP production, and promotes radiation-induced genotoxic stress response and a tumor permissive phenotype [124,126,127,180,181]. There is a negative correlation between ROS generated by complex 1 in the ETC and lifespan, and bypassing complex 1 increases lifespan in the fruit fly by mechanisms that are uncertain, but may involve altered sirtuins and cellular NAD^+ levels [178,182]. Given the "mitochondrial gatekeeper" role of SIRT3 for post-translational modification of mitochondrial proteins, not surprisingly SIRT3 is implicated in modulating mitochondrial metabolism. For example, Bass and colleagues demonstrated that circadian control of SIRT3 activity resulted in rhythms in the acetylation and activity of oxidative enzymes and respiration in isolated mitochondria, and that NAD^+ supplementation restored mitochondrial protein deacetylation and augmented OCR in circadian mutant mice [183]. Mitochondrial NAD^+ levels are also regulated by SIRT3 activity [182]. Lower levels of NAD^+ due to aging have also been found to produce a hypoxic-like state that inhibits intracellular signaling [184]. There is some evidence that simply replacing the cellular NAD^+ pool promotes recovery of cells from the aging metabolic phenotype [169]. PGC-1α-dependent SIRT3 signaling prevents complex 1 damage and preserves ETC function [185]. Increased PGC-1α levels have also been implicated in mitochondrial biogenesis, via a serine protease Omi-dependent mechanism [186]. Loss of SIRT3 can exacerbate the Parkinson's phenotype in mice through inhibition of complex 1, leading to excess ROS production and mtDNA damage, resulting in neuronal death [143].

Other SIRTs, especially SIRT1, may also have important roles in mitochondrial metabolism. Cells and tissues from old animals exhibit an increase of SIRT1 expression that is associated with decreased SIRT1 activity, NAD^+ levels, and ETC activity and augmented levels of nuclear p53, PARP, FOXO1, and oxidation of proteins, DNA, and lipids [178,187,188]. Despite SIRT3's key mitochondrial function, there is some evidence suggesting that its activity is highly dependent upon the activity of the nuclear-localized SIRT1 effects on RELB [173]. Additional studies are necessary to better understand the roles of SIRT3 and other sirtuins on AEC mitochondrial metabolism in the setting of oxidative stress as well as the translational significance in human lung diseases.

6. Conclusions

The available evidence reviewed herein convincingly shows that AEC mtDNA plays a key role in modulating mitochondrial function and apoptosis. Furthermore, AEC mtDNA damage following oxidative or environmental stress may be important in promoting pro-fibrotic signaling as can be seen in IPF, asbestosis, and other fibrotic lung diseases. A hypothetical model of AEC mtDNA damage in mediating intrinsic apoptosis that we reviewed is shown in Figure 2. Furthermore, we explored the data implicating that ongoing mtDNA damage may also be important in promoting other degenerative conditions, aging, and cancer (Figure 1). Emerging findings also suggest that SIRT3 and mitochondrial metabolism may be important in attenuating the deleterious effects of oxidative stress in a variety of cell types and murine models of degenerative diseases. Thus, the mitochondria clearly function not only as the "powerhouse" of the cell, but also regulate important cellular functions and signaling that determine cell life and death decisions. The role of OGG1, ACO-2, and small molecule SIRT3 inducers in modulating mtDNA damage in AEC as well as other cells and how this translates into disease pathophysiology await further study. We reason that the OGG1/ACO-2/SIRT3/mtDNA axis is important in regulating complex cell signaling that promotes pulmonary fibrosis as well as other degenerative disease of the lungs and tumor development.

Acknowledgments

This work was supported by VA Merit and NIH grant RO1 ES020357 to David W. Kamp, and NIH/NHLBI training grant 2T32HL076139-11A1 to Renea P. Jablonski.

Author Contributions

Seok-Jo Kim: Wrote sections of the manuscript, prepared figures and references, and edited the document. Paul Cheresh: Wrote sections of the manuscript. Renea P. Jablonski: Wrote sections of the manuscript. David B. Williams: Wrote sections of the manuscript. David W. Kamp: Wrote sections of the manuscript and edited the document.

References

1. Selman, M.; Pardo, A. Revealing the pathogenic and aging-related mechanisms of the enigmatic idiopathic pulmonary fibrosis. An integral model. *Am. J. Respir. Crit. Care Med.* **2014**, *189*, 1161–1172.

2. Trifunovic, A.; Wredenberg, A.; Falkenberg, M.; Spelbrink, J.N.; Rovio, A.T.; Bruder, C.E.; Bohlooly, Y.M.; Gidlof, S.; Oldfors, A.; Wibom, R.; *et al.* Premature ageing in mice expressing defective mitochondrial DNA polymerase. *Nature* **2004**, *429*, 417–423.

3. Held, N.M.; Houtkooper, R.H. Mitochondrial quality control pathways as determinants of metabolic health. *Bioessays* **2015**, *37*, 867–876.

4. Miller, F.J.; Rosenfeldt, F.L.; Zhang, C.; Linnane, A.W.; Nagley, P. Precise determination of mitochondrial DNA copy number in human skeletal and cardiac muscle by a pcr-based assay: Lack of change of copy number with age. *Nucleic Acids Res.* **2003**, *31*, e61, doi:10.1093/nar/gng060.

5. Bell, O.; Tiwari, V.K.; Thoma, N.H.; Schubeler, D. Determinants and dynamics of genome accessibility. *Nat. Rev. Genet.* **2011**, *12*, 554–564.

6. Reeve, A.K.; Krishnan, K.J.; Turnbull, D. Mitochondrial DNA mutations in disease, aging, and neurodegeneration. *Ann. N. Y. Acad. Sci.* **2008**, *1147*, 21–29.

7.   Wallace, D.C. A mitochondrial bioenergetic etiology of disease. *J. Clin. Investig.* **2013**, *123*, 1405–1412.

8.   Kim, S.J.; Cheresh, P.; Williams, D.; Cheng, Y.; Ridge, K.; Schumacker, P.T.; Weitzman, S.; Bohr, V.A.; Kamp, D.W. Mitochondria-targeted Ogg1 and aconitase-2 prevent oxidant-induced mitochondrial DNA damage in alveolar epithelial cells. *J. Biol. Chem.* **2014**, *289*, 6165–6176.

9.   Panduri, V.; Liu, G.; Surapureddi, S.; Kondapalli, J.; Soberanes, S.; de Souza-Pinto, N.C.; Bohr, V.A.; Budinger, G.R.; Schumacker, P.T.; Weitzman, S.A.; *et al.* Role of mitochondrial hOGG1 and aconitase in oxidant-induced lung epithelial cell apoptosis. *Free Radic. Biol. Med.* **2009**, *47*, 750–759.

10. Nakabeppu, Y. Regulation of intracellular localization of human MTH1, OGG1, and MYH proteins for repair of oxidative DNA damage. *Prog. Nucleic Acid. Res. Mol. Biol.* **2001**, *68*, 75–94.

11. Vartanian, V.; Lowell, B.; Minko, I.G.; Wood, T.G.; Ceci, J.D.; George, S.; Ballinger, S.W.; Corless, C.L.; McCullough, A.K.; Lloyd, R.S. The metabolic syndrome resulting from a knockout of the NEIL1 DNA glycosylase. *Proc. Natl. Acad. Sci. USA* **2006**, *103*, 1864–1869.

12. Schumacker, P.T.; Gillespie, M.N.; Nakahira, K.; Choi, A.M.; Crouser, E.D.; Piantadosi, C.A.; Bhattacharya, J. Mitochondria in lung biology and pathology: More than just a powerhouse. *Am. J. Physiol. Lung. Cell Mol. Physiol.* **2014**, *306*, L962–L974.

13. Chouteau, J.M.; Obiako, B.; Gorodnya, O.M.; Pastukh, V.M.; Ruchko, M.V.; Wright, A.J.; Wilson, G.L.; Gillespie, M.N. Mitochondrial DNA integrity may be a determinant of endothelial barrier properties in oxidant-challenged rat lungs. *Am. J. Physiol. Lung Cell Mol. Physiol.* **2011**, *301*, L892–L898.

14. Cerritelli, S.M.; Frolova, E.G.; Feng, C.; Grinberg, A.; Love, P.E.; Crouch, R.J. Failure to produce mitochondrial DNA results in embryonic lethality in Rnaseh1 null mice. *Mol. Cell* **2003**, *11*, 807–815.

15. Simsek, D.; Furda, A.; Gao, Y.; Artus, J.; Brunet, E.; Hadjantonakis, A.K.; van Houten, B.; Shuman, S.; McKinnon, P.J.; Jasin, M. Crucial role for DNA ligase III in mitochondria but not in Xrcc1-dependent repair. *Nature* **2011**, *471*, 245–248.

16. Ballinger, S.W.; Patterson, C.; Yan, C.N.; Doan, R.; Burow, D.L.; Young, C.G.; Yakes, F.M.; van Houten, B.; Ballinger, C.A.; Freeman, B.A.; *et al.* Hydrogen peroxide- and peroxynitrite-induced mitochondrial DNA damage and dysfunction in vascular endothelial and smooth muscle cells. *Circ. Res.* **2000**, *86*, 960–966.

17. Yakes, F.M.; van Houten, B. Mitochondrial DNA damage is more extensive and persists longer than nuclear DNA damage in human cells following oxidative stress. *Proc. Natl. Acad. Sci. USA* **1997**, *94*, 514–519.

18. Bohr, V.A.; Stevnsner, T.; de Souza-Pinto, N.C. Mitochondrial DNA repair of oxidative damage in mammalian cells. *Gene* **2002**, *286*, 127–134.

19. Kroemer, G.; Galluzzi, L.; Brenner, C. Mitochondrial membrane permeabilization in cell death. *Physiol. Rev.* **2007**, *87*, 99–163.

20. Enns, G.M. The contribution of mitochondria to common disorders. *Mol. Genet. Metab.* **2003**, *80*, 11–26.

21. Brandon, M.; Baldi, P.; Wallace, D.C. Mitochondrial mutations in cancer. *Oncogene* **2006**, *25*, 4647–4662.

22. Cline, S.D. Mitochondrial DNA damage and its consequences for mitochondrial gene expression. *Biochim. Biophys. Acta* **2012**, *1819*, 979–991.

23. Tuppen, H.A.; Blakely, E.L.; Turnbull, D.M.; Taylor, R.W. Mitochondrial DNA mutations and human disease. *Biochim. Biophys. Acta* **2010**, *1797*, 113–128.

24. Van Houten, B.; Woshner, V.; Santos, J.H. Role of mitochondrial DNA in toxic responses to oxidative stress. *DNA Repair* **2006**, *5*, 145–152.

25. Figueira, T.R.; Barros, M.H.; Camargo, A.A.; Castilho, R.F.; Ferreira, J.C.; Kowaltowski, A.J.; Sluse, F.E.; Souza-Pinto, N.C.; Vercesi, A.E. Mitochondria as a source of reactive oxygen and nitrogen species: From molecular mechanisms to human health. *Antioxid. Redox Signal.* **2013**, *18*, 2029–2074.

26. Balaban, R.S.; Nemoto, S.; Finkel, T. Mitochondria, oxidants, and aging. *Cell* **2005**, *120*, 483–495.

27. Lin, M.T.; Beal, M.F. Mitochondrial dysfunction and oxidative stress in neurodegenerative diseases. *Nature* **2006**, *443*, 787–795.

28. Turrens, J.F. Mitochondrial formation of reactive oxygen species. *J. Physiol.* **2003**, *552*, 335–344.

29. Aaij, R.; Abellan Beteta, C.; Adeva, B.; Adinolfi, M.; Adrover, C.; Affolder, A.; Ajaltouni, Z.; Albrecht, J.; Alessio, F.; Alexander, M.; *et al.* First observation of *CP* violation in the decays of B_s^0 mesons. *Phys. Rev. Lett.* **2013**, *110*, 221601, doi:10.1103/PhysRevLett.110.221601.

30. Kenney, M.C.; Chwa, M.; Atilano, S.R.; Falatoonzadeh, P.; Ramirez, C.; Malik, D.; Tarek, M.; Caceres-del-Carpio, J.; Nesburn, A.B.; Boyer, D.S.; *et al.* Inherited mitochondrial DNA variants can affect complement, inflammation and apoptosis pathways: Insights into mitochondrial-nuclear interactions. *Hum. Mol. Genet.* **2014**, *23*, 3537–3551.

31. Kamp, D.W.; Graceffa, P.; Pryor, W.A.; Weitzman, S.A. The role of free radicals in asbestos-induced diseases. *Free Radic. Biol. Med.* **1992**, *12*, 293–315.

32. Turci, F.; Tomatis, M.; Lesci, I.G.; Roveri, N.; Fubini, B. The iron-related molecular toxicity mechanism of synthetic asbestos nanofibres: A model study for high-aspect-ratio nanoparticles. *Chemistry* **2011**, *17*, 350–358.

33. Faner, R.; Rojas, M.; Macnee, W.; Agusti, A. Abnormal lung aging in chronic obstructive pulmonary disease and idiopathic pulmonary fibrosis. *Am. J. Respir. Crit. Care Med.* **2012**, *186*, 306–313.

34. Kliment, C.R.; Oury, T.D. Oxidative stress, extracellular matrix targets, and idiopathic pulmonary fibrosis. *Free Radic. Biol. Med.* **2010**, *49*, 707–717.

35. Cheresh, P.; Kim, S.J.; Tulasiram, S.; Kamp, D.W. Oxidative stress and pulmonary fibrosis. *Biochim. Biophys. Acta* **2013**, *1832*, 1028–1040.

36. Gazdhar, A.; Lebrecht, D.; Roth, M.; Tamm, M.; Venhoff, N.; Foocharoen, C.; Geiser, T.; Walker, U.A. Time-dependent and somatically acquired mitochondrial DNA mutagenesis and respiratory chain dysfunction in a scleroderma model of lung fibrosis. *Sci. Rep.* **2014**, *4*, 5336, doi:10.1038/srep05336.

37. Liu, G.; Cheresh, P.; Kamp, D.W. Molecular basis of asbestos-induced lung disease. *Annu. Rev. Pathol.* **2013**, *8*, 161–187.

38. Oury, T.D.; Thakker, K.; Menache, M.; Chang, L.Y.; Crapo, J.D.; Day, B.J. Attenuation of bleomycin-induced pulmonary fibrosis by a catalytic antioxidant metalloporphyrin. *Am. J. Respir. Cell Mol. Biol.* **2001**, *25*, 164–169.

39. Osborn-Heaford, H.L.; Ryan, A.J.; Murthy, S.; Racila, A.M.; He, C.; Sieren, J.C.; Spitz, D.R.; Carter, A.B. Mitochondrial Rac1 GTPase import and electron transfer from cytochrome c are required for pulmonary fibrosis. *J. Biol. Chem.* **2012**, *287*, 3301–3312.

40. Murthy, S.; Ryan, A.; He, C.; Mallampalli, R.K.; Carter, A.B. Rac1-mediated mitochondrial H2O2 generation regulates *MMP-9* gene expression in macrophages via inhibition of SP-1 and AP-1. *J. Biol. Chem.* **2010**, *285*, 25062–25073.

41. Murthy, S.; Adamcakova-Dodd, A.; Perry, S.S.; Tephly, L.A.; Keller, R.M.; Metwali, N.; Meyerholz, D.K.; Wang, Y.; Glogauer, M.; Thorne, P.S.; *et al.* Modulation of reactive oxygen species by rac1 or catalase prevents asbestos-induced pulmonary fibrosis. *Am. J. Physiol. Lung Cell Mol. Physiol.* **2009**, *297*, L846–L855.

42. He, C.; Murthy, S.; McCormick, M.L.; Spitz, D.R.; Ryan, A.J.; Carter, A.B. Mitochondrial Cu, Zn-superoxide dismutase mediates pulmonary fibrosis by augmenting H2O2 generation. *J. Biol. Chem.* **2011**, *286*, 15597–15607.

43. Mossman, B.T.; Marsh, J.P.; Sesko, A.; Hill, S.; Shatos, M.A.; Doherty, J.; Petruska, J.; Adler, K.B.; Hemenway, D.; Mickey, R.; *et al.* Inhibition of lung injury, inflammation, and interstitial pulmonary fibrosis by polyethylene glycol-conjugated catalase in a rapid inhalation model of asbestosis. *Am. Rev. Respir. Dis.* **1990**, *141*, 1266–1271.

44. Gao, F.; Kinnula, V.L.; Myllarniemi, M.; Oury, T.D. Extracellular superoxide dismutase in pulmonary fibrosis. *Antioxid. Redox Signal.* **2008**, *10*, 343–354.

45. Cantin, A.M.; Hubbard, R.C.; Crystal, R.G. Glutathione deficiency in the epithelial lining fluid of the lower respiratory tract in idiopathic pulmonary fibrosis. *Am. Rev. Respir. Dis.* **1989**, *139*, 370–372.

46. Waghray, M.; Cui, Z.; Horowitz, J.C.; Subramanian, I.M.; Martinez, F.J.; Toews, G.B.; Thannickal, V.J. Hydrogen peroxide is a diffusible paracrine signal for the induction of epithelial cell death by activated myofibroblasts. *FASEB J.* **2005**, *19*, 854–856.

47. Hagiwara, S.I.; Ishii, Y.; Kitamura, S. Aerosolized administration of *N*-acetylcysteine attenuates lung fibrosis induced by bleomycin in mice. *Am. J. Respir. Crit. Care Med.* **2000**, *162*, 225–231.

48. Martinez, F.J.; de Andrade, J.A.; Anstrom, K.J.; King, T.E., Jr.; Raghu, G. Randomized trial of acetylcysteine in idiopathic pulmonary fibrosis. *N. Engl. J. Med.* **2014**, *370*, 2093–2101.

49. Crestani, B.; Besnard, V.; Boczkowski, J. Signalling pathways from NADPH oxidase-4 to idiopathic pulmonary fibrosis. *Int. J. Biochem. Cell Biol.* **2011**, *43*, 1086–1089.

50. Hecker, L.; Cheng, J.; Thannickal, V.J. Targeting nox enzymes in pulmonary fibrosis. *Cell Mol. Life Sci.* **2012**, *69*, 2365–2371.

51. Hecker, L.; Vittal, R.; Jones, T.; Jagirdar, R.; Luckhardt, T.R.; Horowitz, J.C.; Pennathur, S.; Martinez, F.J.; Thannickal, V.J. NADPH oxidase-4 mediates myofibroblast activation and fibrogenic responses to lung injury. *Nat. Med.* **2009**, *15*, 1077–1081.

52. Carnesecchi, S.; Deffert, C.; Donati, Y.; Basset, O.; Hinz, B.; Preynat-Seauve, O.; Guichard, C.; Arbiser, J.L.; Banfi, B.; Pache, J.C.; *et al.* A key role for NOX4 in epithelial cell death during development of lung fibrosis. *Antioxid. Redox Signal.* **2011**, *15*, 607–619.

53. Hecker, L.; Logsdon, N.J.; Kurundkar, D.; Kurundkar, A.; Bernard, K.; Hock, T.; Meldrum, E.; Sanders, Y.Y.; Thannickal, V.J. Reversal of persistent fibrosis in aging by targeting Nox4-Nrf2 redox imbalance. *Sci. Transl. Med.* **2014**, *6*, 231ra247, doi:10.1126/scitranslmed.3008182.

54. Thannickal, V.J. Mechanistic links between aging and lung fibrosis. *Biogerontology* **2013**, *14*, 609–615.

55. Lopez-Otin, C.; Blasco, M.A.; Partridge, L.; Serrano, M.; Kroemer, G. The hallmarks of aging. *Cell* **2013**, *153*, 1194–1217.

56. Uhal, B.D.; Nguyen, H. The Witschi Hypothesis revisited after 35 years: Genetic proof from SP-C BRICHOS domain mutations. *Am. J. Physiol. Lung Cell Mol. Physiol.* **2013**, *305*, L906–L911.

57. Mossman, B.T.; Lippmann, M.; Hesterberg, T.W.; Kelsey, K.T.; Barchowsky, A.; Bonner, J.C. Pulmonary endpoints (lung carcinomas and asbestosis) following inhalation exposure to asbestos. *J. Toxicol. Environ. Health B Crit. Rev.* **2011**, *14*, 76–121.

58. Noble, P.W.; Barkauskas, C.E.; Jiang, D. Pulmonary fibrosis: Patterns and perpetrators. *J. Clin. Investig.* **2012**, *122*, 2756–2762.

59. Tanjore, H.; Blackwell, T.S.; Lawson, W.E. Emerging evidence for endoplasmic reticulum stress in the pathogenesis of idiopathic pulmonary fibrosis. *Am. J. Physiol. Lung Cell Mol. Physiol.* **2012**, *302*, L721–L729.

60. Weiss, C.H.; Budinger, G.R.; Mutlu, G.M.; Jain, M. Proteasomal regulation of pulmonary fibrosis. *Proc. Am. Thorac. Soc.* **2010**, *7*, 77–83.

61. Brody, A.R.; Overby, L.H. Incorporation of tritiated thymidine by epithelial and interstitial cells in bronchiolar-alveolar regions of asbestos-exposed rats. *Am. J. Pathol.* **1989**, *134*, 133–140.

62. Shukla, A.; Jung, M.; Stern, M.; Fukagawa, N.K.; Taatjes, D.J.; Sawyer, D.; van Houten, B.; Mossman, B.T. Asbestos induces mitochondrial DNA damage and dysfunction linked to the development of apoptosis. *Am. J. Physiol. Lung Cell Mol. Physiol.* **2003**, *285*, L1018–L1025.

63. Fingerlin, T.E.; Murphy, E.; Zhang, W.; Peljto, A.L.; Brown, K.K.; Steele, M.P.; Loyd, J.E.; Cosgrove, G.P.; Lynch, D.; Groshong, S.; *et al.* Genome-wide association study identifies multiple susceptibility loci for pulmonary fibrosis. *Nat. Genet.* **2013**, *45*, 613–620.

64. Kropski, J.A.; Pritchett, J.M.; Zoz, D.F.; Crossno, P.F.; Markin, C.; Garnett, E.T.; Degryse, A.L.; Mitchell, D.B.; Polosukhin, V.V.; Rickman, O.B.; *et al.* Extensive phenotyping of individuals at risk for familial interstitial pneumonia reveals clues to the pathogenesis of interstitial lung disease. *Am. J. Respir. Crit. Care Med.* **2015**, *191*, 417–426.

65. Cogan, J.D.; Kropski, J.A.; Zhao, M.; Mitchell, D.B.; Rives, L.; Markin, C.; Garnett, E.T.; Montgomery, K.H.; Mason, W.R.; McKean, D.F.; *et al.* Rare variants in RTEL1 are associated with familial interstitial pneumonia. *Am. J. Respir. Crit. Care Med.* **2015**, *191*, 646–655.

66. Wallace, D.C.; Chalkia, D. Mitochondrial DNA genetics and the heteroplasmy conundrum in evolution and disease. *Cold Spring Harb. Perspect. Med.* **2013**, *5*, a021220, doi:10.1101/cshperspect.a021220.

67. Galluzzi, L.; Vitale, I.; Abrams, J.M.; Alnemri, E.S.; Baehrecke, E.H.; Blagosklonny, M.V.; Dawson, T.M.; Dawson, V.L.; El-Deiry, W.S.; Fulda, S.; *et al.* Molecular definitions of cell death subroutines: Recommendations of the nomenclature committee on cell death 2012. *Cell Death Differ.* **2012**, *19*, 107–120.

68. Huang, S.X.; Jaurand, M.C.; Kamp, D.W.; Whysner, J.; Hei, T.K. Role of mutagenicity in asbestos fiber-induced carcinogenicity and other diseases. *J. Toxicol. Environ. Health B Crit. Rev.* **2011**, *14*, 179–245.

69. Anathy, V.; Roberson, E.C.; Guala, A.S.; Godburn, K.E.; Budd, R.C.; Janssen-Heininger, Y.M. Redox-based regulation of apoptosis: S-glutathionylation as a regulatory mechanism to control cell death. *Antioxid. Redox Signal.* **2012**, *16*, 496–505.

70. Anathy, V.; Roberson, E.; Cunniff, B.; Nolin, J.D.; Hoffman, S.; Spiess, P.; Guala, A.S.; Lahue, K.G.; Goldman, D.; Flemer, S.; *et al.* Oxidative processing of latent fas in the endoplasmic reticulum controls the strength of apoptosis. *Mol. Cell. Biol.* **2012**, *32*, 3464–3478.

71. Horan, G.S.; Wood, S.; Ona, V.; Li, D.J.; Lukashev, M.E.; Weinreb, P.H.; Simon, K.J.; Hahm, K.; Allaire, N.E.; Rinaldi, N.J.; *et al.* Partial inhibition of integrin αvβ6 prevents pulmonary fibrosis without exacerbating inflammation. *Am. J. Respir. Crit. Care Med.* **2008**, *177*, 56–65.

72. Armanios, M. Telomerase and idiopathic pulmonary fibrosis. *Mutat. Res.* **2012**, *730*, 52–58.

73. Alder, J.K.; Chen, J.J.; Lancaster, L.; Danoff, S.; Su, S.C.; Cogan, J.D.; Vulto, I.; Xie, M.; Qi, X.; Tuder, R.M.; *et al.* Short telomeres are a risk factor for idiopathic pulmonary fibrosis. *Proc. Natl. Acad. Sci. USA* **2008**, *105*, 13051–13056.

74. Passos, J.F.; Saretzki, G.; Ahmed, S.; Nelson, G.; Richter, T.; Peters, H.; Wappler, I.; Birket, M.J.; Harold, G.; Schaeuble, K.; *et al.* Mitochondrial dysfunction accounts for the stochastic heterogeneity in telomere-dependent senescence. *PLoS Biol.* **2007**, *5*, e110.

75. Degryse, A.L.; Xu, X.C.; Newman, J.L.; Mitchell, D.B.; Tanjore, H.; Polosukhin, V.V.; Jones, B.R.; McMahon, F.B.; Gleaves, L.A.; Phillips, J.A., 3rd; *et al.* Telomerase deficiency does not alter bleomycin-induced fibrosis in mice. *Exp. Lung Res.* **2012**, *38*, 124–134.

76. Santos, J.H.; Hunakova, L.; Chen, Y.; Bortner, C.; van Houten, B. Cell sorting experiments link persistent mitochondrial DNA damage with loss of mitochondrial membrane potential and apoptotic cell death. *J. Biol. Chem.* **2003**, *278*, 1728–1734.

77. Budinger, G.R.; Mutlu, G.M.; Eisenbart, J.; Fuller, A.C.; Bellmeyer, A.A.; Baker, C.M.; Wilson, M.; Ridge, K.; Barrett, T.A.; Lee, V.Y.; *et al.* Proapoptotic bid is required for pulmonary fibrosis. *Proc. Natl. Acad. Sci. USA.* **2006**, *103*, 4604–4609.

78. Bueno, M.; Lai, Y.C.; Romero, Y.; Brands, J.; St Croix, C.M.; Kamga, C.; Corey, C.; Herazo-Maya, J.D.; Sembrat, J.; Lee, J.S.; *et al.* Pink1 deficiency impairs mitochondrial homeostasis and promotes lung fibrosis. *J. Clin. Investig.* **2015**, *125*, 521–538.

79. Patel, A.S.; Song, J.W.; Chu, S.G.; Mizumura, K.; Osorio, J.C.; Shi, Y.; El-Chemaly, S.; Lee, C.G.; Rosas, I.O.; Elias, J.A.; *et al.* Epithelial cell mitochondrial dysfunction and pink1 are induced by transforming growth factor-beta1 in pulmonary fibrosis. *PLoS ONE* **2015**, *10*, e0121246.

80. Lounsbury, K.M.; Stern, M.; Taatjes, D.; Jaken, S.; Mossman, B.T. Increased localization and substrate activation of protein kinase Cδ in lung epithelial cells following exposure to asbestos. *Am. J. Pathol.* **2002**, *160*, 1991–2000.

81. Buder-Hoffmann, S.A.; Shukla, A.; Barrett, T.F.; MacPherson, M.B.; Lounsbury, K.M.; Mossman, B.T. A protein kinase Cδ-dependent protein kinase D pathway modulates ERK1/2 and JNK1/2 phosphorylation and Bim-associated apoptosis by asbestos. *Am. J. Pathol.* **2009**, *174*, 449–459.

82. Corral-Debrinski, M.; Horton, T.; Lott, M.T.; Shoffner, J.M.; Beal, M.F.; Wallace, D.C. Mitochondrial DNA deletions in human brain: Regional variability and increase with advanced age. *Nat. Genet.* **1992**, *2*, 324–329.

83. Michikawa, Y.; Mazzucchelli, F.; Bresolin, N.; Scarlato, G.; Attardi, G. Aging-dependent large accumulation of point mutations in the human mtDNA control region for replication. *Science* **1999**, *286*, 774–779.

84. Kujoth, G.C.; Hiona, A.; Pugh, T.D.; Someya, S.; Panzer, K.; Wohlgemuth, S.E.; Hofer, T.; Seo, A.Y.; Sullivan, R.; Jobling, W.A.; *et al.* Mitochondrial DNA mutations, oxidative stress, and apoptosis in mammalian aging. *Science* **2005**, *309*, 481–484.

85. DeBerardinis, R.J.; Mancuso, A.; Daikhin, E.; Nissim, I.; Yudkoff, M.; Wehrli, S.; Thompson, C.B. Beyond aerobic glycolysis: Transformed cells can engage in glutamine metabolism that exceeds the requirement for protein and nucleotide synthesis. *Proc. Natl. Acad. Sci. USA* **2007**, *104*, 19345–19350.

86. Vander Heiden, M.G.; Cantley, L.C.; Thompson, C.B. Understanding the warburg effect: The metabolic requirements of cell proliferation. *Science* **2009**, *324*, 1029–1033.

87. Fliss, M.S.; Usadel, H.; Caballero, O.L.; Wu, L.; Buta, M.R.; Eleff, S.M.; Jen, J.; Sidransky, D. Facile detection of mitochondrial DNA mutations in tumors and bodily fluids. *Science* **2000**, *287*, 2017–2019.

88. Wang, Z.; Choi, S.; Lee, J.; Huang, Y.T.; Chen, F.; Zhao, Y.; Lin, X.; Neuberg, D.; Kim, J.; Christiani, D.C. Mitochondrial variations in non-small cell lung cancer (NSCLC) survival. *Cancer Inform.* **2015**, *14*, 1–9.

89. Ishikawa, K.; Takenaga, K.; Akimoto, M.; Koshikawa, N.; Yamaguchi, A.; Imanishi, H.; Nakada, K.; Honma, Y.; Hayashi, J. Ros-generating mitochondrial DNA mutations can regulate tumor cell metastasis. *Science* **2008**, *320*, 661–664.

90. King, M.P.; Attardi, G. Injection of mitochondria into human cells leads to a rapid replacement of the endogenous mitochondrial DNA. *Cell* **1988**, *52*, 811–819.

91. Tan, A.S.; Baty, J.W.; Dong, L.F.; Bezawork-Geleta, A.; Endaya, B.; Goodwin, J.; Bajzikova, M.; Kovarova, J.; Peterka, M.; Yan, B.; *et al.* Mitochondrial genome acquisition restores respiratory function and tumorigenic potential of cancer cells without mitochondrial DNA. *Cell Metab.* **2015**, *21*, 81–94.

92. Chevillard, S.; Radicella, J.P.; Levalois, C.; Lebeau, J.; Poupon, M.F.; Oudard, S.; Dutrillaux, B.; Boiteux, S. Mutations in *OGG1*, a gene involved in the repair of oxidative DNA damage, are found in human lung and kidney tumours. *Oncogene* **1998**, *16*, 3083–3086.

93. Youn, C.K.; Song, P.I.; Kim, M.H.; Kim, J.S.; Hyun, J.W.; Choi, S.J.; Yoon, S.P.; Chung, M.H.; Chang, I.Y.; You, H.J. Human 8-oxoguanine DNA glycosylase suppresses the oxidative stress induced apoptosis through a p53-mediated signaling pathway in human fibroblasts. *Mol. Cancer Res.* **2007**, *5*, 1083–1098.

94. Ruchko, M.; Gorodnya, O.; LeDoux, S.P.; Alexeyev, M.F.; Al-Mehdi, A.B.; Gillespie, M.N. Mitochondrial DNA damage triggers mitochondrial dysfunction and apoptosis in oxidant-challenged lung endothelial cells. *Am. J. Physiol. Lung Cell Mol. Physiol.* **2005**, *288*, L530–L535.

95. Hashiguchi, K.; Stuart, J.A.; de Souza-Pinto, N.C.; Bohr, V.A. The C-terminal aO helix of human Ogg1 is essential for 8-oxoguanine DNA glycosylase activity: The mitochondrial β-Ogg1 lacks this domain and does not have glycosylase activity. *Nucleic Acids Res.* **2004**, *32*, 5596–5608.

96. Bulteau, A.L.; Ikeda-Saito, M.; Szweda, L.I. Redox-dependent modulation of aconitase activity in intact mitochondria. *Biochemistry* **2003**, *42*, 14846–14855.

97. Chen, X.J.; Wang, X.; Kaufman, B.A.; Butow, R.A. Aconitase couples metabolic regulation to mitochondrial DNA maintenance. *Science* **2005**, *307*, 714–717.

98. Cheresh, P.; Morales-Nebreda, L.; Kim, S.J.; Yeldandi, A.; Williams, D.B.; Cheng, Y.; Mutlu, G.M.; Budinger, G.R.; Ridge, K.; Schumacker, P.T.; *et al.* Asbestos-induced pulmonary fibrosis is augmented in 8-oxoguanine DNA glycosylase knockout mice. *Am. J. Respir. Cell Mol. Biol.* **2015**, *52*, 25–36.

99. Park, L.C.; Albers, D.S.; Xu, H.; Lindsay, J.G.; Beal, M.F.; Gibson, G.E. Mitochondrial impairment in the cerebellum of the patients with progressive supranuclear palsy. *J. Neurosci. Res.* **2001**, *66*, 1028–1034.

100. Przybylowska, K.; Kabzinski, J.; Sygut, A.; Dziki, L.; Dziki, A.; Majsterek, I. An association selected polymorphisms of *XRCC1*, *OGG1* and *MUTYH* gene and the level of efficiency oxidative DNA damage repair with a risk of colorectal cancer. *Mutat. Res.* **2013**, *745–746*, 6–15.

101. Duan, W.X.; Hua, R.X.; Yi, W.; Shen, L.J.; Jin, Z.X.; Zhao, Y.H.; Yi, D.H.; Chen, W.S.; Yu, S.Q. The association between *OGG1* Ser326Cys polymorphism and lung cancer susceptibility: A meta-analysis of 27 studies. *PLoS ONE* **2012**, *7*, e35970.

102. Elahi, A.; Zheng, Z.; Park, J.; Eyring, K.; McCaffrey, T.; Lazarus, P. The human OGG1 DNA repair enzyme and its association with orolaryngeal cancer risk. *Carcinogenesis* **2002**, *23*, 1229–1234.

103. Wang, J.; Wang, Q.; Watson, L.J.; Jones, S.P.; Epstein, P.N. Cardiac overexpression of 8-oxoguanine DNA glycosylase 1 protects mitochondrial DNA and reduces cardiac fibrosis following transaortic constriction. *Am. J. Physiol. Heart Circ. Physiol.* **2011**, *301*, H2073–H2080.

104. Tsutsui, H. Oxidative stress in heart failure: The role of mitochondria. *Intern. Med.* **2001**, *40*, 1177–1182.

105. Ding, Z.; Liu, S.; Wang, X.; Khaidakov, M.; Dai, Y.; Mehta, J.L. Oxidant stress in mitochondrial DNA damage, autophagy and inflammation in atherosclerosis. *Sci. Rep.* **2013**, *3*, 1077, doi:10.1038/srep01077.

106. Picard, M.; Jung, B.; Liang, F.; Azuelos, I.; Hussain, S.; Goldberg, P.; Godin, R.; Danialou, G.; Chaturvedi, R.; Rygiel, K.; *et al.* Mitochondrial dysfunction and lipid accumulation in the human diaphragm during mechanical ventilation. *Am. J. Respir. Crit. Care Med.* **2012**, *186*, 1140–1149.

107. Hashizume, M.; Mouner, M.; Chouteau, J.M.; Gorodnya, O.M.; Ruchko, M.V.; Potter, B.J.; Wilson, G.L.; Gillespie, M.N.; Parker, J.C. Mitochondrial-targeted DNA repair enzyme 8-oxoguanine DNA glycosylase 1 protects against ventilator-induced lung injury in intact mice. *Am. J. Physiol. Lung Cell Mol. Physiol.* **2013**, *304*, L287–L297.

108. Tsui, K.H.; Feng, T.H.; Lin, Y.F.; Chang, P.L.; Juang, H.H. P53 downregulates the gene expression of mitochondrial aconitase in human prostate carcinoma cells. *Prostate* **2011**, *71*, 62–70.

109. Koczor, C.A.; Torres, R.A.; Fields, E.J.; Boyd, A.; Lewis, W. Mitochondrial matrix P53 sensitizes cells to oxidative stress. *Mitochondrion* **2013**, *13*, 277–281.

110. Marudamuthu, A.S.; Bhandary, Y.P.; Shetty, S.K.; Fu, J.; Sathish, V.; Prakash, Y.; Shetty, S. Role of the urokinase-fibrinolytic system in epithelial-mesenchymal transition during lung injury. *Am. J. Pathol.* **2015**, *185*, 55–68.

111. Marudamuthu, A.S.; Shetty, S.K.; Bhandary, Y.P.; Karandashova, S.; Thompson, M.; Sathish, V.; Florova, G.; Hogan, T.B.; Pabelick, C.M.; Prakash, Y.S.; *et al.* Plasminogen activator inhibitor-1 suppresses profibrotic responses in fibroblasts from fibrotic lungs. *J. Biol. Chem.* **2015**, *290*, 9428–9441.

112. Bhandary, Y.P.; Shetty, S.K.; Marudamuthu, A.S.; Fu, J.; Pinson, B.M.; Levin, J.; Shetty, S. Role of p53-fibrinolytic system cross-talk in the regulation of quartz-induced lung injury. *Toxicol. Appl. Pharmacol.* **2015**, *283*, 92–98.

113. Huang, W.T.; Akhter, H.; Jiang, C.; MacEwen, M.; Ding, Q.; Antony, V.; Thannickal, V.J.; Liu, R.M. Plasminogen activator inhibitor 1, fibroblast apoptosis resistance, and aging-related susceptibility to lung fibrosis. *Exp. Gerontol.* **2015**, *61*, 62–75.

114. Cassel, S.L.; Eisenbarth, S.C.; Iyer, S.S.; Sadler, J.J.; Colegio, O.R.; Tephly, L.A.; Carter, A.B.; Rothman, P.B.; Flavell, R.A.; Sutterwala, F.S. The Nalp3 inflammasome is essential for the development of silicosis. *Proc. Natl. Acad. Sci. USA* **2008**, *105*, 9035–9040.

115. Zhou, R.; Yazdi, A.S.; Menu, P.; Tschopp, J. A role for mitochondria in Nlrp3 inflammasome activation. *Nature* **2011**, *469*, 221–225.

116. Kirillov, V.; Siler, J.T.; Ramadass, M.; Ge, L.; Davis, J.; Grant, G.; Nathan, S.D.; Jarai, G.; Trujillo, G. Sustained activation of toll-like receptor 9 induces an invasive phenotype in lung fibroblasts: Possible implications in idiopathic pulmonary fibrosis. *Am. J. Pathol.* **2015**, *185*, 943–957.

117. Gu, X.; Wu, G.; Yao, Y.; Zeng, J.; Shi, D.; Lv, T.; Luo, L.; Song, Y. Intratracheal administration of mitochondrial DNA directly provokes lung inflammation through the TLR9-p38 mapk pathway. *Free Radic. Biol. Med.* **2015**, *83*, 149–158.

118. Kuck, J.L.; Obiako, B.O.; Gorodnya, O.M.; Pastukh, V.M.; Kua, J.; Simmons, J.D.; Gillespie, M.N. Mitochondrial DNA damage-associated molecular patterns mediate a feed-forward cycle of bacteria-induced vascular injury in perfused rat lungs. *Am. J. Physiol. Lung Cell Mol. Physiol.* **2015**, *308*, L1078–L1085.

119. Dos Santos, G.; Rogel, M.R.; Baker, M.A.; Troken, J.R.; Urich, D.; Morales-Nebreda, L.; Sennello, J.A.; Kutuzov, M.A.; Sitikov, A.; Davis, J.M.; *et al.* Vimentin regulates activation of the Nlrp3 inflammasome. *Nat. Commun.* **2015**, *6*, 6574, doi:10.1038/ncomms7574.

120. Vaquero, A. The conserved role of sirtuins in chromatin regulation. *Int. J. Dev. Biol.* **2009**, *53*, 303–322.

121. Verdin, E.; Hirschey, M.D.; Finley, L.W.; Haigis, M.C. Sirtuin regulation of mitochondria: Energy production, apoptosis, and signaling. *Trends Biochem. Sci.* **2010**, *35*, 669–675.

122. Bosch-Presegue, L.; Vaquero, A. Sirtuins in stress response: Guardians of the genome. *Oncogene* **2014**, *33*, 3764–3775.

123. Kaniak-Golik, A.; Skoneczna, A. Mitochondria-nucleus network for genome stability. *Free Radic. Biol. Med.* **2015**, *82*, 73–104.

124. Kincaid, B.; Bossy-Wetzel, E. Forever young: SIRT3 a shield against mitochondrial meltdown, aging, and neurodegeneration. *Front. Aging Neurosci.* **2013**, *5*, 48, doi:10.3389/fnagi.2013.00048.

125. Bellizzi, D.; Rose, G.; Cavalcante, P.; Covello, G.; Dato, S.; de Rango, F.; Greco, V.; Maggiolini, M.; Feraco, E.; Mari, V.; *et al.* A novel vntr enhancer within the *SIRT3* gene, a human homologue of *SIR2*, is associated with survival at oldest ages. *Genomics* **2005**, *85*, 258–263.

126. Cheng, Y.; Ren, X.; Gowda, A.S.; Shan, Y.; Zhang, L.; Yuan, Y.S.; Patel, R.; Wu, H.; Huber-Keener, K.; Yang, J.W.; *et al.* Interaction of Sirt3 with OGG1 contributes to repair of mitochondrial DNA and protects from apoptotic cell death under oxidative stress. *Cell Death Dis.* **2013**, *4*, e731, doi:10.1038/cddis.2013.254.

127. Chen, Y.; Fu, L.L.; Wen, X.; Wang, X.Y.; Liu, J.; Cheng, Y.; Huang, J. Sirtuin-3 (sirt3), a therapeutic target with oncogenic and tumor-suppressive function in cancer. *Cell Death Dis.* **2014**, *5*, e1047, doi:10.1038/cddis.2014.14.

128. Shulga, N.; Pastorino, J.G. Ethanol sensitizes mitochondria to the permeability transition by inhibiting deacetylation of cyclophilin-d mediated by sirtuin-3. *J. Cell Sci.* **2010**, *123*, 4117–4127.

129. Sundaresan, N.R.; Samant, S.A.; Pillai, V.B.; Rajamohan, S.B.; Gupta, M.P. SIRT3 is a stress-responsive deacetylase in cardiomyocytes that protects cells from stress-mediated cell death by deacetylation of Ku70. *Mol. Cell. Biol.* **2008**, *28*, 6384–6401.

130. Li, S.; Banck, M.; Mujtaba, S.; Zhou, M.M.; Sugrue, M.M.; Walsh, M.J. P53-induced growth arrest is regulated by the mitochondrial sirt3 deacetylase. *PLoS ONE* **2010**, *5*, e10486.

131. Kawamura, Y.; Uchijima, Y.; Horike, N.; Tonami, K.; Nishiyama, K.; Amano, T.; Asano, T.; Kurihara, Y.; Kurihara, H. Sirt3 protects *in vitro*-fertilized mouse preimplantation embryos against oxidative stress-induced p53-mediated developmental arrest. *J. Clin. Investig.* **2010**, *120*, 2817–2828.

132. D'Aquila, P.; Rose, G.; Panno, M.L.; Passarino, G.; Bellizzi, D. *SIRT3* gene expression: A link between inherited mitochondrial DNA variants and oxidative stress. *Gene* **2012**, *497*, 323–329.

133. Wu, Y.T.; Lee, H.C.; Liao, C.C.; Wei, Y.H. Regulation of mitochondrial F_0F_1ATPase activity by Sirt3-catalyzed deacetylation and its deficiency in human cells harboring 4977bp deletion of mitochondrial DNA. *Biochim. Biophys. Acta* **2013**, *1832*, 216–227.

134. Bause, A.S.; Matsui, M.S.; Haigis, M.C. The protein deacetylase SIRT3 prevents oxidative stress-induced keratinocyte differentiation. *J. Biol. Chem.* **2013**, *288*, 36484–36491.

135. Shadel, G.S. Mitochondrial DNA, aconitase "wraps" it up. *Trends Biochem. Sci.* **2005**, *30*, 294–296.

136. Gibellini, L.; Pinti, M.; Beretti, F.; Pierri, C.L.; Onofrio, A.; Riccio, M.; Carnevale, G.; de Biasi, S.; Nasi, M.; Torelli, F.; *et al.* Sirtuin 3 interacts with lon protease and regulates its acetylation status. *Mitochondrion* **2014**, *18*, 76–81.

137. Sundaresan, N.R.; Gupta, M.; Kim, G.; Rajamohan, S.B.; Isbatan, A.; Gupta, M.P. Sirt3 blocks the cardiac hypertrophic response by augmenting Foxo3a-dependent antioxidant defense mechanisms in mice. *J. Clin. Investig.* **2009**, *119*, 2758–2771.

138. Someya, S.; Xu, J.; Kondo, K.; Ding, D.; Salvi, R.J.; Yamasoba, T.; Rabinovitch, P.S.; Weindruch, R.; Leeuwenburgh, C.; Tanokura, M.; *et al.* Age-related hearing loss in C57BL/6J mice is mediated by Bak-dependent mitochondrial apoptosis. *Proc. Natl. Acad. Sci. USA* **2009**, *106*, 19432–19437.

139. Someya, S.; Yu, W.; Hallows, W.C.; Xu, J.; Vann, J.M.; Leeuwenburgh, C.; Tanokura, M.; Denu, J.M.; Prolla, T.A. Sirt3 mediates reduction of oxidative damage and prevention of age-related hearing loss under caloric restriction. *Cell* **2010**, *143*, 802–812.

140. Coleman, M.C.; Olivier, A.K.; Jacobus, J.A.; Mapuskar, K.A.; Mao, G.; Martin, S.M.; Riley, D.P.; Gius, D.; Spitz, D.R. Superoxide mediates acute liver injury in irradiated mice lacking sirtuin 3. *Antioxid. Redox Signal.* **2014**, *20*, 1423–1435.

141. Morigi, M.; Perico, L.; Rota, C.; Longaretti, L.; Conti, S.; Rottoli, D.; Novelli, R.; Remuzzi, G.; Benigni, A. Sirtuin 3-dependent mitochondrial dynamic improvements protect against acute kidney injury. *J. Clin. Investig.* **2015**, *125*, 715–726.

142. Chen, T.; Li, J.; Liu, J.; Li, N.; Wang, S.; Liu, H.; Zeng, M.; Zhang, Y.; Bu, P. Activation of SIRT3 by resveratrol ameliorates cardiac fibrosis and improves cardiac function via the TGF-β/Smad3 pathway. *Am. J. Physiol. Heart Circ. Physiol.* **2015**, *308*, H424–H434.

143. Liu, L.; Peritore, C.; Ginsberg, J.; Kayhan, M.; Donmez, G. SIRT3 attenuates MPTP-induced nigrostriatal degeneration via enhancing mitochondrial antioxidant capacity. *Neurochem. Res.* **2015**, *40*, 600–608.

144. Wang, X.Q.; Shao, Y.; Ma, C.Y.; Chen, W.; Sun, L.; Liu, W.; Zhang, D.Y.; Fu, B.C.; Liu, K.Y.; Jia, Z.B.; *et al.* Decreased SIRT3 in aged human mesenchymal stromal/stem cells increases cellular susceptibility to oxidative stress. *J. Cell Mol. Med.* **2014**, *18*, 2298–2310.

145. Huang, K.; Kang, X.; Wang, X.; Wu, S.; Xiao, J.; Li, Z.; Wu, X.; Zhang, W. Conversion of bone marrow mesenchymal stem cells into type II alveolar epithelial cells reduces pulmonary fibrosis by decreasing oxidative stress in rats. *Mol. Med. Rep.* **2015**, *11*, 1685–1692.

146. Johnson, M.L.; Irving, B.A.; Lanza, I.R.; Vendelbo, M.H.; Konopka, A.R.; Robinson, M.M.; Henderson, G.C.; Klaus, K.A.; Morse, D.M.; Heppelmann, C.; *et al.* Differential effect of endurance training on mitochondrial protein damage, degradation, and acetylation in the context of aging. *J. Gerontol. A Biol. Sci. Med. Sci.* **2014**, doi:10.1093/gerona/glu221.

147. Dai, S.H.; Chen, T.; Wang, Y.H.; Zhu, J.; Luo, P.; Rao, W.; Yang, Y.F.; Fei, Z.; Jiang, X.F. Sirt3 protects cortical neurons against oxidative stress via regulating mitochondrial Ca^{2+} and mitochondrial biogenesis. *Int. J. Mol. Sci.* **2014**, *15*, 14591–14609.

148. Rato, L.; Duarte, A.I.; Tomas, G.D.; Santos, M.S.; Moreira, P.I.; Socorro, S.; Cavaco, J.E.; Alves, M.G.; Oliveira, P.F. Pre-diabetes alters testicular PGC1-α/SIRT3 axis modulating mitochondrial bioenergetics and oxidative stress. *Biochim. Biophys. Acta* **2014**, *1837*, 335–344.

149. Kim, M.; Lee, J.S.; Oh, J.E.; Nan, J.; Lee, H.; Jung, H.S.; Chung, S.S.; Park, K.S. SIRT3 overexpression attenuates palmitate-induced pancreatic β-cell dysfunction. *PLoS ONE* **2015**, *10*, e0124744.

150. Choudhary, C.; Kumar, C.; Gnad, F.; Nielsen, M.L.; Rehman, M.; Walther, T.C.; Olsen, J.V.; Mann, M. Lysine acetylation targets protein complexes and co-regulates major cellular functions. *Science* **2009**, *325*, 834–840.

151. Haigis, M.C.; Deng, C.X.; Finley, L.W.; Kim, H.S.; Gius, D. SIRT3 is a mitochondrial tumor suppressor: A scientific tale that connects aberrant cellular ROS, the warburg effect, and carcinogenesis. *Cancer Res.* **2012**, *72*, 2468–2472.

152. Lombard, D.B.; Alt, F.W.; Cheng, H.L.; Bunkenborg, J.; Streeper, R.S.; Mostoslavsky, R.; Kim, J.; Yancopoulos, G.; Valenzuela, D.; Murphy, A.; *et al.* Mammalian Sir2 homolog SIRT3 regulates global mitochondrial lysine acetylation. *Mol. Cell. Biol.* **2007**, *27*, 8807–8814.

153. Koentges, C.; Pfeil, K.; Schnick, T.; Wiese, S.; Dahlbock, R.; Cimolai, M.C.; Meyer-Steenbuck, M.; Cenkerova, K.; Hoffmann, M.M.; Jaeger, C.; *et al.* SIRT3 deficiency impairs mitochondrial and contractile function in the heart. *Basic Res. Cardiol.* **2015**, *110*, 493, doi:10.1007/s00395-015-0493-6.

154. Paulin, R.; Dromparis, P.; Sutendra, G.; Gurtu, V.; Zervopoulos, S.; Bowers, L.; Haromy, A.; Webster, L.; Provencher, S.; Bonnet, S.; *et al.* Sirtuin 3 deficiency is associated with inhibited mitochondrial function and pulmonary arterial hypertension in rodents and humans. *Cell Metab.* **2014**, *20*, 827–839.

155. Zeng, L.; Yang, Y.; Hu, Y.; Sun, Y.; Du, Z.; Xie, Z.; Zhou, T.; Kong, W. Age-related decrease in the mitochondrial sirtuin deacetylase Sirt3 expression associated with ROS accumulation in the auditory cortex of the mimetic aging rat model. *PLoS ONE* **2014**, *9*, e88019.

156. Marques-Aleixo, I.; Santos-Alves, E.; Mariani, D.; Rizo-Roca, D.; Padrao, A.I.; Rocha-Rodrigues, S.; Viscor, G.; Torrella, J.R.; Ferreira, R.; Oliveira, P.J.; *et al.* Physical exercise prior and during treatment reduces sub-chronic doxorubicin-induced mitochondrial toxicity and oxidative stress. *Mitochondrion* **2015**, *20*, 22–33.

157. Wood, J.G.; Rogina, B.; Lavu, S.; Howitz, K.; Helfand, S.L.; Tatar, M.; Sinclair, D. Sirtuin activators mimic caloric restriction and delay ageing in metazoans. *Nature* **2004**, *430*, 686–689.

158. Desquiret-Dumas, V.; Gueguen, N.; Leman, G.; Baron, S.; Nivet-Antoine, V.; Chupin, S.; Chevrollier, A.; Vessieres, E.; Ayer, A.; Ferre, M.; *et al.* Resveratrol induces a mitochondrial complex I-dependent increase in NADH oxidation responsible for sirtuin activation in liver cells. *J. Biol. Chem.* **2013**, *288*, 36662–36675.

159. Royce, S.G.; Dang, W.; Yuan, G.; Tran, J.; El Osta, A.; Karagiannis, T.C.; Tang, M.L. Resveratrol has protective effects against airway remodeling and airway hyperreactivity in a murine model of allergic airways disease. *Pathobiol. Aging Age Relat. Dis.* **2011**, *1*, doi:10.3402/PBA.v1i0.7134.

160. Haohao, Z.; Guijun, Q.; Juan, Z.; Wen, K.; Lulu, C. Resveratrol improves high-fat diet induced insulin resistance by rebalancing subsarcolemmal mitochondrial oxidation and antioxidantion. *J. Physiol. Biochem.* **2015**, *71*, 121–131.

161. Sener, G.; Topaloglu, N.; Sehirli, A.O.; Ercan, F.; Gedik, N. Resveratrol alleviates bleomycin-induced lung injury in rats. *Pulm. Pharmacol. Ther.* **2007**, *20*, 642–649.

162. Zghonda, N.; Yoshida, S.; Ezaki, S.; Otake, Y.; Murakami, C.; Mliki, A.; Ghorbel, A.; Miyazaki, H. Epsilon-viniferin is more effective than its monomer resveratrol in improving the functions of vascular endothelial cells and the heart. *Biosci. Biotechnol. Biochem.* **2012**, *76*, 954–960.

163. Fu, J.; Jin, J.; Cichewicz, R.H.; Hageman, S.A.; Ellis, T.K.; Xiang, L.; Peng, Q.; Jiang, M.; Arbez, N.; Hotaling, K.; *et al.* Trans-(–)-ε-viniferin increases mitochondrial sirtuin 3 (SIRT3), activates AMP-activated protein kinase (AMPK), and protects cells in models of huntington disease. *J. Biol. Chem.* **2012**, *287*, 24460–24472.

164. Pillai, V.B.; Samant, S.; Sundaresan, N.R.; Raghuraman, H.; Kim, G.; Bonner, M.Y.; Arbiser, J.L.; Walker, D.I.; Jones, D.P.; Gius, D.; *et al.* Honokiol blocks and reverses cardiac hypertrophy in mice by activating mitochondrial Sirt3. *Nat. Commun.* **2015**, *6*, 6656, doi:10.1038/ncomms7656.

165. Nunnari, J.; Suomalainen, A. Mitochondria: In sickness and in health. *Cell* **2012**, *148*, 1145–1159.

166. Aon, M.A.; Tocchetti, C.G.; Bhatt, N.; Paolocci, N.; Cortassa, S. Protective mechanisms of mitochondria and heart function in diabetes. *Antioxid. Redox Signal.* **2015**, *22*, 1563–1586.

167. Gatenby, R.A.; Gillies, R.J. Why do cancers have high aerobic glycolysis? *Nat. Rev. Cancer* **2004**, *4*, 891–899.

168. Chen, W.; Wang, Q.; Bai, L.; Chen, W.; Wang, X.; Tellez, C.S.; Leng, S.; Padilla, M.T.; Nyunoya, T.; Belinsky, S.A.; *et al.* RIP1 maintains DNA integrity and cell proliferation by regulating PGC-1α-mediated mitochondrial oxidative phosphorylation and glycolysis. *Cell Death Differ.* **2014**, *21*, 1061–1070.

169. Mendelsohn, A.R.; Larrick, J.W. Partial reversal of skeletal muscle aging by restoration of normal NAD$^+$ levels. *Rejuv. Res.* **2014**, *17*, 62–69.

170. Metodiev, M.D.; Gerber, S.; Hubert, L.; Delahodde, A.; Chretien, D.; Gerard, X.; Amati-Bonneau, P.; Giacomotto, M.C.; Boddaert, N.; Kaminska, A.; *et al.* Mutations in the tricarboxylic acid cycle enzyme, aconitase 2, cause either isolated or syndromic optic neuropathy with encephalopathy and cerebellar atrophy. *J. Med. Genet.* **2014**, *51*, 834–838.

171. Cha, M.Y.; Kim, D.K.; Mook-Jung, I. The role of mitochondrial DNA mutation on neurodegenerative diseases. *Exp. Mol. Med.* **2015**, *47*, e150.

172. Van Waveren, C.; Sun, Y.; Cheung, H.S.; Moraes, C.T. Oxidative phosphorylation dysfunction modulates expression of extracellular matrix—Remodeling genes and invasion. *Carcinogenesis* **2006**, *27*, 409–418.

173. Liu, T.F.; Vachharajani, V.; Millet, P.; Bharadwaj, M.S.; Molina, A.J.; McCall, C.E. Sequential actions of SIRT1-RELB-SIRT3 coordinate nuclear-mitochondrial communication during immunometabolic adaptation to acute inflammation and sepsis. *J. Biol. Chem.* **2015**, *290*, 396–408.

174. Ashrafi, G.; Schwarz, T.L. The pathways of mitophagy for quality control and clearance of mitochondria. *Cell Death Differ.* **2013**, *20*, 31–42.

175. Ayala-Pena, S. Role of oxidative DNA damage in mitochondrial dysfunction and huntington's disease pathogenesis. *Free Radic. Biol. Med.* **2013**, *62*, 102–110.

176. Diebold, I.; Hennigs, J.K.; Miyagawa, K.; Li, C.G.; Nickel, N.P.; Kaschwich, M.; Cao, A.; Wang, L.; Reddy, S.; Chen, P.I.; *et al.* BMPR2 preserves mitochondrial function and DNA during reoxygenation to promote endothelial cell survival and reverse pulmonary hypertension. *Cell Metab.* **2015**, *21*, 596–608.

177. De Cavanagh, E.M.; Inserra, F.; Ferder, L. Angiotensin II blockade: A strategy to slow ageing by protecting mitochondria? *Cardiovasc Res.* **2011**, *89*, 31–40.

178. Radak, Z.; Koltai, E.; Taylor, A.W.; Higuchi, M.; Kumagai, S.; Ohno, H.; Goto, S.; Boldogh, I. Redox-regulating sirtuins in aging, caloric restriction, and exercise. *Free Radic. Biol. Med.* **2013**, *58*, 87–97.

179. Boyette, L.B.; Tuan, R.S. Adult stem cells and diseases of aging. *J. Clin. Med.* **2014**, *3*, 88–134.

180. Tao, R.; Coleman, M.C.; Pennington, J.D.; Ozden, O.; Park, S.H.; Jiang, H.; Kim, H.S.; Flynn, C.R.; Hill, S.; Hayes McDonald, W.; *et al.* Sirt3-mediated deacetylation of evolutionarily conserved lysine 122 regulates MNSoD activity in response to stress. *Mol. Cell* **2010**, *40*, 893–904.

181. Kim, H.S.; Patel, K.; Muldoon-Jacobs, K.; Bisht, K.S.; Aykin-Burns, N.; Pennington, J.D.; van der Meer, R.; Nguyen, P.; Savage, J.; Owens, K.M.; *et al.* SIRT3 is a mitochondria-localized tumor suppressor required for maintenance of mitochondrial integrity and metabolism during stress. *Cancer Cell* **2010**, *17*, 41–52.

182. Stefanatos, R.; Sanz, A. Mitochondrial complex I: A central regulator of the aging process. *Cell Cycle* **2011**, *10*, 1528–1532.

183. Peek, C.B.; Affinati, A.H.; Ramsey, K.M.; Kuo, H.Y.; Yu, W.; Sena, L.A.; Ilkayeva, O.; Marcheva, B.; Kobayashi, Y.; Omura, C.; *et al.* Circadian clock NAD+ cycle drives mitochondrial oxidative metabolism in mice. *Science* **2013**, *342*, 1243417, doi:10.1126/science.1243417.

184. Gomes, A.P.; Price, N.L.; Ling, A.J.; Moslehi, J.J.; Montgomery, M.K.; Rajman, L.; White, J.P.; Teodoro, J.S.; Wrann, C.D.; Hubbard, B.P.; *et al.* Declining NAD+ induces a pseudohypoxic state disrupting nuclear-mitochondrial communication during aging. *Cell* **2013**, *155*, 1624–1638.

185. Zhou, X.; Chen, M.; Zeng, X.; Yang, J.; Deng, H.; Yi, L.; Mi, M.T. Resveratrol regulates mitochondrial reactive oxygen species homeostasis through Sirt3 signaling pathway in human vascular endothelial cells. *Cell Death Dis.* **2014**, *5*, e1576, doi:10.1038/cddis.2014.530.

186. Xu, R.; Hu, Q.; Ma, Q.; Liu, C.; Wang, G. The protease Omi regulates mitochondrial biogenesis through the GSK3β/PGC-1α pathway. *Cell Death Dis.* **2014**, *5*, e1373, doi:10.1038/cddis.2014.328.

187. Massudi, H.; Grant, R.; Braidy, N.; Guest, J.; Farnsworth, B.; Guillemin, G.J. Age-associated changes in oxidative stress and NAD+ metabolism in human tissue. *PLoS ONE* **2012**, *7*, e42357.

188. Braidy, N.; Guillemin, G.J.; Mansour, H.; Chan-Ling, T.; Poljak, A.; Grant, R. Age related changes in NAD+ metabolism oxidative stress and sirt1 activity in wistar rats. *PLoS ONE* **2011**, *6*, e19194.

5

Mitochondrial Oxidative Stress, Mitochondrial DNA Damage and their Role in Age-Related Vascular Dysfunction

Yuliya Mikhed [1,†], **Andreas Daiber** [1,†,*] **and Sebastian Steven** [1,2,†]

1   2nd Medical Clinic, Medical Center of the Johannes Gutenberg-University,
    Mainz 55131, Germany; E-Mails: yuliya.mikhed@unimedizin-mainz.de (Y.M.);
    sebastiansteven@gmx.de (S.S.)
2   Center for Thrombosis and Hemostasis, Medical Center of the Johannes Gutenberg-University,
    Mainz 55131, Germany

†   These authors contributed equally to this work.

*   Author to whom correspondence should be addressed; E-Mail: daiber@uni-mainz.de

Academic Editors: Lars Olson, Jaime M. Ross and Giuseppe Coppotelli

---

Abstract: The prevalence of cardiovascular diseases is significantly increased in the older population. Risk factors and predictors of future cardiovascular events such as hypertension, atherosclerosis, or diabetes are observed with higher frequency in elderly individuals. A major determinant of vascular aging is endothelial dysfunction, characterized by impaired endothelium-dependent signaling processes. Increased production of reactive oxygen species (ROS) leads to oxidative stress, loss of nitric oxide (·NO) signaling, loss of endothelial barrier function and infiltration of leukocytes to the vascular wall, explaining the low-grade inflammation characteristic for the aged vasculature. We here discuss the importance of different sources of ROS for vascular aging and their contribution to the increased cardiovascular risk in the elderly population with special emphasis on mitochondrial ROS formation and oxidative damage of mitochondrial DNA. Also the interaction (crosstalk) of mitochondria with nicotinamide adenosine dinucleotide phosphate (NADPH) oxidases is highlighted. Current concepts of vascular aging, consequences for the development of cardiovascular events and the particular role of ROS are evaluated on the basis of cell culture experiments, animal studies and clinical trials.

Present data point to a more important role of oxidative stress for the maximal healthspan (healthy aging) than for the maximal lifespan.

Keywords: aging; mitochondrial oxidative stress; mitochondrial DNA damage; vascular dysfunction

---

1. Introduction

Demographic change is an emerging issue in the Western world. The proportion of people older than 65 years will dramatically increase within the next decades [1]. Besides its negative effects on the costs for retirement funds, an increasing average age will amplify the economic burden for healthcare costs in these countries. Cardiovascular diseases (CVD) are a main cause of morbidity and mortality in elderly people and their incidence is closely correlated with age [2] (Figure 1A). The term "vascular aging" outlines all changes in vessels, which are associated with aging. Smooth muscle cells and endothelial cells are involved in these changes during vascular aging. Progressive aging leads to arterial stiffness and endothelial dysfunction, which is known to correlate with future cardiovascular events in humans [3]. Furthermore, aged vessels are more prone to develop atherosclerotic lesions, vascular injury, impaired angiogenesis and calcification [4]. Consequently, the incidence and frequency of cardiovascular diseases such as atherosclerosis and its late complications such as coronary artery disease or stroke, increase substantially with age [5]. However, endothelial dysfunction in the elderly is not only associated with CVD, but also with other disorders related to aging, such as erectile dysfunction, renal dysfunction, Alzheimer's disease or retinopathy [6–9]. Since the CVD burden is predicted to increase dramatically in Western societies and the knowledge about vascular aging is limited, there is urgent need for research in this field in order to reduce morbidity and mortality in the aging population. Within the last years, scientists identified three key players in the vascular aging process: nitric oxide signaling, oxidative stress and inflammation [10]. It should be noted, that these players do not stand alone as they affect and influence each other. Especially pathophysiological convergence of different organ diseases with associated comorbidities increases at higher age and represents another important field of research that needs to be addressed in the future [11–13].

Nitric oxide ($^\bullet$NO) is essential for a functional endothelium and diminished $^\bullet$NO bioavailability leads to endothelial dysfunction [14,15]. In aged vessels the bioavailability of $^\bullet$NO is reduced, whereas production of reactive oxygen species (ROS) is increased [10,16,17]. It is not only the reaction of $^\bullet$NO with superoxide anion ($O_2^{\bullet-}$), leading in turn to production of peroxynitrite ($ONOO^-$) [17], which reduces $^\bullet$NO bioavailability. Also dysregulation of the endothelial nitric oxide synthase (eNOS), known as eNOS uncoupling, results in impaired $^\bullet$NO release from the endothelium and leads instead to increased superoxide production [18]. The mechanisms of this uncoupling process are complex and multiple. They include decreased availability of the eNOS substrate L-arginine or the cofactor tetrahydrobiopterin (BH4), but also phosphorylation state (Ser1177, Thr495, Tyr657) or S-glutathionlyation of the protein (for review see [19]). All of them play an important role for the coupling state of the enzyme and many of them were identified in the vascular aging process [16,20–22]. Imbalance of $^\bullet$NO bioavailability by ROS is not only induced by eNOS itself. Increased oxidative stress from mitochondria and other enzymatic sources are observed in aged animals and affect the coupling state of eNOS [23]. This observation points to a strong correlation between aging, oxidative stress, and as a consequence of imbalanced 'NO bioavailability, the development of endothelial dysfunction (Figure 1B) [24]. The impact of vascular oxidative stress on endothelial function and the predictive value of this parameter was previously shown by a large clinical trial demonstrating better cardiovascular prognosis in patients with lower burden of vascular oxidative stress (less pronounced effect of vitamin C infusion on flow-mediated dilation) (Figure 1C) [25].

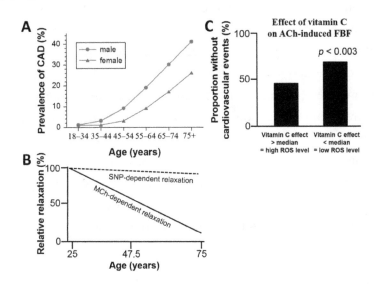

Figure 1. (**A**) Prevalence of coronary artery diseases (CAD) increases with progressing age and gender in Germany. Drawn from results of the Detect Study [26,27] and figure adopted from [28] with permission of the publisher. © Springer Science+Business Media, LLC 2010; (**B**) Correlation between age and endothelium-dependent (methacholine (MCh), solid line) and -independent (sodium nitroprusside (SNP), broken line) relaxation. Healthy individuals with an age of 25–70 years were tested for MCh- and SNP-dependent vasodilation. Endothelium-dependent relaxation was impaired with age ($r = 0.81, p < 0.001$, r is the correlation coefficient), whereas endothelium-independent relaxation was decreased only by trend in older individuals ($r = 0.1$, not significant). According to [24]; and (**C**) Results from Kaplan-Meier-analysis for the cardiovascular event rate in two cohorts of patients displaying either pronounced or weak effect of vitamin C on endothelial function (measured by forearm plethysmography after infusion of acetylcholine (ACh)) over a time period of more than 6 years. The take-home message is: Higher levels of vascular oxidative stress (free radicals) are associated with a more pronounced beneficial effect of the radical scavenger vitamin C on endothelial function and an increased cardiovascular event rate. FBF means forearm blood flow. According to Heitzer *et al.*, Circulation 2001 [25].

There is good evidence that mitochondria represent a major source of ROS in aging tissues [29,30]. Mitochondrial DNA damage accumulates in the aging cell leading to mitochondrial dysfunction [31] and aging-related cardiovascular and neurodegenerative disease [10,32]. The present review will discuss the impact of mitochondrial oxidative stress and mitochondrial DNA damage on vascular dysfunction in the aging process.

2. The Cardiovascular System

The cardiovascular system is a closed network containing arteries, veins and capillaries. The center of this network is the heart. Transportation is one of the most important functions of the human cardiovascular system. By every heartbeat nutrients, oxygen, carbon dioxide and hormones are distributed to all parts of the body. Furthermore, the cardiovascular system is involved in host defense by the inflammatory system and hemostasis by the coagulation system. As the interface between blood and vessel wall, the endothelium plays a crucial role as a specialized monolayered squamous epithelium that lines the interior surface of blood vessels. Preserving the blood barrier function and thereby preventing adhesion of immune cells is a defense against infiltration of immune cells such as monocytes into lesion-prone areas of the endothelium, an essential step in the development of atherosclerotic plaques [33,34]. There are over 2 billion heartbeats in one human life and every heartbeat is associated with increased sheer stress and elongation of the vessel. The endothelial cell layer has to control the vascular tone under all circumstances by nitric oxide ('NO), endothelium-derived hyperpolarizing factor, prostacyclin or natriuretic peptides. Furthermore, these mediators released by the endothelium have antiaggregatory properties and suppress thrombus formation, vascular stenosis [35] and cardiac hypertrophy. On the other hand, the endothelium acts synergistically with a regulatory system, which consists of vasoconstrictors such as catecholamines and other vasoactive peptides (*i.e.*, angiotensin, vasopressin, endothelin).

The aging endothelium is more and more unable to fulfill all these tasks. In elderly people a significant impairment of endothelium-dependent relaxation (endothelial dysfunction) can be found [36,37]. This dysfunction promotes thrombosis, vasoconstriction, leukocyte infiltration and cell proliferation in the vessel wall. Thus, endothelial dysfunction in aging is an early predictor for the development of atherosclerosis, hypertension and future cardiovascular events. Besides this interaction during the aging process, this correlation was also proven by a meta-analysis of 23 studies [3], which nicely demonstrates flow-mediated dilation (FMD) of the brachial artery as a prognostic marker for cardiovascular events. Although this study cannot prove endothelial dysfunction as the cause of increased cardiovascular morbidity, it demonstrates that endothelial dysfunction is a precursor of cardiovascular disease. Not only are macrovessels, like aorta or coronary arteries, affected by aging-dependent endothelial dysfunction and oxidative stress but the microcirculation (resistance vessels) are especially affected by vascular aging (for review see [38]). Studies of Mayhan *et al.* demonstrated impaired eNOS-dependent reactivity of cerebral arterioles, which was associated with increased oxidative stress [39]. Similar evidence for endothelial dysfunction could be found for retinal vessels during the aging process [40] and its contribution to neurodegenerative disease is very likely [41,42] Our group and many others revealed impaired 'NO signaling, vascular inflammation and oxidative stress as key players in the pathogenesis of aging dependent endothelial dysfunction (for review see [28]).

3. Aging and Oxidative Stress

As early as in 1954, Harman expressed for the first time the free radical theory of aging [43]. This idea was based on the observations, that aging is a universal phenomenon, and its contributing factors must be present in every living organism. His first hypothesis emphasized the importance of the hydroxyl radical, as well as molecular oxygen in the aging process [44]. Later, this concept was extended to mitochondria which are the most abundant cellular source of ROS. Mitochondrial ROS formation probably contributes to the high mutation rate of the mitochondrial genome. In general, assembly of the respiratory chain components requires the contribution of two spatially separated genomes, the nuclear DNA and the maternally inherited mtDNA [45]. Malfunctioning of the mitochondrial genome is directly correlated with impaired mitochondrial physiology and depleted ATP-synthesis, which are accompanied by enhanced ROS formation and increased apoptosis [29]. Age-dependent impairment of vascular redox regulation is demonstrated by the bioavailability of another free radical species –'NO. Nitric oxide is not only involved in vasodilation, but also in vascular smooth muscle cell proliferation, inhibition of platelet aggregation and several others [46]. It has been postulated that 'NO is gradually reduced with age and might serve as an applicable biomarker for age-dependent endothelial dysfunction. The prevailing paradigm is that an age-dependent increase in superoxide rapidly consumes 'NO, consequently reduces its endothelial levels and thereby leads to impaired vasorelaxation [24,47].

Oxidative stress burden usually correlates with cellular thiol levels or vice versa cellular thiol/disulfide ratio is a well-accepted indicator of the redox state of a cell. Therefore, thiols and thiol-dependent enzymes were in the focus of oxidative stress and aging-related research. Cellular thiols possess significant antioxidant effects and affect the organismal healthspan. Glutathione peroxidases (GPx) belong to the class of enzymes responsible for the removal of H_2O_2 from the intracellular compartments. *GPx* deficiency leads to increased levels of oxidative stress, pronounced vascular dysfunction [16] and increased senescence of fibroblasts [48]. Even though genetic depletion of either *GPx-1* or *GPx-4* has no effect on the lifespan of the experimental animals, their effect on the process of healthy aging cannot be disputed [16]. Thioredoxins (Trx) are another class of antioxidant enzymes that can directly react with peroxides and eliminate damage caused by peroxides via reduction of disulfides and methionine sulfoxides [49]. Complete knock-out of the mitochondrial Trx isoform ($Trx2^{-/-}$) is embryonically lethal and partial knock-out ($Trx2^{+/-}$) mice show elevated levels of lipid peroxides, oxidized nucleobases and proteins [50]. Although $Trx2^{+/-}$ mice exhibited reduction in their lifespan by trend, a further increase of the significance power would require higher number of animals. On the other hand, genetic knock-in of the cytosolic isoform of thioredoxin, *Trx1*, showed considerable increase in mice longevity and stronger resistance to oxidative stress inducers, like UV-light or ischemia/reperfusion, further supporting the previous notion of the importance of antioxidant enzymes [51].

The impact of antioxidant defense enzymes on aging-related cardiovascular complications is well established and has been previously demonstrated for the mitochondrial superoxide dismutase 2 (SOD2) [52], the cytosolic superoxide dismutase (SOD1) [47,53], the extracellular superoxide dismutase (ecSOD), and the thioredoxin-1 protein (Trx) [49]. Considering the fact that superoxide is the major contributing factor to the endothelial dysfunction in the aging vasculature further investigations of the antioxidant systems have been conducted in order to understand why these defense mechanisms are not able to combat increasing levels of the oxidative stress. On the example of SOD2, it has been shown that in aging vessels, MnSOD has been heavily nitrated, most probably by peroxynitrite, as indicated by increased staining for 3-nitrotyrosine [54]. Inhibition of this protective enzyme results in the activation of the vicious cycle of increased oxidative burden. On the other hand, no direct correlation between lifespan and deletion of or overexpression of most antioxidant enzymes ($SOD2^{+/-}$ or transgenic overexpression of *SOD2* ($SOD2^{tg}$), $GPx-1^{-/-}$, $GPx-4^{-/-}$ or $MsrA^{-/-}$, transgenic overexpression of *SOD1*

(*SOD1^tg*), transgenic overexpression of catalase (*catalase^tg*)) could affect the longevity [55]. Only *SOD1^{-/-}* mice and mice with double gene ablation combinations showed reduced life expectancy [55,56]. It is worth to mention that mice completely deficient in *SOD2* show lethality at the embryo stage or a few weeks after birth, once again stressing the importance of these antioxidant enzymes in the normal physiology [57,58]. Of note, overexpression of *Trx1* increased the lifespan and stress resistance [51]. Although there is only a limited role for oxidative stress as a direct determinant for accelerated aging or decreased lifespan [55,56,59], there is substantial evidence for a contribution of oxidative stress to detrimental effects on physiological organ function during the aging process preventing healthy aging [60–63].

The observation that antioxidant enzymes have a significant effect on the healthspan of animals during normal aging (e.g., indicated by decreased aging-associated cardiovascular complications during the sunset years) and also on the resistance to stress conditions is of high clinical importance [51]. Previously, we demonstrated that genetic deletion of the mitochondrial antioxidant proteins aldehyde dehydrogenase-2 (*ALDH-2*) and manganese superoxide dismutase (*Mn-SOD*) leads to vascular dysfunction and mitochondrial oxidative stress with increasing age [23]. These data support the concept that oxidative stress in general and mitochondrial ROS formation in particular, despite not playing a key role for the lifespan, have significant impact on the quality of aging, the healthspan [60–63].

4. Vascular Function, Oxidative Stress and ˙NO Bioavailability in Aging

Endothelial dysfunction was found in several animal models of hypertension or atherosclerosis, both representing important cardiovascular risk factors (for review see [19]). Furthermore, patients with endothelial dysfunction display a higher burden of oxidative stress and have increased risk factors for cardiovascular disease and events (see Figure 1). Endothelial dysfunction and most cardiovascular disease are characterized by increased levels of ROS formation due to an imbalance between pro-oxidative enzymes (xanthine oxidase, NADPH oxidase, uncoupled eNOS or enzymes of mitochondrial respiration) and antioxidant enzymes (Cu, Zn-SOD, Mn-SOD and extracellular SOD), resulting in a deviation of cellular redox environment from the normal [64]. A similar pattern of vascular dysregulation can be found in aging tissues (for review see [28]) and was first described in 1956 by Harman *et al.* ("free radical theory of aging").

Irreversible oxidations and accumulation of oxidized biological macromolecules (e.g., DNA mutations, oxidized proteins) appear in biological systems, which are suffering from chronic oxidative stress. Besides these long-term consequences, ROS interfere rapidly with nitric oxide (˙NO) signaling. The accepted concept for reduced ˙NO bioavailability is the reaction of superoxide with ˙NO under formation of peroxynitrite ($ONOO^-$) [65]. Not only is reduced bioavailability of the important vasodilator ˙NO problematic for the vascular system, $ONOO^-$ itself has the ability to disturb the enzymatic function of proteins by nitration of tyrosine residues and oxidation of cysteine-thiol-groups [66–68]. Among others, the mitochondrial isoform of superoxide dismutase, Mn-SOD, is affected by nitration and becomes inactivated which further reduces antioxidant capacity of the cell [69].

The ˙NO producing enzyme eNOS itself is highly susceptible to damage by increased oxidative stress [15]. Tetrahydrobiopterin (BH4), a cofactor of eNOS, can be oxidized by $ONOO^-$ and the latter can potentially uncouple eNOS [70,71]. BH4 is a redox cofactor of eNOS and regulates the catalytic activity. In aged animals reduced vascular BH4 levels were shown [72], but the results in the literature are controversial [73].

Nevertheless, pharmacological supplementation of BH4 improves endothelial function in aged humans compared to young subjects [22]. This shortage of cofactor leads to a conformational change in eNOS resulting in uncoupling. Besides BH4, eNOS has several other redox switches that may lead to dysfunction/uncoupling in a ROS-dependent fashion: it can be S-glutathionylated [74], inhibited by asymmetric dimethylarginine (ADMA) and phosphorylated in a protein kinase C (PKC) or protein tyrosine kinase (PYK-2) dependent manner at Thr495 or Tyr657 [75]. Likewise, the zinc-sulfur-complex at the dimer-binding-interface can be oxidatively disrupted [76].

Uncoupling of eNOS switches the enzyme from good to evil [77]. In the uncoupled state, eNOS is generating ROS, which further oxidize BH4 and reduce ˙NO bioavailability [71]. This vicious circle is an established concept and part of the pathogenesis of endothelial dysfunction in aged vessels [24,36]. Several groups reported on increased eNOS expression levels in aging, which might be a counter-regulatory effect to compensate for decreased ˙NO bioavailability. In contrast, other groups found no change of eNOS expression in aging, but observed decreased Akt-dependent phosphorylation of eNOS at Ser1177 with increasing age as a potential explanation for an impaired endothelial dysfunction in the elderly [78]. Our group just recently provided evidence for S-glutathionylation and adverse phosphorylation of eNOS at Thr495 and Tyr657 by redox-sensitive PKC and PYK-2, respectively, as important mechanisms in the process of aging-induced vascular dysfunction [16].

NADPH oxidase (Nox) is a major source of ROS in the cardiovascular system [79,80]. Isoforms 1, 2, 4 and 5 are significantly expressed in heart and vessels. Nox2 and Nox4 are known to be upregulated in vascular tissue of aged mice [81]. In addition, these enzymes are regulated by tumor necrosis factor-α (TNF-α), which is known to be elevated in aged animals and humans [82,83]. The cytokine TNF-α plays an important role in many inflammatory disorders and vascular dysfunction is closely linked to inflammatory processes [84]. In fact, administration of TNF-α can promote oxidative stress by activation of Nox, endothelial dysfunction, endothelial apoptosis, and upregulation of proatherogenic inflammatory mediators, like inducible nitric oxide synthase (iNOS) and adhesion molecules [85,86]. Furthermore, TNF-α stimulates mitochondrial superoxide production in human retinal endothelial cells [87]. Chronic TNF-α inhibition improves flow-mediated arterial dilation in resistance arteries of aged animals, while reducing iNOS and intercellular adhesion molecule-1 (ICAM-1) expression [88]. All the mentioned effects are similar to functional alterations of the aged vascular endothelium. Not only TNF-α, but also interleukins (IL-1β, IL-6, IL-17) and C-reactive protein (CRP) are elevated in aging independent to other risk factors (e.g., smoking) [89]. Since, infiltrating leukocytes contribute to increased oxidative stress and reduced ˙NO bioavailability in the vessel wall [90,91], cytokine release and chemoattraction of leukocytes by the endothelium are important in the pathogenesis of aging-mediated endothelial dysfunction.

5. Aging, Mitochondrial Oxidative Stress, Mitochondrial DNA Damage and Endothelial Dysfunction

In 1972, Harman modified his "free radical theory of aging" to specify the role of mitochondria [92]. He tried to explain why exogenous supplementation of antioxidants to rodents could not improve their lifespan. His explanation was that these antioxidants do not reach the mitochondrion. He proposed that mitochondria are both the primary origin and target of oxidative stress.

Recently, we demonstrated in two different knock-out models with increased mitochondrial ROS (*ALDH-2*$^{-/-}$, *MnSOD*$^{-/-}$ mice), that mitochondrial ROS formation and oxidative mitochondrial DNA (mtDNA) lesions as well as vascular dysfunction are increasing with age [23] (Figure 2). According to our data, endothelial dysfunction was clearly correlated with mitochondrial oxidative stress. The increase of mitochondrial ROS was more dependent on aging, then on the presence or absence of antioxidant proteins. The correlation between mtROS and mtDNA strand breaks, led us to speculate that the mitochondrial DNA damage could induce even more mtROS. Since the mitochondrial DNA mainly encodes for proteins of the mitochondrial respiration chain, one could assume that impaired mtDNA translation leads to mitochondrial uncoupling with secondary increase in mtROS formation.

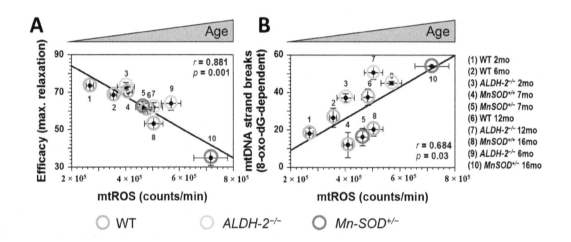

Figure 2. Correlations between mitochondrial oxidative stress (mtROS), mitochondrial DNA (mtDNA) damage and vascular (endothelial) function (ACh-induced maximal relaxation). (**A**) mtROS formation was plotted for all age-groups and mouse strains *versus* the corresponding maximal efficacy in response to acetylcholine (ACh); (**B**) mtROS was plotted for all age-groups and mouse strains *versus* the corresponding mtDNA damage. ROS were measured using L-012 (100 μM) enhanced chemiluminescence in isolated cardiac mitochondria upon stimulation with succinate (5 mM). *r* is the correlation coefficient. The groups are: 1 = B6 WT, 2mo; 2 = B6 WT, 6mo; 3 = *ALDH-2*$^{-/-}$, 2mo; 4 = *MnSOD*$^{+/+}$, 7mo; 5 = *MnSOD*$^{+/-}$, 7mo; 6 = WT B6, 12mo; 7 = *ALDH-2*$^{-/-}$, 12mo; 8 = *MnSOD*$^{+/+}$, 16mo; 9 = *ALDH-2*$^{-/-}$, 6mo; 10 = *MnSOD*$^{+/-}$, 16mo. The age of measured groups increases from the left to the right. Adopted from Wenzel *et al.*, Cardiovasc. Res. 2008 [23]. With permission of the European Society of Cardiology. All rights reserved. © The Author and Oxford University Press 2008.

Previous reports highlighted increased mitochondrial and systemic oxidative stress in mice with genetic deficiency in glutathione peroxidase-1 (*GPx-1*) [48]. In addition, *GPx-1* deficiency showed synergistic negative effects on vascular function in the setting of diabetes [93], hyperlipidemia [94], and hypertension [95]. Moreover, increased senescence was reported for fibroblasts from *GPx-1*$^{-/-}$ mice [48]. Most importantly, a correlation between cardiovascular risk and GPx-1 activity in blood cells was previously reported conferring high clinical relevance to the expression/activity of GPx-1 [96] and again supporting the concept that antioxidant enzymes and oxidative stress might contribute significantly to the healthspan and comorbidity of the elderly [60–63].

Recently, we demonstrated for the first time that aging per se leads to eNOS dysfunction and eNOS uncoupling via increased adverse phosphorylation and *S*-glutathionylation of the enzyme (Figure 3B) [16]. We also established that *GPx-1* deficiency resulted in a phenotype of endothelial and vascular dysfunction, which was substantially potentiated by the aging process (Figure 3A). By using oxidative stress-prone $GPx-1^{-/-}$ mice (a model representing decreased break-down of cellular hydrogen peroxide) in a study of the aging process, we can provide a strong mechanistic link between oxidative stress, eNOS dysfunction and vascular dysfunction in aging animals (Figure 3). Most importantly, ˙NO bioavailability was also significantly decreased in aged $GPx-1^{-/-}$ mice (Figure 4) supporting a dysregulation of eNOS and/or increased oxidative degradation of ˙NO during the aging process in general and in animals with decreased antioxidant defense in particular.

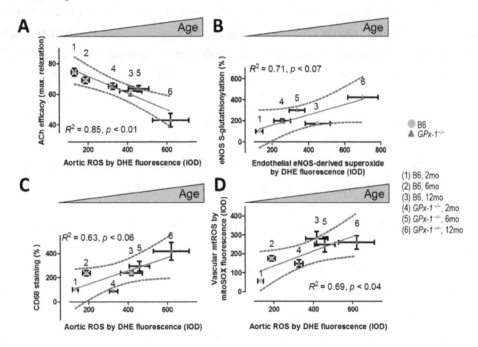

Figure 3. (**A**) Correlation between endothelium (ACh)-dependent relaxation (isometric tension measurement in isolated aortic ring segments) and aortic ROS formation (DHE staining of the aortic wall). Linear regression: $p < 0.01$, $R^2 = 0.85$; (**B**) Correlation between eNOS uncoupling marker (*S*-glutathionylated eNOS) and endothelial (eNOS-derived) superoxide formation (endothelial DHE staining). Linear regression: $p < 0.07$, $R^2 = 0.71$; (**C**) Correlation between inflammation (CD68 staining) and aortic ROS formation (DHE staining of the aortic wall). Linear regression: $p < 0.06$, $R^2 = 0.63$; and (**D**) Correlation between mitochondrial ROS formation (mitoSOX staining) and aortic ROS formation (DHE staining of the aortic wall). Linear regression: $p < 0.04$, $R^2 = 0.69$. Linear regressions were performed with GraphPad Prism 6 for Windows (version 6.02). All data were collected from our previous work [16]. Each data point was based on measurement of 4–10 animals. B6 means C57/BL6 wild type control; $GPx-1^{-/-}$ means glutathione peroxidase-1 knockout mice on C57/BL6 background. The age of measured groups increases from the left to the right. The solid red lines are simple linear regression fits to the data. Blue lines are the 95% confidence intervals on the estimated means. With permission of Wolters Kluwer Health, Inc. Copyright © 2014, Wolters Kluwer Health.

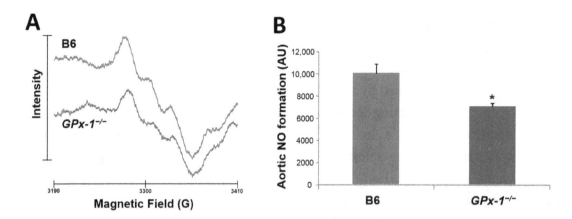

Figure 4. Nitric oxide formation in isolated aortic ring segments in old (12 mo) wild type (WT) and *GPx-1* knockout mice. ˙NO was measured in aortic ring segments (1 thoracic aorta for each measurement) upon stimulation with calcium ionophore (A23187, 10 μM) for 60 min at 37 °C in the presence of freshly prepared lipophilic spin trap Fe(II)(DETC)$_2$. ˙NO bound to the spin trap generates a stable paramagnetic nitrosyl-iron species that yield a typical triplet signal when measured by electron spin resonance (EPR) spectroscopy in liquid nitrogen. The detailed method was published in [97,98] and samples were used from a published study [16]. (**A**) Representative spectra and (**B**) quantification of signal intensity. Data are mean ± SEM of 9 mice per group. *, $p < 0.05$ *versus* wild type.

As a proof of endothelial and vascular dysfunction, we showed that both, endothelium-dependent and -independent relaxation was impaired in aged *GPx-1*$^{-/-}$ mice [16]. Altered eNOS function by inactivating or uncoupling phosphorylation, PKC-dependent at Thr495 [99,100] or PYK-2-dependent at Tyr657 [101], and *S*-glutathionylation [74] leading to diminished ˙NO bioavailability are plausible explanations for this phenotype. The deregulatory modifications of eNOS were also translated to increased uncoupling of the enzyme as envisaged by endothelial superoxide formation, which increased with age, was more pronounced in the *GPx-1*$^{-/-}$ group and nicely correlated with *S*-glutathionylation as a marker of uncoupled eNOS (Figure 3B) [16]. Since the ˙NO target enzyme soluble guanylyl cyclase (sGC) is also subject to oxidative inactivation (*S*-oxidation, *S*-nitrosation, heme-oxidation) [102–108], it might be speculated that the aging process will lead to an inactivation or at least desensitization of the enzyme. At least decreased expression of sGC subunits have been reported in tissues of old animals [109–111]. Future studies with sGC activators will prove whether apo-sGC or heme-oxidized sGC play a role for aging-induced vascular dysfunction.

In cultured endothelial cells we demonstrated that *GPx-1* silencing increased adhesion of leukocytes, which may contribute to the observed endothelial/vascular dysfunction (e.g., by increased oxidative breakdown of ˙NO and/or impairment of the ˙NO-cGMP signaling cascade by infiltrated leukocytes) [16]. Furthermore, we observed an appreciable increase in cardiovascular oxidative stress and mild vascular remodeling, as detected by Sirius red and Masson's trichrome staining (indicative for increased fibrosis of the intima and thus a decrease in intima/media ratio) [16].

GPx-1 deficiency has been demonstrated to increase the susceptibility of cultured endothelial cells to lipopolysaccharide (LPS) by enforcing TLR4/CD14 signaling [112]. In conductance vessels, sustained overproduction of vasodilators (e.g., ˙NO by iNOS) may reduce the responsiveness of the vasculature to these messengers because of a desensitization of the ˙NO/cGMP pathway [113]. Indeed, increased iNOS expression and activity has been demonstrated for selenium-deficient RAW cell macrophages [114] and selenium is the precursor for selenocysteine synthesis forming the active site of GPx-1. iNOS-derived ˙NO formation could also provide the basis for extensive protein tyrosine nitration as reported for old mice in general and *GPx-1* deficient mice in particular [16]. In summary, the progressing phenotype of low-grade inflammation in GPx-1 deficient mice during the aging process was nicely reflected by the correlation of the marker of inflammation (CD68 staining) with the overall vascular ROS formation (dihydroethidine staining (DHE staining)) in dependence of age and antioxidant defense state of the animals (Figure 3C) [16]. Since global vascular ROS formation was nicely correlated with mitochondrial ROS formation (Figure 3D), and all other parameters were linked to global vascular ROS formation, one can assume that mtROS formation has significant impact on eNOS dysregulation/uncoupling, vascular function and low-grade inflammation during the aging process [16]. This assumption is in good accordance to the reports on mtROS-driven activation of the inflammasome and expression of proinflammatory cytokines [115–118].

We observed a moderate but consistent decline in reduced thiol groups in aged GPx-$1^{-/-}$ mice as compared to only a minor tendency of this decline in the aged B6 wild type mice [16]. Overall, the majority of literature supports a trend of decrease in reduced thiols during the aging process, which could affect the *S*-glutathionylation pattern and accordingly the coupling state of eNOS. Smith *et al.* showed in 2006 that the decline in endothelial GSH may contribute to a change of eNOS phosphorylation pattern (decline in P-Ser1176 and increase in P-Thr494) that was associated with a loss of vascular ˙NO bioavailability, increased proinflammatory cytokines and impaired endothelium-dependent vasodilation [119]. Recent work by Crabtree and coworkers even described an interplay of BH4 deficiency and eNOS *S*-glutathionylation in cells with diminished GTP-cyclohydrolase-1 expression providing a functional link between these two routes of eNOS uncoupling [120] that could be of relevance for the aging process as well.

According to our own previous data, mitochondrial oxidative stress increases with age and is a strong trigger of age-related endothelial/vascular dysfunction (Figure 2A) [23,28]. Using two genetic mouse models with ablated mitochondrial aldehyde dehydrogenase ($ALDH$-$2^{-/-}$) or mitochondrial superoxide dismutase ($MnSOD^{+/-}$), both important antioxidant enzymes, we could show that increased mitochondrial oxidative stress is associated with augmented oxidative mtDNA lesions (Figure 2B). Outcome from studies in genetic animal models with increased mitochondrial ROS formation (e.g., *MnSOD*- or *Trx-2*-deficiency) strongly supports an important link between cellular aging and mitochondrial dysfunction. Of note, overexpression of mitochondria-targeted catalase enhanced protection of mitochondria from ROS-induced damage and extended life span in mice [121].

Mitochondria represent an important source of reactive oxygen species, caused by electron leakage in the respiratory chain that results in univalent reduction of oxygen into $O_2^{\cdot-}$. The steady state concentration of superoxide in the mitochondrial matrix is about 5- to 10-fold higher than that in the cytosolic and nuclear spaces. These apparently high mitochondrial superoxide formation rates correlate well with the reported mitochondrial oxidative DNA lesions being 10- to 20-fold higher in mitochondrial compared to nuclear DNA [29]. Cadenas and Davies proposed that susceptibility of mtDNA to oxidative damage may be ascribed to a combination of factors besides the higher superoxide formation rate in the mitochondrial matrix: unlike nuclear DNA, mitochondrial DNA lacks protective histones and enjoys only a relatively low DNA repair activity [29]. Therefore, mitochondrial 8-oxo-deoxyguanosine (8-oxo-dG) DNA lesion could represent an interesting marker for the burden of oxidative stress during the aging process [122]. According to Sastre *et al.* "mitochondrial oxidative stress should be considered a hallmark of cellular aging" [123]. The impact of mitochondrial ROS production on longevity may involve direct signal transduction pathways that are sensitive to oxidative stress, and indirect pathways related to the accumulation of oxidative damage to mitochondrial DNA, proteins, and lipids. Of note, the majority of mtDNA encodes for proteins of the mitochondrial respiratory chain and accumulation of mtDNA lesions might contribute to further uncoupling of mitochondrial electron flow at the expense of oxygen reduction to water but instead favor the formation of superoxide [124].

The free radical hypothesis of aging highlights that reactive oxygen species are responsible for the accumulation of altered biological macromolecules such as DNA, over an organism's lifespan [31]. Nucleic acid, in particular mitochondrial DNA (mtDNA), is regarded as a highly susceptible target for oxidant-induced mutations and deletions, which causes progressive deterioration of mitochondrial function over time (Figure 5). mtDNA deterioration belongs to a destructive cycle in which mitochondrial dysfunction further increases oxidative burden resulting in loss of cellular functions and finally apoptosis and necrosis. One of the major oxidative modifications of the mtDNA is 8-oxo-deoxyguanosine (8-oxo-dG) [125,126]. 8-oxo-dG is a mutagenic lesion and its accumulation is directly correlated with the development of pathological processes [127]. The correlation of lifespan with oxidant-induced mtDNA damage was demonstrated for the first time by Barja and co-workers [122]. These authors showed that in short-lived animals 8-oxo-dG content in nuclear and mitochondrial DNA was increased in cardiac tissue (Figure 6). These findings could be attributed to higher burden of oxidative stress in these short-lived animals (due to higher metabolic rate, less efficient antioxidant defense and/or less efficient DNA repair machinery). However, when brain tissue was investigated, accumulation of 8-oxo-dG in nuclear DNA was more pronounced in the long-lived animals (data not shown) [122]. This important study demonstrates that accumulation of oxidative DNA damage cannot per se be assumed for more living years among all different animal species, but each of them obviously has distinct kinetics of formation and repair of DNA damage, which, on top of this, depends on the specific tissue used for the quantification.

This assumption was later expanded in genetically modified mice with a proofreading-deficient mitochondrial polymerase-γ (Polyγ). These mice accumulated severe mtDNA mutations, leading to mitochondrial dysfunction, increase in apoptosis and premature aging [31,128]. One of the more recent studies clearly depicted that a transgenic mouse with cardiac tissue-specific overexpression of mutated human Poly [129] developed early aging symptoms. Elevated ROS generation and severe cardiomyopathy, typical for the "mtDNA-mutator mouse", was also observed in these animals. Our current knowledge of maternally inherited human diseases [130], e.g., DAD-syndrome (Leu-UUR tRNA = diabetes mellitus and deafness), MELAS- (mitochondrial encephalomyopathy, lactic acidosis, and stroke-like syndrome) [131–133] or KSS- (Kearns-Sayre syndrome) [131,133], highlight the importance of mtDNA. Various mutations or deletions, especially in tissues with high oxygen and energy consumption such as the myocardium, increase the rate of apoptosis, free radical species formation, leading to the functional impairment of the specific organ [131,134]. Therefore, mutated mtDNA is commonly regarded as a major contributor to vascular aging and various cardiovascular disorders [131,134].

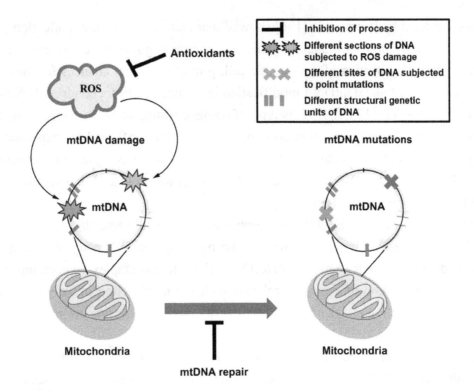

Figure 5. Schematic representation of mitochondrial DNA (mtDNA) damage by reactive oxygen species (ROS) leading to mtDNA mutations. Deleterious activity of ROS can be prevented by the administration of antioxidants. Damaged mtDNA can be repaired by the appropriate mtDNA repair pathway.

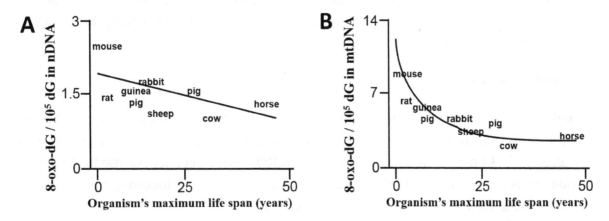

Figure 6. Correlation of an organism's life span with the content of 8-oxo-dG in nuclear (**A**) or mitochondrial (**B**) DNA in cardiac tissue. Surprisingly, oxidative DNA lesions do not per se accumulate with increasing number of living years but show distinct kinetics among different animal species, tissues and probably the underlying burden of oxidative stress, efficiency of the antioxidant system and DNA repair machinery. According to Barja *et al.* [122].

Considering that mtDNA damage accumulation with age is already widely accepted, more profound molecular explanations were provided during the last years. It has been recently shown that the observed mtDNA mutations might be mainly ascribed to errors in the replication process, to unrepaired damages, or to the spontaneous deamination of the nucleobases, indicating effects of ROS only as concomitant [135].

Investigations conducted by Itsara *et al.* [136] showed that malfunction of the replication process leads to a high accumulation of mtDNA mutations. This observation might be based on the fact that mtDNA propagates throughout the lifespan of the somatic cell, providing higher chances for the occurrence of mtDNA damage [137]. A typical mtDNA modification introduced by mitochondrial ROS is 8-hydroxy-deoxyguanosine (8-oxo-dG) [125,126]. This type of damage results in G:C to T:A transversions after DNA replication [138]. Nonetheless, this concept has not been confirmed by experimental studies, detecting only 10% of all mutations to be G:C to T:A transversions, having no correlation with the age of the animals. The most prevailing type of detected mutation was G:C to A:T transitions, attributed to the imperfect activity of mtDNA polymerase γ.

Another study by Kennedy *et al.* [139], utilizing a more clinically relevant experimental model of aging human brain, showed that mtDNA mutations during aging consist mostly of transition mutations (G:C to A:T), as depicted by ultra-sensitive detection technique and Duplex Sequencing methodology. These mtDNA mutations showed a nice correlation with the malfunction of Polγ or deamination of cytidine resulting in uracil and adenosine deamination, yielding inosine as the major mutagenic contributors in mtDNA.

Several recent papers that were summarized in the review by Cha *et al.* [140], highlight the direct correlation of mitochondrial DNA mutations with neurodegenerative diseases, in particular Huntington's, Parkinson's, Alzheimer's diseases and amyotrophic lateral sclerosis (ALS). The incidence of these neurodegenerative disease increases with higher age [32]. In the setting of Alzheimer's diseases (AD) it has been shown that post-mortem brain tissues of AD patients have elevated levels of degraded mtDNA [141] and defective base excision repair [142]. Another group was able to show that patients suffering from AD have an increased number of cytochrome C oxidase deficient neurons [143], supporting the above mentioned concept that accumulating mtDNA damage during the aging process leads to impaired biosynthesis of the respiratory chain proteins.

6. Aging and Mitochondrial DNA Repair

Not only the particular damage of the mtDNA molecule itself, but also the lifetime of mtDNA lesions has profound effects on the progression and characteristics of the aging phenotype. The accumulation of mtDNA damage is not only determined by the higher mtROS formation rates but also by the activity or expression levels of mitochondrial DNA repair systems. Therefore, the following part of the review concentrates on the impact of aging on the DNA repair machinery.

Taking into account the highly oxidizing environment of the mitochondria, malfunctioning of the Polγ and peculiarity of the mtDNA replication process would ultimately lead to the accumulation of mtDNA lesions. During mtDNA replication, the lagging strand is kept in the single-stranded condition for a prolonged period of time, and thereby the chances are increased for impairment of the replication. For this reason, mitochondrial protein machinery evolutionary created a multi-layered DNA repair system that is able to resolve such complex challenges [144].

One of the most extensively studied DNA repair pathways in mitochondria is base excision repair (BER) [145]. Its enzymatic pathways are identical to the ones that take place in the nucleus, starting with the modified base identification by specific glycosylase, followed by its excision, insertion of the correct nucleotide and finishing with the DNA strand ligation [146]. The family of glycosylases involved in mitochondrial BER consists of several members: OGG1 that is able to remove the most common and the most mutagenic modification introduced to the mtDNA—8-oxo-dG [147]; UNG1, which is responsible for the removal of uracil, resulting from the spontaneous deamination of the cytosine [148]; NTH1-dichotomous enzyme, possessing glycosylase and AP lyase activities, that excises pyrimidine lesions (ThyGly, FapyG and FapyA) [149]; NEIL1 and NEIL2 that are also involved in the removal of FapyG and FapyA [150]; MYH, enzyme that detects adenine placed opposite to 8-oxo-dG [151]. After specific glycosylases have identified and extracted the damaged base, the abasic sites are resolved by APE endonuclease that prepares the DNA molecule for the Polγ mediated repair process by cleaving 3′-hydroxyl and 5′-deoxyribose-5-phosphate sites [152]. Afterwards, the newly synthesized section of DNA is ligated to the rest of the molecule by DNA ligase III.

In case that the incorrect base has not been identified by BER and the replication process actually resulted in the formation of a mismatch, the adequate mismatch repair pathway (MMR) can be activated. There has been a lot of dispute in the field about the existence of this repair mechanism, since mitochondria doesn't possess classical players of MMR, like MSH3, MSH6 or MLH1 [153]. Though recently, with the help of specific mass spectrometry analysis, a novel MMR repair protein has been identified. Y-box binding protein (YB-1) has been shown to efficiently bind DNA containing mismatches [154]. This finding was further supported by identifying 3′ and 5′-exonuclease activity of YB-1 on single stranded DNA and weak endonuclease activity on double-stranded DNA. Depletion of this enzyme by siRNA showed increased levels of mtDNA mutagenesis, confirming the presence of a unique mitochondrial MMR pathway. In contrast to the nucleus, mitochondrion doesn't possess a nucleotide excision repair. This limitation leads to the accumulation of unrepaired bulky pyrimidine dimers, as observed upon UV irradiation.

Enzymatic reactants of the homologous recombination (HR) or non-homologous end joining (NHEJ) that are quite abundantly involved in the DNA repair inside the nucleus have not been precisely identified in the mitochondria. So far, only products of their reactivity have been detected by super-resolution and transmission electron microscopy. Among them are the following ones: 1. mtDNA deletions, which are attributed to the exo- and endonucleases activity; 2. Holiday junctions, detected in the mtDNA of the human heart and brain [155]; 3. Formation of diverse brunched structures and multiple-way junctions. All three of them are indicative of the active homologous recombination process [156]. The identification of the novel single strand annealing enzyme Mgm101 further supports this notion [157].

Recent findings on the expression levels of DNA repair systems in the matrix of aging mitochondria are quite specific for the different DNA repair systems [158]. For example, it has been shown that incidents of the homologous recombination become more abundant with the progress of aging, being strongly correlated with linear increase in the mtDNA damage [159]. Alternatively, the specific DNA glycosylase, OGG1, has been shown to be down-regulated with the onset of aging, augmenting the deleterious effects of the oxidative stress burden in the mitochondrial environment and accelerating the process of cellular senescence [160].

7. Crosstalk between Mitochondrial and NADPH Oxidase-Generated Reactive Oxygen and Nitrogen Species and Impact on Endothelial Function

Primary mtROS not only cause direct oxidative damage to cellular structures but may also contribute to the activation of secondary ROS sources such as the NADPH oxidases. In a feed-forward fashion, this crosstalk initiates a vicious cycle that finally may lead to eNOS dysfunction/uncoupling and impairment of endothelial function [75]. Previously, we reported on the crosstalk between mtROS and cytosolic ROS in the model of nitroglycerin-induced nitrate tolerance that is associated with increased mitochondrial oxidative stress. Nitrate tolerance is an excellent model of vascular dysfunction and oxidative stress in general [161] and mitochondrial oxidative stress and dysfunction in particular [162–164]. Two distinct ROS sources could be identified: endothelial dysfunction was linked to activation of NADPH oxidases, whereas vascular dysfunction was associated with mitochondrial oxidative stress [165]. Cyclosporine A, the mitochondrial permeability transition pore inhibitor, blocked this interaction (crosstalk) between mitochondrial and NADPH-dependent ROS formation and selectively improved endothelial dysfunction, whereas nitrate tolerance was not affected. In support of this observation, $gp91phox^{-/-}$ and $p47phox^{-/-}$ mice developed tolerance under nitroglycerin treatment but no endothelial dysfunction. In contrast, endothelial dysfunction and tolerance was improved by the respiratory complex I inhibitor rotenone (preventing complex I-derived ROS formation by reverse electron transfer [166]). Likewise, administration of the K_{ATP} opener diazoxide caused a nitrate tolerance-like phenomenon in control animals, whereas tolerance phenomenon was improved by the K_{ATP} inhibitor glibenclamide.

Very similar effects of these compounds have been recently demonstrated in animal and cell culture models of angiotensin-II induced hypertension [167,168]. NADPH oxidase-driven activation of mitochondrial ROS formation via K_{ATP} channels (acting as a redox switch) and changes in the membrane potential was previously proposed [169,170] and later confirmed [167]. The proposed mechanism for mtROS-driven activation of NADPH oxidase is redox-sensitive stimulation of protein kinases such as PKC and cSrc in a calcium-dependent process [97,166,171]. Synergistic formation of mtROS and NADPH oxidase derived ROS lead to uncoupling of eNOS, nitration of prostacyclin synthase and desensitization sGC [19]. Recently, we showed that this interaction (crosstalk) plays an essential role in angiotensin-II induced hypertension, vascular oxidative stress and endothelial dysfunction (envisaged by eNOS S-glutathionylation) [97]. In support of this proposed mechanism, increased oxidative stress per se is able to activate NADPH oxidase in a positive feedback fashion [172].

We and others propose a similar crosstalk between mitochondrial and NADPH oxidase-dependent ROS formation in the aging vasculature leading to age-related vascular dysfunction (Figure 7) [23,28,97,173]. This proposal is based on the finding that mtROS formation increases with age (and is higher in $MnSOD^{+/-}$ mice) and endothelial function is impaired with age (to a higher extent in $MnSOD^{+/-}$ mice) [23]. Of note, we and others also showed that mtROS participate in the activation of immune cells via stimulation of the phagocytic NADPH oxidase (Nox2) [97,174]. mtROS have also been reported to participate in the activation of the inflammasome and trigger the expression of proinflammatory cytokines [115–118]. In summary these data support a proinflammatory role of mtROS for progression of low-grade inflammation in the aging vasculature.

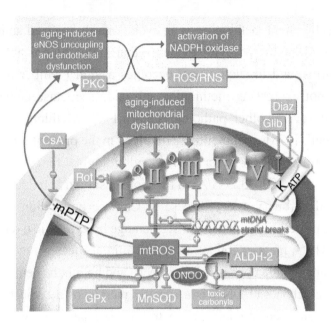

Figure 7. Hypothetic scheme of aging-induced vascular dysfunction and the role of mitochondria in this process. Aging-induced mitochondrial dysfunction triggers mitochondrial reactive oxygen species (mtROS) formation from respiratory complexes I, II, and III (Q = ubiquinone), whereas respiratory complexes IV and V were not reported to contribute to mtROS formation directly. Break-down of mtROS is catalyzed by glutathione peroxidase (GPx, for H_2O_2) or manganese superoxide dismutase (MnSOD), the latter is in turn inhibited by mitochondrial peroxynitrite (ONOO$^-$) formation. mtROS increase the levels of toxic aldehydes and inhibit the mitochondrial aldehyde dehydrogenase (ALDH-2), the detoxifying enzyme of those aldehydes. Increase in mtROS and toxic aldehydes also leads to mtDNA strand breaks which leads to augmented dysfunction in respiratory chain complexes and further increase in mtROS since mtDNA encodes mainly for those respiratory complexes. mtROS also activates mitochondrial permeability transition pore (mPTP), which upon opening releases mtROS to the cytosol leading to protein kinase C (PKC)-dependent NADPH oxidase activation, eNOS uncoupling and finally to endothelial dysfunction [165]. Cytosolic reactive oxygen and nitrogen species (ROS/RNS) in turn were demonstrated to activate K_{ATP} channels, which causes alterations in mitochondrial membrane potential (C) and further augments mtROS levels [167]. Effects of rotenone (Rot), cyclosporine A (CsA), diazoxide (Diaz) and glibenclamide (Glib) have been recently demonstrated in related models of vascular dysfunction and oxidative stress, nitroglycerin-induced nitrate tolerance and angiotensin-II triggered hypertension [165,167]. + means promotion of pathways; − means inhibition of pathways. Adopted from Wenzel *et al.*, Cardiovasc. Res. 2008 [23]. With permission of the European Society of Cardiology. All rights reserved. © The Author and Oxford University Press 2008.

8. Emerging Concepts of Aging

Moosmann and coworkers have published an interesting concept, based on the observation that intramembrane accumulation of methionine exhibits antioxidant and cytoprotective properties in living cells [175]. Their findings highlight methionine as an evolutionarily selected antioxidant of the respiratory chain complexes. On top of that they provide evidence that methionine is able to redox-cycle between oxidized and reduced forms, and in such a way becomes a vital member of the antioxidant defense system. Knockout mice not expressing methionine sulfoxide reductase enzyme are characterized by a decreased lifespan and several other pathologies [176,177]. Methionine sulfoxide reductases are expressed in endothelial cells [178], are potentially involved in the prevention of endothelial dysfunction via regulation of RUNX2 transcription factor activity and biological function in endothelial cells [179]. The functional polymorphism (rs10903323 G/A) in methionine sulfoxide reductase A shows an association with the increased risk of coronary artery disease in Chinese population [180]. Moreover, vascular smooth muscle cells were protected against oxidative damage by cytosolic overexpression of methionine sulfoxide reductase A [181]. A meta-examination of 248 animal species genome sequences with known maximum lifespan, including mammals, birds, fish, insects, and helminths demonstrated that the frequency of cysteine encoded by mitochondrial DNA is a specific marker of aerobic longevity [182]: long-lived organisms synthesize respiratory chain complexes with low abundance of cysteine. These results provide distinct (indirect) support for the free radical theory of aging.

Another explanation for worsening of the physical condition with age is based on a profound role of the mitochondrial enzyme p66Shc as an adaptor protein which is implicated in mitochondrial reactive oxygen species generation and translation of oxidative signals into apoptosis [183]. Mice deficient in $p66Shc^{-/-}$ gene produce decreased quantities of intracellular oxidants and display 30% longer life span. In order to elucidate the function of p66Shc and its possible implication in age-associated cardiovascular diseases, a series of studies were initiated. Extensive research revealed that $p66Shc^{-/-}$ mice are protected from age-dependent endothelial dysfunction [184] as well as age-related risk factors such as diabetes and hypercholesterolemia. The review of Camici et al. focused on deciphering the novel role of the p66Shc adaptor protein and its involvement in the age-associated cardiovascular disease and pathophysiology of aging. One of the major findings of these authors is that p66Shc N terminus is activated through reversible tetramerization by forming two disulfide bonds, as a result of which it forms a redox module responsible for apoptosis initiation that is tightly associated with senescence [185]. Other systems that are involved in p66Shc regulation are two antioxidant enzymatic classes—glutathione and thioredoxin enzymes that can inactivate p66Shc through a reduction mechanism. Consequently, this forms a thiol-based redox sensor system and initiates apoptosis once cellular protection systems cannot ameliorate cellular stress anymore. Protein kinase C β and prolyl isomerase 1 effectively regulates the mitochondrial effects of the longevity-associated stimulator-p66Shc [186]. Recently, highly specialized signaling pathways leading to mitochondrial import of p66Shc that are responsible for its proapoptotic activity upon oxidative stress were analyzed [187]. In contrast, advantages for diabetic cardiovascular complications [188] and age-associated endothelial ˙NO formation [189] were reported for genetic deletion of $p66Shc$. Last, but not least, it was validated that a p53-p66Shc signaling pathway controls intracellular redox status and contributes to increased levels of oxidative DNA damage [190] and mitochondrial oxidative stress [191]. The important role of p66Shc for vascular function is supported by recent findings that p66Shc expression correlates with the prognosis of stroke patients and post-ischemic inhibition of p66Shc reduces ischemia/reperfusion brain injury [192].

Another emerging concept in the field of aging is based on the contribution of epigenetic pathways. Epigenetic mechanisms that are involved in the aging process include alterations of the DNA methylation status, modifications of the histone tails (mainly acetylation and methylation) and changes in the expression of non-coding RNAs [193]. With increasing age, global DNA demethylation processes have been detected, leading to a DNA hypomethylation condition. This has been mostly observed on the CpG islands, which constitute regions of the DNA consisting for more than 50% of cytosine and guanine repeats [194]. On the other hand, there is a lot of information regarding sequestered, locus specific DNA hypermethylation. These nuclear regions are called senescence-associated heterochromatin foci (SAHF) [195]. The presence of such DNA segments is of high interest since they are at variance with the generally accepted fact that aging is associated with a more relaxed state of chromatin, called euchromatin [196].

One of the major epigenetic hallmarks of aging is the increased acetylation level of the histone tails. Such state is mostly attributed to the decreased level of histone deacetylases, in particular NAD^+-dependent sirtuins [197]. The most disputed histone modification that is associated with aging is the methylation status of lysine terminal ends. Recent data support a trend of increasing tri- and di-methylation of lysine 4 and lysine 36 on the histone variant 3 (H3K4me2/3 and H3K36me3), which are considered to be gene activating marks, during the aging process. Likewise, a trend of decreasing methylation levels of lysine 27 and lysine 9 on the histone variant 3 (H3K27me3, H3K9me2/3), which are known to be gene repressing marks, was reported for the aging process. These observations support a relaxed chromatin state, which is transcriptionally active [196]. Such epigenetic and genetic alterations of the coding nucleic acid molecules might at least partially explain the increased inflammation levels due to the transcriptional gene activation that are associated with the aging process.

The field of non-coding RNAs, especially in the context of aging is currently one of the least discovered. The class of non-coding RNAs consists of microRNA, long non-coding RNAs and piwiRNA. The role of non-coding RNAs in the senescence mechanisms has been much appreciated in the form of biomarkers [198]. The novel microRNA—miR-34a, was documented as an aging marker in several tissues. Boon and colleagues have shown that miR-34a is induced in a cardiac aging model, particularly in cardiac tissue. miR-34a involvement has been also shown in acute myocardial infarction (MI). miR-34a inhibition reduces cell death and fibrosis associated with post MI conditions [199]. Investigations of Boon *et al.* clearly highlighted miR-34a and its target PNUTS as a key molecule regulating heart contractile function during the aging process by inducing DNA damage responses and telomere shortening.

Finally, the aging process is closely linked to immunosenescence and low-grade inflammation contributing to higher prevalence of metabolic syndrome, diabetes and associated cardiovascular complications [200]. Since the risk factors for cardiovascular diseases and diabetes show a clear overlap, especially at the level of inflammation, the latter could represent a key player for aging-associated disorders and increased comorbidity in the elderly [11–13]. Therefore, targeting of the chronic inflammatory phenotype in the elderly could represent a promising strategy to normalize the increased prevalence of comorbidities in the elderly and increase their healthspan [201]. mtROS formation is augmented with increasing age [28] and mtROS can lead to the activation of immune cells and their phagocytic NADPH oxidase, induce the inflammasome and trigger cytokine release [97,115–118,174]. Therefore, targeting mitochondrial oxidative stress in the elderly could represent another strategy to suppress the chronic inflammatory phenotype and adverse effects of the aging process. This was recently shown in an animal model for metformin-dependent AMP-activated protein kinase activation that suppressed oxidative damage and chronic inflammation in old animals and increased their lifespan and healthspan [202].

9. Clinical Impact

The link between endothelial dysfunction, oxidative stress and aging has not only been defined in animal models. Hypertension, dyslipidemia and atherosclerosis are precursors of cardiovascular events, like stroke or myocardial infarction [203,204]. Oxidative stress and reduced ˙NO bioavailability impair vascular protective function of the endothelium [205]. In patients, non-invasive flow-mediated dilation (FMD) of the forearm brachial artery or plethysmography (acetylcholine-dependent vasodilation) are used to determine endothelial function *in vivo* [24] and are a predictor for cardiovascular events [3]. In patients with well-defined risk factors such as dyslipidemia or smoking, a significantly impaired acetylcholine-triggered endothelium-dependent vasodilation was observed and both risk factors are known to be associated with oxidative stress. Endothelial dysfunction of coronary arteries is directly associated with an increased risk of myocardial infarction [206]. Furthermore, Heitzer *et al.* demonstrated that patients who showed improved endothelial function after vitamin C infusion had a worse prognosis for cardiovascular events as compared to patients with low vitamin C effects (Figure 1C) [25]. These findings indicate that oxidative stress is not only a key player in the pathogenesis of endothelial dysfunction *in vivo*, but furthermore also reflects the prognosis of patients with established coronary artery disease. The concept of an increased burden of oxidative stress is broadly accepted, but nevertheless results from clinical trials investigating antioxidant vitamins like B, C, E and folic acid are disappointing (for review see [207]) and for vitamin E even increased mortality and numbers of heart failure were found (HOPE and HOPE-TOO). These findings prove what Harman already postulated in 1975 with his modified "free radical theory of aging" – that site-specific formation of ROS (e.g., in mitochondria) might be the key to understand the obvious discrepancy between association of most cardiovascular disease with oxidative stress but failure of antioxidant therapy so far. The reasons for the failure of large clinical trials on antioxidant therapy to display profound beneficial effects could be, among others, that this secondary prevention is applied to patients with already irreversible tissue/organ damage. In addition, secondary antioxidant prevention does not specifically target the defective defense and repair mechanisms (e.g., it could interfere with important intrinsic protective mechanisms such as ischemic preconditioning). Finally, the concentrations of the antioxidants reached at the sites of ROS formation could be too low (e.g., compliance was not controlled by measurement of plasma levels of the administrated antioxidants) [208]. The controversial and even contradictory results from antioxidant clinical trials or experiments manipulating antioxidants by pharmacological (or genetic approaches) suggest that aging is a complex and multifaceted process that cannot be explained by a single theory.

In humans, the incidence of hypertension, diabetes and atherosclerosis correlates with age (Figure 1A) [26,27]. In parallel, endothelial dysfunction manifests with age (Figure 1B) [24], together with oxidative stress from mitochondria and other enzymatic sources [209,210]. Aging is an independent risk factor for cardiovascular disease, which is mainly caused by endothelial dysfunction due to oxidative stress and low-grade inflammation [24,211]. Recent data provided evidence for changes in high-density lipoprotein composition and function in dependence of age [212]. Therefore, the quality of high density lipoprotein (HDL) may be another future target for therapeutic intervention in and/or diagnosis of age-related cardiovascular disease [213] because HDL quality decreases with age and this will negatively influence the endothelial function. Recently, the nitrovasodilator pentaerithrityl tetranitrate was demonstrated to provide heritable blood pressure lowering effects in hypertensive rats associated with enhanced H3K27ac and H3K4me3 and transcriptional activation of cardioprotective genes such as *eNOS*, *SOD2*, *GPx-1*, and *HO-1* [214]. Drugs like pentaerithrityl tetranitrate could represent the prototype of future epigenetic drugs that could also improve the healthspan in general and cardiovascular aging in particular. Mitochondria-targeted antioxidants could represent another promising therapeutic strategy to combat the "side effects" of the aging process. Mito-quinone improved age-related endothelial dysfunction in mice [215]. Since aging cannot be stopped like smoking [216] and unspecific antioxidant treatment using vitamins is not effective, aging-induced mitochondrial ROS formation may become a target for diagnosis and treatment of cardiovascular disease in the elderly.

10. Perspective

In the present review, we have provided strong evidence from our own and others studies that mitochondrial oxidative stress plays a key determinant for aging-induced impairment of cellular signaling and as a consequence cell death. There is a large body of evidence for the association of cellular aging with mitochondrial dysfunction based on genetic animal models with increased mitochondrial reactive oxygen species (ROS) formation (e.g., $MnSOD^{+/-}$ or $Trx-2$-deficiency). Interestingly, overexpression of catalase, another enzyme crucially involved in the antioxidant defense, enhanced protection of mitochondria from ROS, led to an extended life span in mice [121]. The increase in life span was much more pronounced when catalase was targeted to mitochondria as compared to overexpression in peroxisomes or in the nucleus. There is also evidence for an interaction (crosstalk) between mitochondrial oxidative stress and cytosolic sources of oxidative stress providing a direct link between aging and vascular dysfunction. Therefore, a better understanding of the role of mitochondria in the aging process may lead to specifically designed therapies to interfere with mitochondrial dysfunction and to delay the aging process for longevity. Since regulation of the vascular tone largely depends on a redox-balance in favor of a more reductive milieu, increased oxidative stress impairs vascular function and leads to endothelial dysfunction, atherosclerosis and other cardiovascular complications. Therefore, therapeutic intervention at the level of mitochondrial dysfunction would not only beneficially influence the aging process but also most kinds of cardiovascular diseases. The hyperacetylation state of the histone tails and impaired DNA repair capacity in aged tissues imply a therapeutic modulation of the aging process by epigenetic drugs and improved DNA repair. Since cardiovascular diseases are the main reason for mortality in the Western world and their prevalence increases with age, development of therapeutic interventions not only promises a prolonged healthspan (maybe even increased lifespan) for a large part of the world population but also represents an appreciable pharmaceutical market.

Acknowledgments

The present work was supported by continuous funding by Stufe1 and NMFZ programs of the Johannes Gutenberg-University Mainz and University Medical Center Mainz as well as Mainzer Herz Foundation (Andreas Daiber). Sebastian Steven holds a Virchow-Fellowship from the Center of

Thrombosis and Hemostasis (Mainz, Germany) funded by the Federal Ministry of Education and Research (BMBF 01EO1003). Yuliya Mikhed holds a stipend from the International PhD Program on the "Dynamics of Gene Regulation, Epigenetics and DNA Damage Response" from the Institute of Molecular Biology gGmbH, (Mainz, Germany) funded by the Boehringer Ingelheim Foundation. All authors of this review were supported by the European Cooperation in Science and Technology (COST Action BM1203/EU-ROS).

References

1. Kelly, D.T. Paul dudley white international lecture. Our future society. A global challenge. *Circulation* **1997**, *95*, 2459–2464.

2. Lakatta, E.G.; Levy, D. Arterial and cardiac aging: Major shareholders in cardiovascular disease enterprises: Part I: Aging arteries: A "set up" for vascular disease. *Circulation* **2003**, *107*, 139–146.

3. Ras, R.T.; Streppel, M.T.; Draijer, R.; Zock, P.L. Flow-mediated dilation and cardiovascular risk prediction: A systematic review with meta-analysis. *Int. J. Cardiol.* **2013**, *168*, 344–351.

4. Herrera, M.D.; Mingorance, C.; Rodriguez-Rodriguez, R.; Alvarez de Sotomayor, M. Endothelial dysfunction and aging: An update. *Ageing Res. Rev.* **2010**, *9*, 142–152.

5. Bischoff, B.; Silber, S.; Richartz, B.M.; Pieper, L.; Klotsche, J.; Wittchen, H.U. Inadequate medical treatment of patients with coronary artery disease by primary care physicians in germany. *Clin. Res. Cardiol.* **2006**, *95*, 405–412.

6. Burnett, A.L. The role of nitric oxide in erectile dysfunction: Implications for medical therapy. *J. Clin. Hypertens.* **2006**, *8*, 53–62.

7. Csiszar, A.; Toth, J.; Peti-Peterdi, J.; Ungvari, Z. The aging kidney: Role of endothelial oxidative stress and inflammation. *Acta Physiol. Hung.* **2007**, *94*, 107–115.

8. Price, J.M.; Hellermann, A.; Hellermann, G.; Sutton, E.T. Aging enhances vascular dysfunction induced by the alzheimer's peptide β-amyloid. *Neurol. Res.* **2004**, *26*, 305–311.

9. Coleman, H.R.; Chan, C.C.; Ferris, F.L., III; Chew, E.Y. Age-related macular degeneration. *Lancet* **2008**, *372*, 1835–1845.

10. El Assar, M.; Angulo, J.; Rodriguez-Manas, L. Oxidative stress and vascular inflammation in aging. *Free Radic. Biol. Med.* **2013**, *65*, 380–401.

11. Cesari, M.; Onder, G.; Russo, A.; Zamboni, V.; Barillaro, C.; Ferrucci, L.; Pahor, M.; Bernabei, R.; Landi, F. Comorbidity and physical function: Results from the aging and longevity study in the Sirente geographic area (iLSIRENTE study). *Gerontology* **2006**, *52*, 24–32.

12. Yancik, R.; Ershler, W.; Satariano, W.; Hazzard, W.; Cohen, H.J.; Ferrucci, L. Report of the national institute on aging task force on comorbidity. *J. Gerontol. Ser. A* **2007**, *62*, 275–280.

13. Wieland, G.D. From bedside to bench: Research in comorbidity and aging. *Sci. Aging Knowl. Environ.* **2005**, *2005*, pe29.

14. Munzel, T.; Daiber, A.; Mulsch, A. Explaining the phenomenon of nitrate tolerance. *Circ. Res.* **2005**, *97*, 618–628.

15. Munzel, T.; Daiber, A.; Ullrich, V.; Mulsch, A. Vascular consequences of endothelial nitric oxide synthase uncoupling for the activity and expression of the soluble guanylyl cyclase and the cGMP-dependent protein kinase. *Arterioscler. Thromb. Vasc. Biol.* **2005**, *25*, 1551–1557.

16. Oelze, M.; Kroller-Schon, S.; Steven, S.; Lubos, E.; Doppler, C.; Hausding, M.; Tobias, S.; Brochhausen, C.; Li, H.; Torzewski, M.; *et al.* Glutathione peroxidase-1 deficiency potentiates dysregulatory modifications of endothelial nitric oxide synthase and vascular dysfunction in aging. *Hypertension* **2014**, *63*, 390–396.

17. Van der Loo, B.; Labugger, R.; Skepper, J.N.; Bachschmid, M.; Kilo, J.; Powell, J.M.; Palacios-Callender, M.; Erusalimsky, J.D.; Quaschning, T.; Malinski, T.; *et al.* Enhanced peroxynitrite formation is associated with vascular aging. *J. Exp. Med.* **2000**, *192*, 1731–1744.

18. Forstermann, U.; Sessa, W.C. Nitric oxide synthases: Regulation and function. *Eur. Heart J.* **2012**, *33*, 829–837.

19. Daiber, A.; Oelze, M.; Daub, S.; Steven, S.; Schuff, A.; Kroller-Schon, S.; Hausding, M.; Wenzel, P.; Schulz, E.; Gori, T.; *et al.* Vascular redox signaling, redox switches in endothelial nitric oxide synthase and endothelial dysfunction. In *Systems Biology of Free Radicals and Antioxidants*; Laher, I., Ed.; Springer-Verlag: Berlin, Germany; Heidelberg, Germany, 2014; pp. 1177–1211.

20. Donato, A.J.; Gano, L.B.; Eskurza, I.; Silver, A.E.; Gates, P.E.; Jablonski, K.; Seals, D.R. Vascular endothelial dysfunction with aging: Endothelin-1 and endothelial nitric oxide synthase. *Am. J. Phys. Heart Circ. Physiol.* **2009**, *297*, H425–H432.

21. Donato, A.J.; Magerko, K.A.; Lawson, B.R.; Durrant, J.R.; Lesniewski, L.A.; Seals, D.R. SIRT-1 and vascular endothelial dysfunction with ageing in mice and humans. *J. Physiol.* **2011**, *589*, 4545–4554.

22. Higashi, Y.; Sasaki, S.; Nakagawa, K.; Kimura, M.; Noma, K.; Hara, K.; Jitsuiki, D.; Goto, C.; Oshima, T.; Chayama, K.; *et al.* Tetrahydrobiopterin improves aging-related impairment of endothelium-dependent vasodilation through increase in nitric oxide production. *Atherosclerosis* **2006**, *186*, 390–395.

23. Wenzel, P.; Schuhmacher, S.; Kienhofer, J.; Muller, J.; Hortmann, M.; Oelze, M.; Schulz, E.; Treiber, N.; Kawamoto, T.; Scharffetter-Kochanek, K.; *et al.* Manganese superoxide dismutase and aldehyde dehydrogenase deficiency increase mitochondrial oxidative stress and aggravate age-dependent vascular dysfunction. *Cardiovasc. Res.* **2008**, *80*, 280–289.

24. Gerhard, M.; Roddy, M.A.; Creager, S.J.; Creager, M.A. Aging progressively impairs endothelium-dependent vasodilation in forearm resistance vessels of humans. *Hypertension* **1996**, *27*, 849–853.

25. Heitzer, T.; Schlinzig, T.; Krohn, K.; Meinertz, T.; Munzel, T. Endothelial dysfunction, oxidative stress, and risk of cardiovascular events in patients with coronary artery disease. *Circulation* **2001**, *104*, 2673–2678.

26. Savji, N.; Rockman, C.B.; Skolnick, A.H.; Guo, Y.; Adelman, M.A.; Riles, T.; Berger, J.S. Association between advanced age and vascular disease in different arterial territories: A population database of over 3.6 million subjects. *J. Am. Coll. Cardiol.* **2013**, *61*, 1736–1743.

27. Ong, K.L.; Cheung, B.M.; Man, Y.B.; Lau, C.P.; Lam, K.S. Prevalence, awareness, treatment, and control of hypertension among united states adults 1999–2004. *Hypertension* **2007**, *49*, 69–75.

28. Daiber, A.; Kienhoefer, J.; Zee, R.; Ullrich, V.; van der Loo, B.; Bachschmid, M. The role of mitochondrial reactive oxygen species formation for age-induced vascular dysfunction. In *Aging and Age-Related Disorders*; Bondy, S.C., Maiese, K., Eds.; Humana Press: Clifton, NJ, USA, 2010; pp. 237–257.

29. Cadenas, E.; Davies, K.J. Mitochondrial free radical generation, oxidative stress, and aging. *Free Radic. Biol. Med.* **2000**, *29*, 222–230.

30. Lenaz, G.; Bovina, C.; D'Aurelio, M.; Fato, R.; Formiggini, G.; Genova, M.L.; Giuliano, G.; Pich, M.M.; Paolucci, U.; Castelli, G.P.; *et al.* Role of mitochondria in oxidative stress and aging. *Ann. N. Y. Acad. Sci.* **2002**, *959*, 199–213.

31. Kujoth, G.C.; Hiona, A.; Pugh, T.D.; Someya, S.; Panzer, K.; Wohlgemuth, S.E.; Hofer, T.; Seo, A.Y.; Sullivan, R.; Jobling, W.A.; *et al.* Mitochondrial DNA mutations, oxidative stress, and apoptosis in mammalian aging. *Science* **2005**, *309*, 481–484.

32. Yin, F.; Boveris, A.; Cadenas, E. Mitochondrial energy metabolism and redox signaling in brain aging and neurodegeneration. *Antioxid. Redox Signal.* **2014**, *20*, 353–371.

33. Cheng, Z.J.; Vapaatalo, H.; Mervaala, E. Angiotensin II and vascular inflammation. *Med. Sci. Monit.* **2005**, *11*, RA194–RA205.

34. Lau, D.; Baldus, S. Myeloperoxidase and its contributory role in inflammatory vascular disease. *Pharmacol. Ther.* **2006**, *111*, 16–26.

35. Willerson, J.T.; Golino, P.; Eidt, J.; Campbell, W.B.; Buja, L.M. Specific platelet mediators and unstable coronary artery lesions. Experimental evidence and potential clinical implications. *Circulation* **1989**, *80*, 198–205.

36. Seals, D.R.; Jablonski, K.L.; Donato, A.J. Aging and vascular endothelial function in humans. *Clin. Sci.* **2011**, *120*, 357–375.

37. Tanaka, H.; Dinenno, F.A.; Seals, D.R. Age-related increase in femoral intima-media thickness in healthy humans. *Arterioscler. Thromb. Vasc. Biol.* **2000**, *20*, 2172.

38. Crimi, E.; Ignarro, L.J.; Napoli, C. Microcirculation and oxidative stress. *Free Radic. Res.* **2007**, *41*, 1364–1375.

39. Mayhan, W.G.; Arrick, D.M.; Sharpe, G.M.; Sun, H. Age-related alterations in reactivity of cerebral arterioles: Role of oxidative stress. *Microcirculation* **2008**, *15*, 225–236.

40. Militante, J.; Lombardini, J.B. Age-related retinal degeneration in animal models of aging: Possible involvement of taurine deficiency and oxidative stress. *Neurochem. Res.* **2004**, *29*, 151–160.

41. Fischer, R.; Maier, O. Interrelation of oxidative stress and inflammation in neurodegenerative disease: Role of TNF. *Oxidative Med. Cell. Longev.* **2015**, *2015*, 610813.

42. Blasiak, J.; Petrovski, G.; Vereb, Z.; Facsko, A.; Kaarniranta, K. Oxidative stress, hypoxia, and autophagy in the neovascular processes of age-related macular degeneration. *BioMed. Res. Int.* **2014**, *2014*, 768026.

43. Harman, D. Aging: A theory based on free radical and radiation chemistry. *J. Gerontol.* **1956**, *11*, 298–300.

44. Waters, W.A. Some recent developments in the chemistry of free radicals. *J. Chem. Soc.* **1946**, 409–415.

45. Rogell, B.; Dean, R.; Lemos, B.; Dowling, D.K. Mito-nuclear interactions as drivers of gene movement on and off the X-chromosome. *BMC Genomics* **2014**, *15*, 330.

46. Thomas, D.D.; Ridnour, L.A.; Isenberg, J.S.; Flores-Santana, W.; Switzer, C.H.; Donzelli, S.; Hussain, P.; Vecoli, C.; Paolocci, N.; Ambs, S.; *et al.* The chemical biology of nitric oxide: Implications in cellular signaling. *Free Radic. Biol. Med.* **2008**, *45*, 18–31.

47. Van der Loo, B.; Bachschmid, M.; Skepper, J.N.; Labugger, R.; Schildknecht, S.; Hahn, R.; Mussig, E.; Gygi, D.; Luscher, T.F. Age-associated cellular relocation of Sod 1 as a self-defense is a futile mechanism to prevent vascular aging. *Biochem. Biophys. Res. Commun.* **2006**, *344*, 972–980.

48. De Haan, J.B.; Bladier, C.; Lotfi-Miri, M.; Taylor, J.; Hutchinson, P.; Crack, P.J.; Hertzog, P.; Kola, I. Fibroblasts derived from Gpx1 knockout mice display senescent-like features and are susceptible to H_2O_2-mediated cell death. *Free Radic. Biol. Med.* **2004**, *36*, 53–64.

49. Altschmied, J.; Haendeler, J. Thioredoxin-1 and endothelial cell aging: Role in cardiovascular diseases. *Antioxid. Redox Signal.* **2009**, *11*, 1733–1740.

50. Go, Y.M.; Jones, D.P. Redox control systems in the nucleus: Mechanisms and functions. *Antioxid. Redox Signal.* **2010**, *13*, 489–509.

51. Salmon, A.B.; Richardson, A.; Perez, V.I. Update on the oxidative stress theory of aging: Does oxidative stress play a role in aging or healthy aging? *Free Radic. Biol. Med.* **2010**, *48*, 642–655.

52. Brown, K.A.; Didion, S.P.; Andresen, J.J.; Faraci, F.M. Effect of aging, MnSOD deficiency, and genetic background on endothelial function: Evidence for MnSOD haploinsufficiency. *Arterioscler. Thromb. Vasc. Biol.* **2007**, *27*, 1941–1946.

53. Didion, S.P.; Kinzenbaw, D.A.; Schrader, L.I.; Faraci, F.M. Heterozygous CuZn superoxide dismutase deficiency produces a vascular phenotype with aging. *Hypertension* **2006**, *48*, 1072–1079.

54. Goldstein, S.; Czapski, G.; Lind, J.; Merenyi, G. Tyrosine nitration by simultaneous generation of ˙NO and O˙2 under physiological conditions. How the radicals do the job. *J. Biol. Chem.* **2000**, *275*, 3031–3036.

55. Perez, V.I.; Bokov, A.; van Remmen, H.; Mele, J.; Ran, Q.; Ikeno, Y.; Richardson, A. Is the oxidative stress theory of aging dead? *Biochim. Biophys. Acta* **2009**, *1790*, 1005–1014.

56. Muller, F.L.; Lustgarten, M.S.; Jang, Y.; Richardson, A.; van Remmen, H. Trends in oxidative aging theories. *Free Radic. Biol. Med.* **2007**, *43*, 477–503.

57. Lebovitz, R.M.; Zhang, H.; Vogel, H.; Cartwright, J., Jr.; Dionne, L.; Lu, N.; Huang, S.; Matzuk, M.M. Neurodegeneration, myocardial injury, and perinatal death in mitochondrial superoxide dismutase-deficient mice. *Proc. Natl. Acad. Sci. USA* **1996**, *93*, 9782–9787.

58. Li, Y.; Huang, T.T.; Carlson, E.J.; Melov, S.; Ursell, P.C.; Olson, J.L.; Noble, L.J.; Yoshimura, M.P.; Berger, C.; Chan, P.H.; *et al.* Dilated cardiomyopathy and neonatal lethality in mutant mice lacking manganese superoxide dismutase. *Nat. Genet.* **1995**, *11*, 376–381.

59. Jang, Y.C.; Remmen, H.V. The mitochondrial theory of aging: Insight from transgenic and knockout mouse models. *Exp. Gerontol.* **2009**, *44*, 256–260.

60. Dai, D.F.; Chiao, Y.A.; Marcinek, D.J.; Szeto, H.H.; Rabinovitch, P.S. Mitochondrial oxidative stress in aging and healthspan. *Longev. Healthspan* **2014**, *3*, 6.

61. Hamilton, R.T.; Walsh, M.E.; van Remmen, H. Mouse models of oxidative stress indicate a role for modulating healthy aging. *J. Clin. Exp. Pathol.* **2012**, doi:10.4172/2161-0681.S4-005.

62. Berry, A.; Cirulli, F. The *p66Shc* gene paves the way for healthspan: Evolutionary and mechanistic perspectives. *Neurosci. Biobehav. Rev.* **2013**, *37*, 790–802.

63. Wanagat, J.; Dai, D.F.; Rabinovitch, P. Mitochondrial oxidative stress and mammalian healthspan. *Mech. Ageing Dev.* **2010**, *131*, 527–535.

64. Sies, H. Oxidative stress: A concept in redox biology and medicine. *Redox Biol.* **2015**, *4*, 180–183.

65. Beckman, J.S.; Koppenol, W.H. Nitric oxide, superoxide, and peroxynitrite: The good, the bad, and ugly. *Am. J. Physiol.* **1996**, *271*, C1424–C1437.

66. Daiber, A.; Bachschmid, M. Enzyme inhibition by peroxynitrite-mediated tyrosine nitration and thiol oxidation. *Curr. Enzym. Inhib.* **2007**, *3*, 103–117.

67. Beckman, J.S. Protein tyrosine nitration and peroxynitrite. *FASEB J.* **2002**, *16*, 1144.

68. Quijano, C.; Alvarez, B.; Gatti, R.M.; Augusto, O.; Radi, R. Pathways of peroxynitrite oxidation of thiol groups. *Biochem. J.* **1997**, *322*, 167–173.

69. MacMillan-Crow, L.A.; Crow, J.P.; Kerby, J.D.; Beckman, J.S.; Thompson, J.A. Nitration and inactivation of manganese superoxide dismutase in chronic rejection of human renal allografts. *Proc. Natl. Acad. Sci. USA* **1996**, *93*, 11853–11858.

70. Kuzkaya, N.; Weissmann, N.; Harrison, D.G.; Dikalov, S. Interactions of peroxynitrite, tetrahydrobiopterin, ascorbic acid, and thiols: Implications for uncoupling endothelial nitric-oxide synthase. *J. Biol. Chem.* **2003**, *278*, 22546–22554.

71. Schulz, E.; Jansen, T.; Wenzel, P.; Daiber, A.; Munzel, T. Nitric oxide, tetrahydrobiopterin, oxidative stress, and endothelial dysfunction in hypertension. *Antioxid. Redox Signal.* **2008**, *10*, 1115–1126.

72. Yoshida, Y.I.; Eda, S.; Masada, M. Alterations of tetrahydrobiopterin biosynthesis and pteridine levels in mouse tissues during growth and aging. *Brain Dev.* **2000**, *22*, S45–S49.

73. Blackwell, K.A.; Sorenson, J.P.; Richardson, D.M.; Smith, L.A.; Suda, O.; Nath, K.; Katusic, Z.S. Mechanisms of aging-induced impairment of endothelium-dependent relaxation: Role of tetrahydrobiopterin. *Am. J. Physiol. Heart Circ. Physiol.* **2004**, *287*, H2448–H2453.

74. Chen, C.A.; Wang, T.Y.; Varadharaj, S.; Reyes, L.A.; Hemann, C.; Talukder, M.A.; Chen, Y.R.; Druhan, L.J.; Zweier, J.L. S-glutathionylation uncouples eNOS and regulates its cellular and vascular function. *Nature* **2010**, *468*, 1115–1118.

75. Schulz, E.; Wenzel, P.; Munzel, T.; Daiber, A. Mitochondrial redox signaling: Interaction of mitochondrial reactive oxygen species with other sources of oxidative stress. *Antioxid. Redox Signal.* **2014**, *20*, 308–324.

76. Zou, M.H.; Shi, C.; Cohen, R.A. Oxidation of the zinc-thiolate complex and uncoupling of endothelial nitric oxide synthase by peroxynitrite. *J. Clin. Investig.* **2002**, *109*, 817–826.

77. Forstermann, U.; Munzel, T. Endothelial nitric oxide synthase in vascular disease: From marvel to menace. *Circulation* **2006**, *113*, 1708–1714.

78. Soucy, K.G.; Ryoo, S.; Benjo, A.; Lim, H.K.; Gupta, G.; Sohi, J.S.; Elser, J.; Aon, M.A.; Nyhan, D.; Shoukas, A.A.; *et al.* Impaired shear stress-induced nitric oxide production through decreased NOS phosphorylation contributes to age-related vascular stiffness. *J. Appl. Physiol.* **2006**, *101*, 1751–1759.

79. Cave, A.C.; Brewer, A.C.; Narayanapanicker, A.; Ray, R.; Grieve, D.J.; Walker, S.; Shah, A.M. Nadph oxidases in cardiovascular health and disease. *Antioxid. Redox signal.* **2006**, *8*, 691–728.

80. Griendling, K.K.; Sorescu, D.; Ushio-Fukai, M. NAD(P)H oxidase: Role in cardiovascular biology and disease. *Circ. Res.* **2000**, *86*, 494–501.

81. Paneni, F.; Osto, E.; Costantino, S.; Mateescu, B.; Briand, S.; Coppolino, G.; Perna, E.; Mocharla, P.; Akhmedov, A.; Kubant, R.; *et al.* Deletion of the activated protein-1 transcription factor JunD induces oxidative stress and accelerates age-related endothelial dysfunction. *Circulation* **2013**, *127*, 1229–1240.

82. Roubenoff, R.; Harris, T.B.; Abad, L.W.; Wilson, P.W.; Dallal, G.E.; Dinarello, C.A. Monocyte cytokine production in an elderly population: Effect of age and inflammation. *J. Gerontol. Ser. A* **1998**, *53*, M20–M26.

83. Moe, K.T.; Aulia, S.; Jiang, F.; Chua, Y.L.; Koh, T.H.; Wong, M.C.; Dusting, G.J. Differential upregulation of Nox homologues of NADPH oxidase by tumor necrosis factor-α in human aortic smooth muscle and embryonic kidney cells. *J. Cell. Mol. Med.* **2006**, *10*, 231–239.

84. Karbach, S.; Wenzel, P.; Waisman, A.; Munzel, T.; Daiber, A. eNOS uncoupling in cardiovascular diseases—The role of oxidative stress and inflammation. *Curr. Pharm. Des.* **2014**, *20*, 3579–3594.

85. Nandi, J.; Saud, B.; Zinkievich, J.M.; Yang, Z.J.; Levine, R.A. TNF-α modulates INOS expression in an experimental rat model of indomethacin-induced jejunoileitis. *Mol. Cell. Biochem.* **2010**, *336*, 17–24.

86. Ungvari, Z.; Csiszar, A.; Edwards, J.G.; Kaminski, P.M.; Wolin, M.S.; Kaley, G.; Koller, A. Increased superoxide production in coronary arteries in hyperhomocysteinemia: Role of tumor necrosis factor-α, NAD(P)H oxidase, and inducible nitric oxide synthase. *Arterioscler. Thromb. Vasc. Biol.* **2003**, *23*, 418–424.

87. Busik, J.V.; Mohr, S.; Grant, M.B. Hyperglycemia-induced reactive oxygen species toxicity to endothelial cells is dependent on paracrine mediators. *Diabetes* **2008**, *57*, 1952–1965.

88. Csiszar, A.; Labinskyy, N.; Smith, K.; Rivera, A.; Orosz, Z.; Ungvari, Z. Vasculoprotective effects of anti-tumor necrosis factor-α treatment in aging. *Am. J. Pathol.* **2007**, *170*, 388–398.

89. Ferrucci, L.; Corsi, A.; Lauretani, F.; Bandinelli, S.; Bartali, B.; Taub, D.D.; Guralnik, J.M.; Longo, D.L. The origins of age-related proinflammatory state. *Blood* **2005**, *105*, 2294–2299.

90. Wenzel, P.; Knorr, M.; Kossmann, S.; Stratmann, J.; Hausding, M.; Schuhmacher, S.; Karbach, S.H.; Schwenk, M.; Yogev, N.; Schulz, E.; *et al.* Lysozyme M-positive monocytes mediate angiotensin II-induced arterial hypertension and vascular dysfunction. *Circulation* **2011**, *124*, 1370–1381.

91. Guzik, T.J.; Hoch, N.E.; Brown, K.A.; McCann, L.A.; Rahman, A.; Dikalov, S.; Goronzy, J.; Weyand, C.; Harrison, D.G. Role of the T cell in the genesis of angiotensin II induced hypertension and vascular dysfunction. *J. Exp. Med.* **2007**, *204*, 2449–2460.

92. Harman, D. The biologic clock: The mitochondria? *J. Am. Geriatr. Soc.* **1972**, *20*, 145–147.

93. Lewis, P.; Stefanovic, N.; Pete, J.; Calkin, A.C.; Giunti, S.; Thallas-Bonke, V.; Jandeleit-Dahm, K.A.; Allen, T.J.; Kola, I.; Cooper, M.E.; *et al.* Lack of the antioxidant enzyme glutathione peroxidase-1 accelerates atherosclerosis in diabetic apolipoprotein e-deficient mice. *Circulation* **2007**, *115*, 2178–2187.

94. Forgione, M.A.; Cap, A.; Liao, R.; Moldovan, N.I.; Eberhardt, R.T.; Lim, C.C.; Jones, J.; Goldschmidt-Clermont, P.J.; Loscalzo, J. Heterozygous cellular glutathione peroxidase deficiency in the mouse: Abnormalities in vascular and cardiac function and structure. *Circulation* **2002**, *106*, 1154–1158.

95. Chrissobolis, S.; Didion, S.P.; Kinzenbaw, D.A.; Schrader, L.I.; Dayal, S.; Lentz, S.R.; Faraci, F.M. Glutathione peroxidase-1 plays a major role in protecting against angiotensin II-induced vascular dysfunction. *Hypertension* **2008**, *51*, 872–877.

96. Blankenberg, S.; Rupprecht, H.J.; Bickel, C.; Torzewski, M.; Hafner, G.; Tiret, L.; Smieja, M.; Cambien, F.; Meyer, J.; Lackner, K.J. Glutathione peroxidase 1 activity and cardiovascular events in patients with coronary artery disease. *N. Engl. J. Med.* **2003**, *349*, 1605–1613.

97. Kroller-Schon, S.; Steven, S.; Kossmann, S.; Scholz, A.; Daub, S.; Oelze, M.; Xia, N.; Hausding, M.; Mikhed, Y.; Zinssius, E.; *et al.* Molecular mechanisms of the crosstalk between mitochondria and NADPH oxidase through reactive oxygen species-studies in white blood cells and in animal models. *Antioxid. Redox Signal.* **2014**, *20*, 247–266.

98. Hausding, M.; Jurk, K.; Daub, S.; Kroller-Schon, S.; Stein, J.; Schwenk, M.; Oelze, M.; Mikhed, Y.; Kerahrodi, J.G.; Kossmann, S.; *et al.* CD40L contributes to angiotensin II-induced pro-thrombotic state, vascular inflammation, oxidative stress and endothelial dysfunction. *Basic Res. Cardiol.* **2013**, *108*, 386.

99. Fleming, I.; Fisslthaler, B.; Dimmeler, S.; Kemp, B.E.; Busse, R. Phosphorylation of Thr[495] regulates Ca^{2+}/calmodulin-dependent endothelial nitric oxide synthase activity. *Circ. Res.* **2001**, *88*, E68–E75.

100. Lin, M.I.; Fulton, D.; Babbitt, R.; Fleming, I.; Busse, R.; Pritchard, K.A., Jr.; Sessa, W.C. Phosphorylation of threonine 497 in endothelial nitric-oxide synthase coordinates the coupling of L-arginine metabolism to efficient nitric oxide production. *J. Biol. Chem.* **2003**, *278*, 44719–44726.

101. Loot, A.E.; Schreiber, J.G.; Fisslthaler, B.; Fleming, I. Angiotensin ii impairs endothelial function via tyrosine phosphorylation of the endothelial nitric oxide synthase. *J. Exp. Med.* **2009**, *206*, 2889–2896.

102. Brune, B.; Schmidt, K.U.; Ullrich, V. Activation of soluble guanylate cyclase by carbon monoxide and inhibition by superoxide anion. *Eur. J. Biochem.* **1990**, *192*, 683–688.

103. Weber, M.; Lauer, N.; Mulsch, A.; Kojda, G. The effect of peroxynitrite on the catalytic activity of soluble guanylyl cyclase. *Free Radic. Biol. Med.* **2001**, *31*, 1360–1367.

104. Artz, J.D.; Schmidt, B.; McCracken, J.L.; Marletta, M.A. Effects of nitroglycerin on soluble guanylate cyclase: Implications for nitrate tolerance. *J. Biol. Chem.* **2002**, *277*, 18253–18256.

105. Crassous, P.A.; Couloubaly, S.; Huang, C.; Zhou, Z.; Baskaran, P.; Kim, D.D.; Papapetropoulos, A.; Fioramonti, X.; Duran, W.N.; Beuve, A. Soluble guanylyl cyclase is a target of angiotensin II-induced nitrosative stress in a hypertensive rat model. *Am. J. Physiol. Heart Circ. Physiol.* **2012**, *303*, H597–H604.

106. Mayer, B.; Kleschyov, A.L.; Stessel, H.; Russwurm, M.; Munzel, T.; Koesling, D.; Schmidt, K. Inactivation of soluble guanylate cyclase by stoichiometric *S*-nitrosation. *Mol. Pharmacol.* **2009**, *75*, 886–891.

107. Sayed, N.; Kim, D.D.; Fioramonti, X.; Iwahashi, T.; Duran, W.N.; Beuve, A. Nitroglycerin-induced *S*-nitrosylation and desensitization of soluble guanylyl cyclase contribute to nitrate tolerance. *Circ. Res.* **2008**, *103*, 606–614.

108. Stasch, J.P.; Schmidt, P.M.; Nedvetsky, P.I.; Nedvetskaya, T.Y.; H S, A.K.; Meurer, S.; Deile, M.; Taye, A.; Knorr, A.; Lapp, H.; *et al.* Targeting the heme-oxidized nitric oxide receptor for selective vasodilatation of diseased blood vessels. *J. Clin. Investig.* **2006**, *116*, 2552–2561.

109. Chen, L.; Daum, G.; Fischer, J.W.; Hawkins, S.; Bochaton-Piallat, M.L.; Gabbiani, G.; Clowes, A.W. Loss of expression of the β subunit of soluble guanylyl cyclase prevents nitric oxide-mediated inhibition of DNA synthesis in smooth muscle cells of old rats. *Circ. Res.* **2000**, *86*, 520–525.

110. Ruetten, H.; Zabel, U.; Linz, W.; Schmidt, H.H. Downregulation of soluble guanylyl cyclase in young and aging spontaneously hypertensive rats. *Circ. Res.* **1999**, *85*, 534–541.

111. Kloss, S.; Bouloumie, A.; Mulsch, A. Aging and chronic hypertension decrease expression of rat aortic soluble guanylyl cyclase. *Hypertension* **2000**, *35*, 43–47.

112. Lubos, E.; Mahoney, C.E.; Leopold, J.A.; Zhang, Y.Y.; Loscalzo, J.; Handy, D.E. Glutathione peroxidase-1 modulates lipopolysaccharide-induced adhesion molecule expression in endothelial cells by altering CD14 expression. *FASEB J.* **2010**, *24*, 2525–2532.

113. Kessler, P.; Bauersachs, J.; Busse, R.; Schini-Kerth, V.B. Inhibition of inducible nitric oxide synthase restores endothelium-dependent relaxations in proinflammatory mediator-induced blood vessels. *Arterioscler. Thromb. Vasc. Biol.* **1997**, *17*, 1746–1755.

114. Prabhu, K.S.; Zamamiri-Davis, F.; Stewart, J.B.; Thompson, J.T.; Sordillo, L.M.; Reddy, C.C. Selenium deficiency increases the expression of inducible nitric oxide synthase in RAW 264.7 macrophages: Role of nuclear factor-κB in up-regulation. *Biochem. J.* **2002**, *366*, 203–209.

115. Bulua, A.C.; Simon, A.; Maddipati, R.; Pelletier, M.; Park, H.; Kim, K.Y.; Sack, M.N.; Kastner, D.L.; Siegel, R.M. Mitochondrial reactive oxygen species promote production of proinflammatory cytokines and are elevated in TNFR1-associated periodic syndrome (TRAPS). *J. Exp. Med.* **2011**, *208*, 519–533.

116. West, A.P.; Brodsky, I.E.; Rahner, C.; Woo, D.K.; Erdjument-Bromage, H.; Tempst, P.; Walsh, M.C.; Choi, Y.; Shadel, G.S.; Ghosh, S. TLR signalling augments macrophage bactericidal activity through mitochondrial ROS. *Nature* **2011**, *472*, 476–480.

117. Zhou, R.; Yazdi, A.S.; Menu, P.; Tschopp, J. A role for mitochondria in NLRP3 inflammasome activation. *Nature* **2011**, *469*, 221–225.

118. Zhou, R.; Tardivel, A.; Thorens, B.; Choi, I.; Tschopp, J. Thioredoxin-interacting protein links oxidative stress to inflammasome activation. *Nat. Immunol.* **2010**, *11*, 136–140.

119. Smith, A.R.; Visioli, F.; Frei, B.; Hagen, T.M. Age-related changes in endothelial nitric oxide synthase phosphorylation and nitric oxide dependent vasodilation: Evidence for a novel mechanism involving sphingomyelinase and ceramide-activated phosphatase 2A. *Aging Cell* **2006**, *5*, 391–400.

120. Crabtree, M.J.; Brixey, R.; Batchelor, H.; Hale, A.B.; Channon, K.M. Integrated redox sensor and effector functions for tetrahydrobiopterin- and glutathionylation-dependent endothelial nitric-oxide synthase uncoupling. *J. Biol. Chem.* **2013**, *288*, 561–569.

121. Schriner, S.E.; Linford, N.J.; Martin, G.M.; Treuting, P.; Ogburn, C.E.; Emond, M.; Coskun, P.E.; Ladiges, W.; Wolf, N.; van Remmen, H.; *et al.* Extension of murine life span by overexpression of catalase targeted to mitochondria. *Science* **2005**, *308*, 1909–1911.

122. Barja, G.; Herrero, A. Oxidative damage to mitochondrial DNA is inversely related to maximum life span in the heart and brain of mammals. *FASEB J.* **2000**, *14*, 312–318.

123. Sastre, J.; Pallardo, F.V.; Vina, J. The role of mitochondrial oxidative stress in aging. *Free Radic. Biol. Med.* **2003**, *35*, 1–8.

124. Madamanchi, N.R.; Runge, M.S. Mitochondrial dysfunction in atherosclerosis. *Circ. Res.* **2007**, *100*, 460–473.

125. De Souza-Pinto, N.C.; Eide, L.; Hogue, B.A.; Thybo, T.; Stevnsner, T.; Seeberg, E.; Klungland, A.; Bohr, V.A. Repair of 8-oxodeoxyguanosine lesions in mitochondrial DNA depends on the oxoguanine DNA glycosylase (OGG1) gene and 8-oxoguanine accumulates in the mitochondrial dna of OGG1-defective mice. *Cancer Res.* **2001**, *61*, 5378–5381.

126. De Souza-Pinto, N.C.; Hogue, B.A.; Bohr, V.A. DNA repair and aging in mouse liver: 8-oxodG glycosylase activity increase in mitochondrial but not in nuclear extracts. *Free Radic. Biol. Med.* **2001**, *30*, 916–923.

127. Souza-Pinto, N.C.; Croteau, D.L.; Hudson, E.K.; Hansford, R.G.; Bohr, V.A. Age-associated increase in 8-oxo-deoxyguanosine glycosylase/ap lyase activity in rat mitochondria. *Nucleic Acids Res.* **1999**, *27*, 1935–1942.

128. Trifunovic, A.; Wredenberg, A.; Falkenberg, M.; Spelbrink, J.N.; Rovio, A.T.; Bruder, C.E.; Bohlooly, Y.M.; Gidlof, S.; Oldfors, A.; Wibom, R.; *et al.* Premature ageing in mice expressing defective mitochondrial DNA polymerase. *Nature* **2004**, *429*, 417–423.

129. Lewis, W.; Day, B.J.; Kohler, J.J.; Hosseini, S.H.; Chan, S.S.; Green, E.C.; Haase, C.P.; Keebaugh, E.S.; Long, R.; Ludaway, T.; *et al.* Decreased mtDNA, oxidative stress, cardiomyopathy, and death from transgenic cardiac targeted human mutant polymerase γ. *Lab. Investig.* **2007**, *87*, 326–335.

130. Finsterer, J. Overview on visceral manifestations of mitochondrial disorders. *Neth. J. Med.* **2006**, *64*, 61–71.

131. Anan, R.; Nakagawa, M.; Miyata, M.; Higuchi, I.; Nakao, S.; Suehara, M.; Osame, M.; Tanaka, H. Cardiac involvement in mitochondrial diseases. A study on 17 patients with documented mitochondrial DNA defects. *Circulation* **1995**, *91*, 955–961.

132. Pinsky, D.J.; Oz, M.C.; Koga, S.; Taha, Z.; Broekman, M.J.; Marcus, A.J.; Liao, H.; Naka, Y.; Brett, J.; Cannon, P.J.; *et al.* Cardiac preservation is enhanced in a heterotopic rat transplant model by supplementing the nitric oxide pathway. *J. Clin. Investig.* **1994**, *93*, 2291–2297.

133. Zeviani, M.; di Donato, S. Mitochondrial disorders. *Brain* **2004**, *127*, 2153–2172.

134. Ballinger, S.W.; Patterson, C.; Knight-Lozano, C.A.; Burow, D.L.; Conklin, C.A.; Hu, Z.; Reuf, J.; Horaist, C.; Lebovitz, R.; Hunter, G.C.; *et al.* Mitochondrial integrity and function in atherogenesis. *Circulation* **2002**, *106*, 544–549.

135. Sevini, F.; Giuliani, C.; Vianello, D.; Giampieri, E.; Santoro, A.; Biondi, F.; Garagnani, P.; Passarino, G.; Luiselli, D.; Capri, M.; *et al.* mtDNA mutations in human aging and longevity: Controversies and new perspectives opened by high-throughput technologies. *Exp.Gerontol.* **2014**, *56*, 234–244.

136. Itsara, L.S.; Kennedy, S.R.; Fox, E.J.; Yu, S.; Hewitt, J.J.; Sanchez-Contreras, M.; Cardozo-Pelaez, F.; Pallanck, L.J. Oxidative stress is not a major contributor to somatic mitochondrial DNA mutations. *PLoS Genet.* **2014**, *10*, e1003974.

137. Larsson, N.G. Somatic mitochondrial DNA mutations in mammalian aging. *Annu. Rev. Biochem.* **2010**, *79*, 683–706.

138. De Bont, R.; van Larebeke, N., Endogenous DNA damage in humans: A review of quantitative data. *Mutagenesis* **2004**, *19*, 169–185.

139. Kennedy, S.R.; Salk, J.J.; Schmitt, M.W.; Loeb, L.A. Ultra-sensitive sequencing reveals an age-related increase in somatic mitochondrial mutations that are inconsistent with oxidative damage. *PLoS Genet.* **2013**, *9*, e1003794.

140. Cha, M.Y.; Kim, D.K.; Mook-Jung, I. The role of mitochondrial DNA mutation on neurodegenerative diseases. *Exp. Mol. Med.* **2015**, *47*, e150.

141. Reddy, P.H. Amyloid β, mitochondrial structural and functional dynamics in alzheimer's disease. *Exp. Neurol.* **2009**, *218*, 286–292.

142. Canugovi, C.; Shamanna, R.A.; Croteau, D.L.; Bohr, V.A. Base excision DNA repair levels in mitochondrial lysates of alzheimer's disease. *Neurobiol. Aging* **2014**, *35*, 1293–1300.

143. Krishnan, K.J.; Ratnaike, T.E.; de Gruyter, H.L.; Jaros, E.; Turnbull, D.M. Mitochondrial DNA deletions cause the biochemical defect observed in alzheimer's disease. *Neurobiol. Aging* **2012**, *33*, 2210–2214.

144. Muftuoglu, M.; Mori, M.P.; de Souza-Pinto, N.C. Formation and repair of oxidative damage in the mitochondrial DNA. *Mitochondrion* **2014**, *17*, 164–181.

145. Liu, P.; Demple, B. DNA repair in mammalian mitochondria: Much more than we thought? *Environ. Mol. Mutagen.* **2010**, *51*, 417–426.

146. Bogenhagen, D.F. Repair of mtDNA in vertebrates. *Am. J. Hum. Genet.* **1999**, *64*, 1276–1281.

147. Nishioka, K.; Ohtsubo, T.; Oda, H.; Fujiwara, T.; Kang, D.; Sugimachi, K.; Nakabeppu, Y. Expression and differential intracellular localization of two major forms of human 8-oxoguanine DNA glycosylase encoded by alternatively spliced OGG1 mRNAs. *Mol. Biol. Cell* **1999**, *10*, 1637–1652.

148. Nilsen, H.; Otterlei, M.; Haug, T.; Solum, K.; Nagelhus, T.A.; Skorpen, F.; Krokan, H.E. Nuclear and mitochondrial uracil-DNA glycosylases are generated by alternative splicing and transcription from different positions in the UNG gene. *Nucleic Acids Res.* **1997**, *25*, 750–755.

149. Ikeda, S.; Kohmoto, T.; Tabata, R.; Seki, Y. Differential intracellular localization of the human and mouse endonuclease III homologs and analysis of the sorting signals. *DNA Repair* **2002**, *1*, 847–854.

150. Hu, J.; de Souza-Pinto, N.C.; Haraguchi, K.; Hogue, B.A.; Jaruga, P.; Greenberg, M.M.; Dizdaroglu, M.; Bohr, V.A. Repair of formamidopyrimidines in DNA involves different glycosylases: Role of the OGG1, NTH1, and NEIL1 enzymes. *J. Biol. Chem.* **2005**, *280*, 40544–40551.

151. Ohtsubo, T.; Nishioka, K.; Imaiso, Y.; Iwai, S.; Shimokawa, H.; Oda, H.; Fujiwara, T.; Nakabeppu, Y. Identification of human muty homolog (hMYH) as a repair enzyme for 2-hydroxyadenine in DNA and detection of multiple forms of hMYH located in nuclei and mitochondria. *Nucleic Acids Res.* **2000**, *28*, 1355–1364.

152. Park, J.S.; Kim, H.L.; Kim, Y.J.; Weon, J.I.; Sung, M.K.; Chung, H.W.; Seo, Y.R. Human AP endonuclease 1: A potential marker for the prediction of environmental carcinogenesis risk. *Oxidative Med. Cell. Longev.* **2014**, *2014*, 730301.

153. Mason, P.A.; Matheson, E.C.; Hall, A.G.; Lightowlers, R.N. Mismatch repair activity in mammalian mitochondria. *Nucleic Acids Res.* **2003**, *31*, 1052–1058.

154. De Souza-Pinto, N.C.; Mason, P.A.; Hashiguchi, K.; Weissman, L.; Tian, J.; Guay, D.; Lebel, M.; Stevnsner, T.V.; Rasmussen, L.J.; Bohr, V.A. Novel DNA mismatch-repair activity involving YB-1 in human mitochondria. *DNA Repair* **2009**, *8*, 704–719.

155. Pohjoismaki, J.L.; Goffart, S.; Tyynismaa, H.; Willcox, S.; Ide, T.; Kang, D.; Suomalainen, A.; Karhunen, P.J.; Griffith, J.D.; Holt, I.J.; *et al.* Human heart mitochondrial DNA is organized in complex catenated networks containing abundant four-way junctions and replication forks. *J. Biol. Chem.* **2009**, *284*, 21446–21457.

156. Chen, X.J. Mechanism of homologous recombination and implications for aging-related deletions in mitochondrial DNA. *Microbiol. Mol. Biol. Rev.* **2013**, *77*, 476–496.

157. Chen, X.J.; Guan, M.X.; Clark-Walker, G.D. MGM101, a nuclear gene involved in maintenance of the mitochondrial genome in saccharomyces cerevisiae. *Nucleic Acids Res.* **1993**, *21*, 3473–3477.

158. Gredilla, R.; Garm, C.; Stevnsner, T. Nuclear and mitochondrial DNA repair in selected eukaryotic aging model systems. *Oxidative Med. Cell. Longev.* **2012**, *2012*, 282438.

159. Bender, A.; Krishnan, K.J.; Morris, C.M.; Taylor, G.A.; Reeve, A.K.; Perry, R.H.; Jaros, E.; Hersheson, J.S.; Betts, J.; Klopstock, T.; *et al.* High levels of mitochondrial DNA deletions in substantia nigra neurons in aging and Parkinson disease. *Nat. Genet.* **2006**, *38*, 515–517.

160. Chen, D.; Cao, G.; Hastings, T.; Feng, Y.; Pei, W.; O'Horo, C.; Chen, J. Age-dependent decline of DNA repair activity for oxidative lesions in rat brain mitochondria. *J. Neurochem.* **2002**, *81*, 1273–1284.

161. Daiber, A.; Oelze, M.; Wenzel, P.; Wickramanayake, J.M.; Schuhmacher, S.; Jansen, T.; Lackner, K.J.; Torzewski, M.; Munzel, T. Nitrate tolerance as a model of vascular dysfunction: Roles for mitochondrial aldehyde dehydrogenase and mitochondrial oxidative stress. *Pharmacol. Rep.* **2009**, *61*, 33–48.

162. Daiber, A.; Oelze, M.; Coldewey, M.; Bachschmid, M.; Wenzel, P.; Sydow, K.; Wendt, M.; Kleschyov, A.L.; Stalleicken, D.; Ullrich, V.; *et al.* Oxidative stress and mitochondrial aldehyde dehydrogenase activity: A comparison of pentaerythritol tetranitrate with other organic nitrates. *Mol. Pharmacol.* **2004**, *66*, 1372–1382.

163. Sydow, K.; Daiber, A.; Oelze, M.; Chen, Z.; August, M.; Wendt, M.; Ullrich, V.; Mulsch, A.; Schulz, E.; Keaney, J.F., Jr.; *et al.* Central role of mitochondrial aldehyde dehydrogenase and reactive oxygen species in nitroglycerin tolerance and cross-tolerance. *J. Clin. Investig.* **2004**, *113*, 482–489.

164. Esplugues, J.V.; Rocha, M.; Nunez, C.; Bosca, I.; Ibiza, S.; Herance, J.R.; Ortega, A.; Serrador, J.M.; D'Ocon, P.; Victor, V.M. Complex I dysfunction and tolerance to nitroglycerin: An approach based on mitochondrial-targeted antioxidants. *Circ. Res.* **2006**, *99*, 1067–1075.

165. Wenzel, P.; Mollnau, H.; Oelze, M.; Schulz, E.; Wickramanayake, J.M.; Muller, J.; Schuhmacher, S.; Hortmann, M.; Baldus, S.; Gori, T.; *et al.* First evidence for a crosstalk between mitochondrial and nadph oxidase-derived reactive oxygen species in nitroglycerin-triggered vascular dysfunction. *Antioxid. Redox Signal.* **2008**, *10*, 1435–1447.

166. Dikalov, S.I.; Nazarewicz, R.R.; Bikineyeva, A.; Hilenski, L.; Lassegue, B.; Griendling, K.K.; Harrison, D.G.; Dikalova, A.E. Nox2-induced production of mitochondrial superoxide in angiotensin II-mediated endothelial oxidative stress and hypertension. *Antioxid. Redox Signal.* **2014**, *20*, 281–294.

167. Doughan, A.K.; Harrison, D.G.; Dikalov, S.I. Molecular mechanisms of angiotensin II-mediated mitochondrial dysfunction: Linking mitochondrial oxidative damage and vascular endothelial dysfunction. *Circ. Res.* **2008**, *102*, 488–496.

168. Nazarewicz, R.R.; Dikalova, A.E.; Bikineyeva, A.; Dikalov, S.I. Nox2 as a potential target of mitochondrial superoxide and its role in endothelial oxidative stress. *Am. J. Physiol. Heart Circ. Physiol.* **2013**, *305*, H1131–H1140.

169. Brandes, R.P. Triggering mitochondrial radical release: A new function for NADPH oxidases. *Hypertension* **2005**, *45*, 847–848.

170. Kimura, S.; Zhang, G.X.; Nishiyama, A.; Shokoji, T.; Yao, L.; Fan, Y.Y.; Rahman, M.; Abe, Y. Mitochondria-derived reactive oxygen species and vascular MAP kinases: Comparison of angiotensin II and diazoxide. *Hypertension* **2005**, *45*, 438–444.

171. Dikalova, A.E.; Bikineyeva, A.T.; Budzyn, K.; Nazarewicz, R.R.; McCann, L.; Lewis, W.; Harrison, D.G.; Dikalov, S.I. Therapeutic targeting of mitochondrial superoxide in hypertension. *Circ. Res.* **2010**, *107*, 106–116.

172. Fukui, T.; Ishizaka, N.; Rajagopalan, S.; Laursen, J.B.; Capers, Q.T.; Taylor, W.R.; Harrison, D.G.; de Leon, H.; Wilcox, J.N.; Griendling, K.K. p22phox mRNA expression and NADPH oxidase activity are increased in aortas from hypertensive rats. *Circ. Res.* **1997**, *80*, 45–51.

173. Cheresh, P.; Kim, S.J.; Tulasiram, S.; Kamp, D.W. Oxidative stress and pulmonary fibrosis. *Biochim. Biophys. Acta* **2013**, *1832*, 1028-1040.

174. Nazarewicz, R.R.; Dikalov, S.I. Mitochondrial ROS in the prohypertensive immune response. *Am. J. Physiol. Regul. Integr. Comp. Physiol.* **2013**, *305*, R98–R100.

175. Bender, A.; Hajieva, P.; Moosmann, B. Adaptive antioxidant methionine accumulation in respiratory chain complexes explains the use of a deviant genetic code in mitochondria. *Proc. Natl. Acad. Sci. USA* **2008**, *105*, 16496–16501.

176. Moskovitz, J.; Bar-Noy, S.; Williams, W.M.; Requena, J.; Berlett, B.S.; Stadtman, E.R. Methionine sulfoxide reductase (MsrA) is a regulator of antioxidant defense and lifespan in mammals. *Proc. Natl. Acad. Sci. USA* **2001**, *98*, 12920–12925.

177. Stadtman, E.R.; Moskovitz, J.; Berlett, B.S.; Levine, R.L. Cyclic oxidation and reduction of protein methionine residues is an important antioxidant mechanism. *Mol. Cell. Biochem.* **2002**, *234–235*, 3–9.

178. Taungjaruwinai, W.M.; Bhawan, J.; Keady, M.; Thiele, J.J. Differential expression of the antioxidant repair enzyme methionine sulfoxide reductase (MSRA and MSRB) in human skin. *Am. J. Dermatopathol.* **2009**, *31*, 427–431.

179. Mochin, M.T.; Underwood, K.F.; Cooper, B.; McLenithan, J.C.; Pierce, A.D.; Nalvarte, C.; Arbiser, J.; Karlsson, A.I.; Moise, A.R.; Moskovitz, J.; *et al.* Hyperglycemia and redox status regulate RUNX2 DNA-binding and an angiogenic phenotype in endothelial cells. *Microvasc. Res.* **2015**, *97*, 55–64.

180. Gu, H.; Chen, W.; Yin, J.; Chen, S.; Zhang, J.; Gong, J. Methionine sulfoxide reductase A rs10903323 G/A polymorphism is associated with increased risk of coronary artery disease in a chinese population. *Clin. Biochem.* **2013**, *46*, 1668–1672.

181. Haenold, R.; Wassef, R.; Brot, N.; Neugebauer, S.; Leipold, E.; Heinemann, S.H.; Hoshi, T. Protection of vascular smooth muscle cells by over-expressed methionine sulphoxide reductase A: Role of intracellular localization and substrate availability. *Free Radic. Res.* **2008**, *42*, 978–988.

182. Moosmann, B.; Behl, C. Mitochondrially encoded cysteine predicts animal lifespan. *Aging Cell* **2008**, *7*, 32–46.

183. Camici, G.G.; Cosentino, F.; Tanner, F.C.; Luscher, T.F. The role of p66Shc deletion in age-associated arterial dysfunction and disease states. *J. Appl. Physiol.* **2008**, *105*, 1628–1631.

184. Francia, P.; delli Gatti, C.; Bachschmid, M.; Martin-Padura, I.; Savoia, C.; Migliaccio, E.; Pelicci, P.G.; Schiavoni, M.; Luscher, T.F.; Volpe, M.; *et al.* Deletion of p66Shc gene protects against age-related endothelial dysfunction. *Circulation* **2004**, *110*, 2889–2895.

185. Gertz, M.; Fischer, F.; Wolters, D.; Steegborn, C. Activation of the lifespan regulator p66Shc through reversible disulfide bond formation. *Proc. Natl. Acad. Sci. USA* **2008**, *105*, 5705–5709.

186. Pinton, P.; Rimessi, A.; Marchi, S.; Orsini, F.; Migliaccio, E.; Giorgio, M.; Contursi, C.; Minucci, S.; Mantovani, F.; Wieckowski, M.R.; *et al.* Protein kinase C β and prolyl isomerase 1 regulate mitochondrial effects of the life-span determinant p66Shc. *Science* **2007**, *315*, 659–663.

187. Pinton, P.; Rizzuto, R. P66Shc, oxidative stress and aging: Importing a lifespan determinant into mitochondria. *Cell. Cycle* **2008**, *7*, 304–308.

188. Rota, M.; LeCapitaine, N.; Hosoda, T.; Boni, A.; De Angelis, A.; Padin-Iruegas, M.E.; Esposito, G.; Vitale, S.; Urbanek, K.; Casarsa, C.; *et al.* Diabetes promotes cardiac stem cell aging and heart failure, which are prevented by deletion of the p66Shc gene. *Circ. Res.* **2006**, *99*, 42–52.

189. Yamamori, T.; White, A.R.; Mattagajasingh, I.; Khanday, F.A.; Haile, A.; Qi, B.; Jeon, B.H.; Bugayenko, A.; Kasuno, K.; Berkowitz, D.E.; *et al.* p66Shc regulates endothelial no production and endothelium-dependent vasorelaxation: Implications for age-associated vascular dysfunction. *J. Mol. Cell. Cardiol.* **2005**, *39*, 992–995.

190. Trinei, M.; Giorgio, M.; Cicalese, A.; Barozzi, S.; Ventura, A.; Migliaccio, E.; Milia, E.; Padura, I.M.; Raker, V.A.; Maccarana, M.; *et al.* A p53-p66Shc signalling pathway controls intracellular redox status, levels of oxidation-damaged DNA and oxidative stress-induced apoptosis. *Oncogene* **2002**, *21*, 3872–3878.

191. Di Lisa, F.; Kaludercic, N.; Carpi, A.; Menabo, R.; Giorgio, M. Mitochondrial pathways for ROS formation and myocardial injury: The relevance of p66Shc and monoamine oxidase. *Basic Res. Cardiol.* **2009**, *104*, 131–139.

192. Spescha, R.D.; Klohs, J.; Semerano, A.; Giacalone, G.; Derungs, R.S.; Reiner, M.F.; Rodriguez Gutierrez, D.; Mendez-Carmona, N.; Glanzmann, M.; Savarese, G.; *et al.* Post-ischaemic silencing of p66Shc reduces ischaemia/reperfusion brain injury and its expression correlates to clinical outcome in stroke. *Eur. Heart J.* **2015**, *36*, 1590–1600.

193. Moskalev, A.A.; Aliper, A.M.; Smit-McBride, Z.; Buzdin, A.; Zhavoronkov, A. Genetics and epigenetics of aging and longevity. *Cell. Cycle* **2014**, *13*, 1063–1077.

194. Barbot, W.; Dupressoir, A.; Lazar, V.; Heidmann, T. Epigenetic regulation of an IAP retrotransposon in the aging mouse: Progressive demethylation and de-silencing of the element by its repetitive induction. *Nucleic Acids Res.* **2002**, *30*, 2365–2373.

195. Narita, M.; Nunez, S.; Heard, E.; Narita, M.; Lin, A.W.; Hearn, S.A.; Spector, D.L.; Hannon, G.J.; Lowe, S.W. Rb-mediated heterochromatin formation and silencing of E2F target genes during cellular senescence. *Cell.* **2003**, *113*, 703–716.

196. Tsurumi, A.; Li, W.X. Global heterochromatin loss: A unifying theory of aging? *Epigenetics* **2012**, *7*, 680–688.

197. McCauley, B.S.; Dang, W. Histone methylation and aging: Lessons learned from model systems. *Biochim. Biophys. Acta* **2014**, *1839*, 1454–1462.

198. Bilsland, A.E.; Revie, J.; Keith, W. Microrna and senescence: The senectome, integration and distributed control. *Crit. Rev. Oncog.* **2013**, *18*, 373–390.

199. Boon, R.A.; Iekushi, K.; Lechner, S.; Seeger, T.; Fischer, A.; Heydt, S.; Kaluza, D.; Treguer, K.; Carmona, G.; Bonauer, A.; *et al.* MicroRNA-34a regulates cardiac ageing and function. *Nature* **2013**, *495*, 107–110.

200. Guarner, V.; Rubio-Ruiz, M.E. Low-grade systemic inflammation connects aging, metabolic syndrome and cardiovascular disease. *Interdiscip. Top. Gerontol.* **2015**, *40*, 99–106.

201. Howcroft, T.K.; Campisi, J.; Louis, G.B.; Smith, M.T.; Wise, B.; Wyss-Coray, T.; Augustine, A.D.; McElhaney, J.E.; Kohanski, R.; Sierra, F. The role of inflammation in age-related disease. *Aging* **2013**, *5*, 84–93.

202. Martin-Montalvo, A.; Mercken, E.M.; Mitchell, S.J.; Palacios, H.H.; Mote, P.L.; Scheibye-Knudsen, M.; Gomes, A.P.; Ward, T.M.; Minor, R.K.; Blouin, M.J.; *et al.* Metformin improves healthspan and lifespan in mice. *Nat. Commun.* **2013**, *4*, 2192.

203. Wilson, P.W. Established risk factors and coronary artery disease: The framingham study. *Am. J. Hypertens.* **1994**, *7*, 7S–12S.

204. Munzel, T.; Sinning, C.; Post, F.; Warnholtz, A.; Schulz, E. Pathophysiology, diagnosis and prognostic implications of endothelial dysfunction. *Ann. Med.* **2008**, *40*, 180–196.

205. Munzel, T.; Gori, T.; Bruno, R.M.; Taddei, S. Is oxidative stress a therapeutic target in cardiovascular disease? *Eur. Heart J.* **2010**, *31*, 2741–2748.

206. Schachinger, V.; Britten, M.B.; Zeiher, A.M. Prognostic impact of coronary vasodilator dysfunction on adverse long-term outcome of coronary heart disease. *Circulation* **2000**, *101*, 1899–1906.

207. Gori, T.; Munzel, T. Oxidative stress and endothelial dysfunction: Therapeutic implications. *Ann. Med.* **2011**, *43*, 259–272.

208. Chen, A.F.; Chen, D.D.; Daiber, A.; Faraci, F.M.; Li, H.; Rembold, C.M.; Laher, I. Free radical biology of the cardiovascular system. *Clin. Sci.* **2012**, *123*, 73–91.

209. Kimura, Y.; Matsumoto, M.; Den, Y.B.; Iwai, K.; Munehira, J.; Hattori, H.; Hoshino, T.; Yamada, K.; Kawanishi, K.; Tsuchiya, H. Impaired endothelial function in hypertensive elderly patients evaluated by high resolution ultrasonography. *Can. J. Cardiol.* **1999**, *15*, 563–568.

210. Wray, D.W.; Nishiyama, S.K.; Harris, R.A.; Zhao, J.; McDaniel, J.; Fjeldstad, A.S.; Witman, M.A.; Ives, S.J.; Barrett-O'Keefe, Z.; Richardson, R.S. Acute reversal of endothelial dysfunction in the elderly after antioxidant consumption. *Hypertension* **2012**, *59*, 818–824.

211. Jousilahti, P.; Vartiainen, E.; Tuomilehto, J.; Puska, P. Sex, age, cardiovascular risk factors, and coronary heart disease: A prospective follow-up study of 14 786 middle-aged men and women in Finland. *Circulation* **1999**, *99*, 1165–1172.

212. Holzer, M.; Trieb, M.; Konya, V.; Wadsack, C.; Heinemann, A.; Marsche, G. Aging affects high-density lipoprotein composition and function. *Biochim. Biophys. Acta* **2013**, *1831*, 1442–1448.

213. Besler, C.; Heinrich, K.; Riwanto, M.; Luscher, T.F.; Landmesser, U. High-density lipoprotein-mediated anti-atherosclerotic and endothelial-protective effects: A potential novel therapeutic target in cardiovascular disease. *Curr. Pharm. Des.* **2010**, *16*, 1480–1493.

214. Wu, Z.; Siuda, D.; Xia, N.; Reifenberg, G.; Daiber, A.; Munzel, T.; Forstermann, U.; Li, H. Maternal treatment of spontaneously hypertensive rats with pentaerythritol tetranitrate reduces blood pressure in female offspring. *Hypertension* **2015**, *65*, 232–237.

215. Gioscia-Ryan, R.A.; LaRocca, T.J.; Sindler, A.L.; Zigler, M.C.; Murphy, M.P.; Seals, D.R. Mitochondria-targeted antioxidant (MitoQ) ameliorates age-related arterial endothelial dysfunction in mice. *J. Physiol.* **2014**, *592*, 2549–2561.

216. Klipstein-Grobusch, K.; Geleijnse, J.M.; den Breeijen, J.H.; Boeing, H.; Hofman, A.; Grobbee, D.E.; Witteman, J.C. Dietary antioxidants and risk of myocardial infarction in the elderly: The rotterdam study. *Am. J. Clin. Nutr.* **1999**, *69*, 261–266.

6

Borrowing Nuclear DNA Helicases to Protect Mitochondrial DNA

Lin Ding and Yilun Liu *

Department of Radiation Biology, Beckman Research Institute, City of Hope, Duarte, CA 91010-3000, USA; E-Mail: lding@coh.org

* Author to whom correspondence should be addressed; E-Mail: yiliu@coh.org

Academic Editors: Jaime M. Ross and Giuseppe Coppotelli

Abstract: In normal cells, mitochondria are the primary organelles that generate energy, which is critical for cellular metabolism. Mitochondrial dysfunction, caused by mitochondrial DNA (mtDNA) mutations or an abnormal mtDNA copy number, is linked to a range of human diseases, including Alzheimer's disease, premature aging and cancer. mtDNA resides in the mitochondrial lumen, and its duplication requires the mtDNA replicative helicase, Twinkle. In addition to Twinkle, many DNA helicases, which are encoded by the nuclear genome and are crucial for nuclear genome integrity, are transported into the mitochondrion to also function in mtDNA replication and repair. To date, these helicases include RecQ-like helicase 4 (RECQ4), petite integration frequency 1 (PIF1), DNA replication helicase/nuclease 2 (DNA2) and suppressor of var1 3-like protein 1 (SUV3). Although the nuclear functions of some of these DNA helicases have been extensively studied, the regulation of their mitochondrial transport and the mechanisms by which they contribute to mtDNA synthesis and maintenance remain largely unknown. In this review, we attempt to summarize recent research progress on the role of mammalian DNA helicases in mitochondrial genome maintenance and the effects on mitochondria-associated diseases.

Keywords: mitochondrial DNA; DNA replication; DNA repair; RECQ4; Twinkle; PIF1; DNA2; SUV3

1. Introduction

The mitochondrion, once an autonomous free-living Proteobacterium, became a part of the eukaryotic cell through endosymbiosis approximately two billion years ago [1]. A symbiotic relationship was established, and now, mitochondria not only serve as the powerhouses of the cell by generating adenosine triphosphate (ATP) via oxidative phosphorylation, but also regulate cellular metabolism through synthesizing heme and steroids, supplying reactive oxygen species (ROS), establishing the membrane potential and controlling calcium and apoptotic signaling [2]. Human mitochondria are maternally inherited organelles, which reside in the cytoplasm. The mitochondrial architecture consists of an outer membrane, an inner membrane, an intermembrane space and the matrix or lumen (Figure 1). The mitochondrial number per cell differs from one cell type to another, and each mitochondrion contains multiple copies of the mitochondrial DNA (mtDNA), ranging from one to 15 copies per mitochondrion [3,4]. mtDNA copy number per cell also varies among different tissues due to the tissue-specific epigenetic regulation of the expression of mtDNA replication polymerase γ (Pol γ) [5]. The human mtDNA resides in the lumen and attaches to the inner membrane [6]. The mtDNA forms a small circle, which consists of 16,569 base pairs that encode two rRNA genes, 22 tRNA genes and 13 protein-encoding genes that produce parts of the electron transport chain and ATP Synthase complexes.

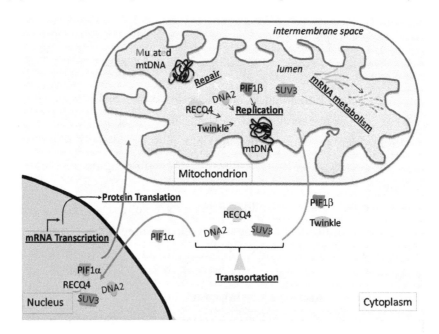

Figure 1. Schematic diagram of the production and the cellular localization of the DNA helicases (Twinkle, purple; RecQ-like helicase 4 (RECQ4), yellow; DNA replication helicase/nuclease 2 (DNA2), green; petite integration frequency 1 (PIF1), red; suppressor of var1 3-like protein 1 (SUV3), blue) that function in the mitochondrion. These DNA helicases are encoded in the nuclear genome, produced in the cytoplasm and transported into the mitochondrial lumen. With the exception of Twinkle, other DNA helicases, including RECQ4, DNA2, PIF1 and SUV3, are transported into the mitochondrial lumen or nucleus depending on the molecular cue. In the mitochondrion, these helicases participate in DNA replication and repair, as well as mRNA metabolism, in order to maintain mtDNA stability.

mtDNA is thought to be duplicated through either strand-displacement replication or RNA incorporation throughout the lagging strand [7]. Interestingly, mtDNA sequences are highly polymorphic, even within an individual. This is due to the fact that somatic mutations in mtDNA, as a result of replication errors, ROS exposure and aging, make mtDNA sequences different from each other, even within the same cell (heteroplasmic), rather than genetically identical (homoplasmic). To safeguard a healthy population of mitochondria in a cell, mitochondria are constantly dividing (fission) and rejoining (fusion). However, should a pathogenic somatic mutation be introduced into the mtDNA genome, the entire mitochondrial population could be affected. Therefore, to maintain mtDNA stability, it is crucial to ensure faithful mtDNA synthesis. In addition, mitochondria employ several DNA repair pathways to restore DNA integrity in response to damage or replication errors [8]. Failure to do so causes mitochondrial morphological changes [9], which may lead to mitochondrial dysfunction, a phenomenon that has been linked to Alzheimer's disease and premature aging [10]. Moreover, recent studies have shown that changes in mtDNA copy number are often associated with human cancers [11,12].

DNA synthesis and DNA repair are sophisticated processes that involve multi-protein complexes. Due to the small size of the mtDNA genome and the limited number of genes it encodes, mitochondria have adapted a mechanism to "borrow" enzymes encoded in the nuclear genome for many of its functions, including mtDNA synthesis and repair. For example, DNA helicases are ATPases that break the hydrogen bonds between DNA base pairs and transiently convert double-stranded DNA (dsDNA) into single-stranded DNA (ssDNA), the latter of which can serve as the template for DNA synthesis or allow the repair of damaged bases or nucleotides. These DNA helicases are transcribed in the nucleus, synthesized in the cytoplasm and imported into the mitochondrial compartment. Mitochondrial transport occurs primarily through either the presequence pathway or the carrier pathway. Both pathways involve interactions with the translocase of the outer membrane (TOM) and the translocase of the inner membrane (TIM) protein complexes, though the protein subunits are different for each pathway [13–15]. The presequence pathway targets the precursor protein to the lumen, where a mitochondrial targeting signal (MTS) located at the *N*-terminus of the precursor protein is then cleaved by a mitochondrial processing peptidase. The precursor proteins that also express hydrophobic sorting signals are either inserted into the inner membrane or released into the inter membrane space. The carrier pathway usually targets the mitochondrial proteins to the inner membrane, and these precursors have a non-cleavable internal targeting signal (ITS) and form complexes with cytosolic chaperones to prevent aggregation. Nonetheless, there are exceptions to these rules; some proteins, such as the tumor suppressor p53, can also be targeted to the mitochondrion via protein-protein interactions [16].

In mammalian cells, mtDNA replication is promoted by the replicative DNA helicase Twinkle, which is encoded by the *C10orf2* gene in the nucleus. In addition to Twinkle, there are many DNA helicases that contribute to mammalian mtDNA integrity. Interestingly, unlike Twinkle, which is known to exclusively function in the mitochondrion, many of these DNA helicases not only are expressed from the nuclear genome, but also are involved in nuclear DNA replication and repair (Figure 1). This raises several questions. How do these DNA helicases balance their distribution and function in the nucleus and mitochondrion? What triggers the translocation of these helicases between different cellular compartments? How do Twinkle and other helicases collaborate in mtDNA replication and repair? In this review, we summarize recent findings on how these nuclear-encoding DNA helicases contribute to mtDNA integrity and associated diseases, and we will try to shine light on future studies in this active field.

2. Mitochondrial Replicative Helicase, Twinkle

Twinkle (for the T7 gp4-like protein with intramitochondrial nucleoid localization or PEO1) was first identified based on a sequence homology search as T7 gene 4 primase/helicase in 2001 [17]. Although Twinkle is conserved in many eukaryotes, such as the mouse, *Drosophila* and zebra fish, it has no orthologs in yeast [18]. It is possible that other yeast helicases compensate for its role in mtDNA replication. Twinkle is essential for embryonic development in mammalian systems, and it is known to unwind mtDNA for mtDNA synthesis by Pol γ [19]. Immunofluorescence microscopy has revealed that Twinkle proteins form punctate foci within mitochondria and colocalize with mitochondrial nucleoids [17], which are aggregates containing mtDNA and proteins that enact mitochondrial genome maintenance and transcription [20,21]. These foci resemble twinkling stars [17]. Human Twinkle, a 684 amino-acid (aa)-long polypeptide with a molecular weight of 77 kDa, oligomerizes to form a hexamer and exhibits 5'–3' helicase activity due to the conserved superfamily 4 (SF4) helicase domain located at its *C*-terminus (Figure 2) [22]. In addition to the conserved SF4 domain, Twinkle also contains a 42-aa MTS for mitochondrial targeting and a non-functional *N*-terminal primase-like domain that connects to the SF4 domain by a linker domain (Figure 2) [22,23]. The linker region is important for the hexamerization of Twinkle and its DNA helicase activity [24]. Recent studies have also found that Twinkle exhibits DNA annealing activity, indicating a possible involvement of Twinkle in recombination-mediated replication initiation or the fork regression pathway of DNA repair [25]. Interestingly, an alternatively-spliced product, Twinky, lacks part of the *C*-terminus, exists as monomers and has no enzymatic activity [23]. The function of Twinky remains unclear, as it cannot localize to the mitochondrial nucleoids [17] nor associate with Twinkle [23], despite the fact that Twinky contains the proposed MTS at the *N*-terminus (Figure 2). This suggests that the unique *C*-terminus of Twinkle may contain an additional sequence that is also important for its mitochondrial localization. Recombinant human Twinkle, combined with Pol γ purified from insect cells, is sufficient to form the minimal mammalian mtDNA replisome [26]. The hexameric Twinkle ring can efficiently bind to the single-stranded region of a closed circular DNA without a helicase loader and support DNA synthesis by Pol γ through the duplex region [26]. The helicase activity of Twinkle is stimulated by mitochondrial single-stranded DNA-binding protein (mtSSB) [22,27].

Given the essential role of Twinkle in mtDNA synthesis, mtDNA stability is greatly influenced by the Twinkle expression level in cells. For example, overexpression of the wild-type Twinkle is associated with increased mtDNA copy number in skeletal muscle in mice and reduced ROS-induced mtDNA mutations [28,29], whereas depletion of the Twinkle protein by small interfering RNA (siRNA) leads to a significant decrease in mtDNA copy number [30]. Furthermore, increasing evidence has linked a set of mutations, which change the stability and enzymatic activity of Twinkle [31], to a wide range of diseases [32], such as mitochondrial myopathy [33] and autosomal dominant progressive external ophthalmoplegia (adPEO) [34]. Individuals suffering from adPEO bear multiple deletions in their mitochondrial genome and exhibit multiple symptoms, including muscle weakening, hearing loss, nerve damage and Parkinsonism [35,36].

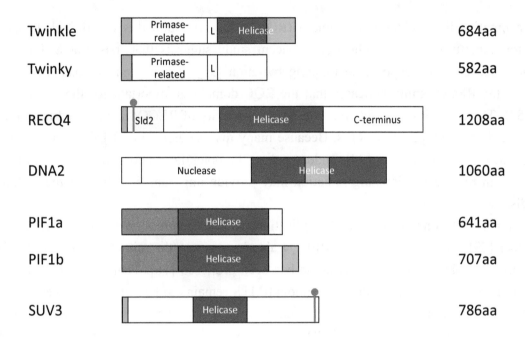

Figure 2. Schematic diagram of the protein domains and alternatively-spliced variants of the human DNA helicases that have known functions in the mitochondrion. Green: mitochondrial targeting sequence (MTS). Red: nuclear localization signal (NLS). Purple: helicase domain. Blue: non-MTS sequence required for mitochondrial localization. Brown: arginine-rich region where potential NLSs reside. Yellow: unique sld2-like domain. L = linker region.

3. The Involvement of the Nuclear DNA Helicases

3.1. RecQ-Like Helicase 4 (RECQ4)

The gene that encodes RecQ-like helicase 4 (RECQ4) was first identified and cloned based on its limited sequence homology to the highly-conserved RECQ family of superfamily 2 (SF2) DNA helicases [37]. RECQ4 mutations were later identified in patients suffering from Rothmund-Thomson syndrome (RTS), Baller-Gerold syndrome and RAPADILINO (RAdial hypo-/aplasia, PAtellae hypo-/aplasia and cleft or highly arched PAlate, DIarrhea and DIslocated joints, LIttle size and LImb malformation, NOse slender and NOrmal intelligence) syndrome, with phenotypes ranging from premature aging to cancer predisposition [38]. *In vitro*, purified recombinant RECQ4 proteins exist as multimeric proteins and unwind DNA in a 3'–5' direction [39]. Interestingly, RECQ4 not only unwinds DNA, but also exhibits strong DNA annealing activity [40]. In addition to the conserved SF2 helicase domain, the vertebrate RECQ4 contains a unique Sld2-like *N*-terminus (Figure 2) that resembles the essential yeast DNA replication initiation factor Sld2 [41]. Researchers have shown that RECQ4 forms a chromatin-specific complex via this Sld2-like *N*-terminal domain with the MCM2-7 replicative helicase complex and participates in nuclear DNA replication initiation [42–47]. This function explains why *recq4* knockout results in embryonic lethality in mice. Furthermore, the expression of a RECQ4 fragment containing only the Sld2-like *N*-terminal domain is sufficient to support embryonic development [48,49]. The *C*-terminus of RECQ4, which is highly conserved among vertebrates, contains a putative RecQ-*C*-terminal domain (RQC) [50]. Although this *C*-terminal domain is not required for unperturbed DNA replication, a recent study suggests that it is crucial for replication elongation when cells are exposed to ionizing radiation [51]. It has been demonstrated with other members of the RECQ family helicases that the RQC domain is important for the DNA unwinding activity [52]. Therefore, it is possible that the helicase activity of RECQ4 is involved in stabilizing or repairing the damaged replication forks. Because many disease-associated RECQ4 mutations disrupt the conserved *C*-terminal domain [38], understanding the potential function of RECQ4 in replication fork stability in response to ionizing radiation may provide important insight into the pathogenicity of these diseases.

In addition to affecting nuclear DNA replication, RECQ4 expression level also affects mtDNA copy number [53]. Consistent with this, RECQ4 also localizes to the mitochondrion [16,53–56], and the existence of a MTS within the first 20 aa has been proposed [16]. That said, whether RECQ4 is targeted to the mitochondrion via the conventional MTS remains to be validated. Given that RECQ4 interacts with the nuclear DNA replicative helicase complex and plays a critical role in nuclear DNA replication [42–47], it is possible that RECQ4 might have a similar role in mtDNA synthesis. Indeed, in a recent study from our laboratory, we reported a weak interaction between RECQ4 and the mitochondrial replicative helicase Twinkle that can be detected in human whole-cell extracts [56]. Perhaps most surprisingly, we found that this interaction between RECQ4 and Twinkle was significantly enhanced in human cells carrying the most common lymphoma-prone RECQ4 mutation: c.1390+2 delT. This mutation produces RECQ4 polypeptides lacking Ala420-Ala463 residues immediately upstream of the conserved helicase domain [56]. As a consequence, there is increased mtDNA synthesis, leading to an increase in the mtDNA copy number and mitochondrial dysfunction in these cells. Clearly, residues Ala420–Ala463, which are missing in this cancer-prone RECQ4 mutant, have an important inhibitory role in mtDNA synthesis, and we further elucidated how this regulation works. We found that residues Ala420–Ala463 of RECQ4 are required for the interaction with p32, and this interaction negatively regulates RECQ4 mitochondrial localization [56]. p32, which resides in both the mitochondrion and the nucleus [56,57], is involved in regulating mitochondrial innate immunity [58], energy production [57,59] and mitochondrial protein translocation [60]. Cells expressing RECQ4 mutants that lack these 44 aa show defective RECQ4-p32 interactions, increased RECQ4 mutant proteins in the mitochondrion and decreased nuclear RECQ4, suggesting that the excess of RECQ4 molecules in the mitochondrion likely results from increased nuclear-mitochondrial transport [56]. Therefore, this work presents a model for the mechanism used by cells to balance the distribution of RECQ4 in the nucleus and mitochondrion via direct protein-protein interaction.

Although mitochondrial localization of RECQ4 is restricted by p32, RECQ4 itself has also been suggested to function as a positive regulator of the mitochondrial transport of the p53 tumor suppressor via a direct protein–protein interaction [16]. Interestingly, mitochondrial localization of p53 can be blocked by the chaperone protein nucleophosmin (NPM) [61], which was found to also interact with RECQ4 in the nucleoplasm [56]. Although the domain of RECQ4 that interacts with NPM remains to be determined, it is tempting to speculate that NPM inhibits the mitochondrial transport of p53 via its interaction with RECQ4 in the nucleus. In summary, RECQ4 is a dynamic interacting protein, and its protein-protein interactions not only govern the rate of nuclear and mitochondrial DNA synthesis, but also regulate its cellular localization.

3.2. DNA Replication Helicase/Nuclease 2 (DNA2)

The DNA replication helicase/nuclease 2 (*DNA2*) gene was first isolated from a genetic screen in budding yeast [62], and the human *DNA2* gene was later identified based on its sequence homology to the yeast counterpart [63]. Human DNA2, a 120-kDa polypeptide, has two independent functional domains: the *N*-terminal nuclease and the *C*-terminal helicase domain (Figure 2). DNA2 is highly conserved among the eukaryotes. As such, expression of either the human or *Xenopus laevis* DNA2 complements the temperature sensitivity of a *DNA2* (*DNA2-1*) mutation in budding yeast [64]. However, the specificity of DNA2 enzymatic activity may vary across species due to the widely divergent sequences of the distal *N*-terminal regions [65,66]. DNA2 proteins purified from human cells and insect cells show that the nuclease domain has both 5'–3' and 3'–5' nuclease activities [65,67], whereas the helicase unwinds dsDNA that contains a 5' flap as a tail [67]. Data from yeast studies suggest that the 5'–3' helicase activity of DNA2 facilitates the production of a 5' flap structure, a substrate of DNA2 nuclease activity *in vitro* [68]. Nonetheless, the yeast helicase activity *in vivo* is dispensable for cell growth under normal conditions [69,70]. It remains to be determined if this is also the case in higher eukaryotes and if other DNA helicases can compensate for the DNA2 helicase activity.

In the nucleus, DNA2 interacts with proliferating cell nuclear antigen, also known as PCNA, a protein that is important for replication processivity and prevents the accumulation of DNA double-strand breaks (DSBs) during replication [71]. In addition, DNA2 interacts with the Fanconi anemia complementation group D2 (FANCD2) protein and functions in the FANCD2-dependent interstrand crosslink repair pathway [72]. Cells with depleted DNA2 show increased DSBs [71], internuclear chromatin bridges [73] and increased sensitivity to interstrand crosslinking agents due to a reduced homologous recombination frequency [72]. Furthermore, DNA2 participates in long-range DNA resection, in concert with the Werner syndrome ATP-dependent helicase (WRN) and the Bloom syndrome protein (BLM), in DSB repair [74–76]. DNA2 also stimulates BLM helicase activity [75]. Recently, DNA2 was also implicated in telomere maintenance based on its ability to cleave G-quadruplex DNA, and heterozygous DNA2 knockout mice were found to be prone to telomeric DNA damage and aneuploidy [77].

Although DNA2 can localize to the nucleus and play a role in nuclear DNA repair, immunofluorescence microscopy data suggest that the majority of the DNA2 molecules are found in the mitochondrion [73,78]. DNA2 does not contain a classical MTS/ITS, but its localization to the mitochondrion requires the sequence located within 734 and 829 aa [78]. It remains unclear how cells regulate the distribution of DNA2 in the mitochondrion and the nucleus in response to either the cell cycle or DNA damage. DNA2 interacts with and stimulates Pol γ in the mitochondrion and is thought to also function in concert with flap structure-specific endonuclease 1 (FEN1) to process 5'-flap intermediates and participate in repairing oxidative lesions in mtDNA by long-range base excision repair [78]. Indeed, DNA2 proteins colocalize with mtDNA nucleoids and Twinkle and through an unknown mechanism; this localization increases in cells carrying some of the adPEO-associated Twinkle mutations [73]. Interestingly, point mutations in the *DNA2* gene itself have also been linked to adPEO, and these patients show progressive myopathy with mitochondrial dysfunction [79]. Importantly, one mutation located within the helicase domain altered the DNA unwinding efficiency [79], suggesting that the helicase activity of DNA2 has an important role in mtDNA maintenance in humans.

Therefore, similar to Twinkle, DNA2 is important for maintaining healthy mitochondrial DNA and preventing related diseases.

3.3. Petite Integration Frequency 1 (PIF1)

PIF1, which stands for petite integration frequency 1, is conserved in both budding yeast and humans [80–83]. PIF1 is a member of the superfamily 1 (SF1) helicase family and has 5'–3' DNA unwinding activity (Figure 2) [84–86]. Similar to RECQ4 and DNA2, PIF1 localizes to both the nucleus and the mitochondrion [83]. However, unlike RECQ4 and DNA2, PIF1 mitochondrial localization in human cells is regulated by alternative splicing, which produces α and β isoforms [83]. Both the α and β isoforms contain the intact helicase domain and the *N*-terminus (Figure 2), which has arginine-rich nuclear localization signals [83] and is important for the interaction with ssDNA [84].

The PIF1 α isoform consists of 641 aa and has a short distal *C*-terminus. This isoform localizes to the nucleus [83], and PIF1 function in the nucleus has been extensively demonstrated [83,85,87,88]. The expression of PIF1 is cell cycle regulated, and the downregulation of PIF1 leads to cell cycle delay [81,83]. Both yeast and human PIF1 bind DNA and promote DNA replication through interaction with G-quadruplex DNA regions [86,87,89–92]. This activity is important for maintaining telomere integrity and for resolving stalled replication forks [85]. Reduction of PIF1α by siRNA knockdown decreases cancer cell survival, but has no impact on non-malignant cells [93], and this is likely due to its role in restarting stalled replication forks [85,94].

The PIF1 β isoform (707 aa) has a long distal *C*-terminus with a lipocalin motif (protein secretion signal; Figure 2). This *C*-terminal region results from alternative splicing and is not present in the α isoform. PIF1β is expected to have similar biochemical properties, compared to PIF1α, as they contain the same helicase domain. However, unlike the α isoform, the majority of this β isoform localizes to the mitochondrion, with some residual nuclear signal [83]. Evidence from yeast studies suggests that PIF1 may associate with mtDNA and mitochondrial inner membranes [95] and contribute to reducing DSBs in mtDNA [96]. Furthermore, it is required for repairing UV- and ethidium bromide-damaged mtDNA [80]. In addition, Twinkle, which cannot efficiently unwind G-quadruplex DNA [97], may rely on PIF1 helicase activity to remove G-quadruplexes, which could potentially lead to mtDNA deletions. Nonetheless, it is unknown how the distal *C*-terminus, which is unique to PIF1β, promotes its mitochondrial localization and how PIF1β protects mtDNA from DSBs. Interestingly, deletion of *PIF1* rescued the lethal phenotype of *DNA2* in budding yeast, suggesting that PIF1 and DNA2 may be involved in similar, but non-redundant pathways in the mitochondrion [98].

3.4. Suppressor of Var1 3-Like Protein 1 (SUV3)

SUV3, a member of the DExH-box helicase family, was first identified in budding yeast as the suppressor of var1 (the small subunit of mitochondrial ribosomal protein) [99], and the gene was later found to be conserved in humans [100]. *SUV3* knockout mice are embryonic lethal, whereas heterozygous mice have shortened lifespan and develop tumors at multiple sites, due to a reduced mtDNA copy number and an elevated number of mtDNA mutations [101]. Reduced SUV3 expression was observed in human breast tumor samples [101]. Nonetheless, unlike RECQ4, PIF1 and DNA2 helicases, the effect of SUV3 deficiency on mtDNA copy number and stability is likely indirect. For example, in the mitochondrion, SUV3 forms a complex with polynucleotide phosphorylase (PNPase) to function in mtRNA degradation [102]. Indeed, analysis using purified recombinant human SUV3 proteins demonstrated that SUV3 is an active ATPase and capable of unwinding not only DNA, but also RNA in a 3'–5' direction [102–104]. This SUV3-PNPase complex transiently associates with the mitochondrial polyadenylation polymerase when the inorganic phosphate level is low in the mitochondrial lumen [105]. The three-component complex is capable of regulating the length of the RNA poly(A) tail. Consistent with this, siRNA knockdown leads to an increase in the amount of mtRNA with shorter poly(A) tails, a reduction in mtDNA copy number [106] and an increase in the rate of apoptosis [107]. In addition, expression of a mutant defective in the ATPase function leads to an abnormally high level of mtRNA, due to the slow mRNA turnover rate [108]. Although it remains unclear how a defect in mtRNA degradation contributes to mtDNA instability in SUV3-deficient cells, it is possible that the abnormal level of mtRNA imposes cellular stress, leading to overproduction of ROS and mtDNA damage.

Early studies suggest that SUV3 localizes to the lumen of the mitochondrion, presumably through cleavage of an MTS localized at the distal *N*-terminus (Figure 2) [103,107]. However, recent studies provide evidence that SUV3 also localizes to the nucleus with a potential nuclear localization signal located between residues 777 and 781 at the *C*-terminus [104,107]. In the nucleus, SUV3 interacts with nuclear DNA replication and repair factors, such as the RECQ helicases BLM and WRN [109], as well as replication protein A (RPA) and FEN1 [104]. Therefore, it is possible that, at least in humans, SUV3 is a key player in nuclear genome maintenance due to its participation in DNA damage repair, whereas it maintains mitochondrial genome integrity by participating in mtRNA metabolism. The reason why cells utilize an mtRNA helicase in nuclear DNA damage repair remains unknown. Interestingly, in mammalian cells, there is an increase in the degradation of mtRNA, but not cytoplasmic RNAs, to protect cells in response to oxidative stress [110]. It is possible that the involvement of SUV3 in nuclear DNA repair provides a mechanism for cells to "sense" oxidative DNA damage and induce mtRNA degradation. Therefore, identifying the molecular switch that balances the localization and the two distinct functions of SUV3 might reveal a novel crosstalk between the nucleus and the mitochondrion in response to DNA damage.

4. Conclusions

Given that mitochondria provide the vital ATP energy source needed by diverse cellular processes that support the development of an organism, it is not surprising that abnormal mtDNA copy number and mitochondrial dysfunction have been correlated with a decline in tissue maintenance and regeneration. Tissue degeneration may contribute to some of the symptoms, such as muscle weakening, hearing loss, nerve damage and Parkinsonism observed in the adPEO1 patients [35,36]. Growing evidence also suggests a close association between mitochondrial dysfunction and age-related bone diseases. For example, osteoporosis is a result of the loss of bone mass and is one of the common symptoms associated with aging [12,111]. Studies in mice indicate that increased apoptosis in osteoblasts, due to the accumulation of ROS generated by damaged mitochondria, is one of the main causes of bone loss [112]. Interestingly, RTS patients with RECQ4 mutations show abnormal bone development and osteoporosis at an early age [113]. Therefore, it is possible that these RTS-associated RECQ4 mutations lead to mitochondrial dysfunction and contribute to the premature aging phenotypes.

In addition to their association with tissue degeneration and developmental defects, mitochondria have recently gained attention for their potential use both as diagnostic tools and as therapeutic targets for cancer treatment [11]. Variations in mtDNA copy number are observed in many cancers and correlate with tumor aggressiveness and survival outcome. For example, mtDNA copy number is significantly elevated in various types of lymphoma, including Burkitt lymphoma and non-Hodgkin lymphoma [114–117]. In addition, highly invasive osteosarcoma cells contain enlarged mitochondria and larger amounts of mtDNA, and inhibiting replication of mtDNA in these cells also effectively slows down tumor growth [118–120]. Because mtDNA copy number correlates with cell growth [121], deregulated mtDNA synthesis could be a risk factor that contributes to cancer pathogenesis or that sustains cancer cell growth. Therefore, reducing aberrant mtDNA synthesis in cancer by targeting enzymes involved in mtDNA synthesis or mtDNA repair may be an effective strategy for controlling tumor progression. It would be of great interest for future studies to explore the possibility that the DNA helicases we have summarized here may be cancer drug targets or biomarkers for cancer diagnosis and prevention.

Acknowledgments

We thank Nancy Linford and Keely Walker for their comments and expert editing of this manuscript. Yilun Liu was supported by funding from the National Cancer Institute (R01 CA151245).

Author Contributions

Lin Ding and Yilun Liu wrote the manuscript.

References

1.   Kurland, C.G.; Andersson, S.G. Origin and evolution of the mitochondrial proteome. *Microb. Mol. Biol. Rev.* **2000**, *64*, 786–820.

2.   Nunnari, J.; Suomalainen, A. Mitochondria: In sickness and in health. *Cell* **2012**, *148*, 1145–1159.

3.   Iborra, F.J.; Kimura, H.; Cook, P.R. The functional organization of mitochondrial genomes in human cells. *BMC Biol.* **2004**, *2*, 9.

4.   Satoh, M.; Kuroiwa, T. Organization of multiple nucleoids and DNA molecules in mitochondria of a human cell. *Exp. Cell Res.* **1991**, *196*, 137–140.

5.   Kelly, R.D.; Mahmud, A.; McKenzie, M.; Trounce, I.A.; St John, J.C. Mitochondrial DNA copy number is regulated in a tissue specific manner by DNA methylation of the nuclear-encoded DNA polymerase gamma A. *Nucleic Acids Res.* **2012**, *40*, 10124–10138.

6. Albring, M.; Griffith, J.; Attardi, G. Association of a protein structure of probable membrane derivation with HeLa cell mitochondrial DNA near its origin of replication. *Proc. Natl. Acad. Sci. USA* **1977**, *74*, 1348–1352.

7. Holt, I.J.; Reyes, A. Human mitochondrial DNA replication. *Cold Spring Harb. Perspect. Biol.* **2012**, *4*, a012971.

8. Kazak, L.; Reyes, A.; Holt, I.J. Minimizing the damage: Repair pathways keep mitochondrial DNA intact. *Nat. Rev. Mol. Cell Biol.* **2012**, *13*, 659–671.

9. Gilkerson, R.W.; Margineantu, D.H.; Capaldi, R.A.; Selker, J.M. Mitochondrial DNA depletion causes morphological changes in the mitochondrial reticulum of cultured human cells. *FEBS Lett.* **2000**, *474*, 1–4.

10. Schapira, A.H. Mitochondrial disease. *Lancet* **2006**, *368*, 70–82.

11. Yu, M. Generation, function and diagnostic value of mitochondrial DNA copy number alterations in human cancers. *Life Sci.* **2011**, *89*, 65–71.

12. Clay Montier, L.L.; Deng, J.J.; Bai, Y. Number matters: Control of mammalian mitochondrial DNA copy number. *J. Genet. Genomics* **2009**, *36*, 125–131.

13. Becker, T.; Bottinger, L.; Pfanner, N. Mitochondrial protein import: From transport pathways to an integrated network. *Trends Biochem. Sci.* **2012**, *37*, 85–91.

14. Schmidt, O.; Pfanner, N.; Meisinger, C. Mitochondrial protein import: From proteomics to functional mechanisms. *Nat. Rev. Mol. Cell Biol.* **2010**, *11*, 655–667.

15. Gebert, N.; Ryan, M.T.; Pfanner, N.; Wiedemann, N.; Stojanovski, D. Mitochondrial protein import machineries and lipids: A functional connection. *Biochim. Biophys. Acta* **2011**, *1808*, 1002–1011.

16. De, S.; Kumari, J.; Mudgal, R.; Modi, P.; Gupta, S.; Futami, K.; Goto, H.; Lindor, N.M.; Furuichi, Y.; Mohanty, D.; *et al.* RECQL4 is essential for the transport of p53 to mitochondria in normal human cells in the absence of exogenous stress. *J. Cell Sci.* **2012**, *125*, 2509–2522.

17. Spelbrink, J.N.; Li, F.Y.; Tiranti, V.; Nikali, K.; Yuan, Q.P.; Tariq, M.; Wanrooij, S.; Garrido, N.; Comi, G.; Morandi, L.; *et al.* Human mitochondrial DNA deletions associated with mutations in the gene encoding Twinkle, a phage T7 gene 4-like protein localized in mitochondria. *Nat. Genet.* **2001**, *28*, 223–231.

18. Westermann, B. Mitochondrial inheritance in yeast. *Biochim. Biophys. Acta* **2014**, *1837*, 1039–1046.

19. Milenkovic, D.; Matic, S.; Kuhl, I.; Ruzzenente, B.; Freyer, C.; Jemt, E.; Park, C.B.; Falkenberg, M.; Larsson, N.G. TWINKLE is an essential mitochondrial helicase required for synthesis of nascent D-loop strands and complete mtDNA replication. *Hum. Mol. Genet.* **2013**, *22*, 1983–1993.

20. Gilkerson, R.; Bravo, L.; Garcia, I.; Gaytan, N.; Herrera, A.; Maldonado, A.; Quintanilla, B. The mitochondrial nucleoid: Integrating mitochondrial DNA into cellular homeostasis. *Cold Spring Harb. Perspect. Biol.* **2013**, *5*, a011080.

21. Bogenhagen, D.F.; Rousseau, D.; Burke, S. The layered structure of human mitochondrial DNA nucleoids. *J. Biol. Chem.* **2008**, *283*, 3665–3675.

22. Korhonen, J.A.; Gaspari, M.; Falkenberg, M. TWINKLE has 5′→3′ DNA helicase activity and is specifically stimulated by mitochondrial single-stranded DNA-binding protein. *J. Biol. Chem.* **2003**, *278*, 48627–48632.

23. Farge, G.; Holmlund, T.; Khvorostova, J.; Rofougaran, R.; Hofer, A.; Falkenberg, M. The *N*-terminal domain of TWINKLE contributes to single-stranded DNA binding and DNA helicase activities. *Nucleic Acids Res.* **2008**, *36*, 393–403.

24. Korhonen, J.A.; Pande, V.; Holmlund, T.; Farge, G.; Pham, X.H.; Nilsson, L.; Falkenberg, M. Structure–function defects of the TWINKLE linker region in progressive external ophthalmoplegia. *J. Mol. Biol.* **2008**, *377*, 691–705.

25. Sen, D.; Nandakumar, D.; Tang, G.Q.; Patel, S.S. Human mitochondrial DNA helicase TWINKLE is both an unwinding and annealing helicase. *J. Biol. Chem.* **2012**, *287*, 14545–14556.

26. Jemt, E.; Farge, G.; Backstrom, S.; Holmlund, T.; Gustafsson, C.M.; Falkenberg, M. The mitochondrial DNA helicase TWINKLE can assemble on a closed circular template and support initiation of DNA synthesis. *Nucleic Acids Res.* **2011**, *39*, 9238–9249.

27. Korhonen, J.A.; Pham, X.H.; Pellegrini, M.; Falkenberg, M. Reconstitution of a minimal mtDNA replisome *in vitro*. *EMBO J.* **2004**, *23*, 2423–2429.

28. Ylikallio, E.; Tyynismaa, H.; Tsutsui, H.; Ide, T.; Suomalainen, A. High mitochondrial DNA copy number has detrimental effects in mice. *Hum. Mol. Genet.* **2010**, *19*, 2695–2705.

29. Pohjoismaki, J.L.; Williams, S.L.; Boettger, T.; Goffart, S.; Kim, J.; Suomalainen, A.; Moraes, C.T.; Braun, T. Over-expression of Twinkle-helicase protects cardiomyocytes from genotoxic stress caused by reactive oxygen species. *Proc. Natl. Acad. Sci. USA* **2013**, *110*, 19408–19013.

30. Tyynismaa, H.; Sembongi, H.; Bokori-Brown, M.; Granycome, C.; Ashley, N.; Poulton, J.; Jalanko, A.; Spelbrink, J.N.; Holt, I.J.; Suomalainen, A. Twinkle helicase is essential for mtDNA maintenance and regulates mtDNA copy number. *Hum. Mol. Genet.* **2004**, *13*, 3219–3227.

31. Longley, M.J.; Humble, M.M.; Sharief, F.S.; Copeland, W.C. Disease variants of the human mitochondrial DNA helicase encoded by C10orf2 differentially alter protein stability, nucleotide hydrolysis, and helicase activity. *J. Biol. Chem.* **2010**, *285*, 29690–29702.

32. Greaves, L.C.; Reeve, A.K.; Taylor, R.W.; Turnbull, D.M. Mitochondrial DNA and disease. *J. Pathol.* **2012**, *226*, 274–286.

33. Arenas, J.; Briem, E.; Dahl, H.; Hutchison, W.; Lewis, S.; Martin, M.A.; Spelbrink, H.; Tiranti, V.; Jacobs, H.; Zeviani, M. The V368i mutation in Twinkle does not segregate with adPEO. *Ann. Neurol.* **2003**, *53*, 278.

34. Li, F.Y.; Tariq, M.; Croxen, R.; Morten, K.; Squier, W.; Newsom-Davis, J.; Beeson, D.; Larsson, C. Mapping of autosomal dominant progressive external ophthalmoplegia to a 7-cM critical region on 10q24. *Neurology* **1999**, *53*, 1265–1271.

35. Zeviani, M.; Servidei, S.; Gellera, C.; Bertini, E.; DiMauro, S.; DiDonato, S. An autosomal dominant disorder with multiple deletions of mitochondrial DNA starting at the D-loop region. *Nature* **1989**, *339*, 309–311.

36. Moslemi, A.R.; Melberg, A.; Holme, E.; Oldfors, A. Autosomal dominant progressive external ophthalmoplegia: Distribution of multiple mitochondrial DNA deletions. *Neurology* **1999**, *53*, 79–84.

37. Kitao, S.; Ohsugi, I.; Ichikawa, K.; Goto, M.; Furuichi, Y.; Shimamoto, A. Cloning of two new human helicase genes of the RecQ family: Biological significance of multiple species in higher eukaryotes. *Genomics* **1998**, *54*, 443–452.

38. Liu, Y. Rothmund-Thomson syndrome helicase, RECQ4: On the crossroad between DNA replication and repair. *DNA Repair. (Amst.)* **2010**, *9*, 325–330.

39. Suzuki, T.; Kohno, T.; Ishimi, Y. DNA helicase activity in purified human RECQL4 protein. *J. Biochem.* **2009**, *146*, 327–335.

40. Xu, X.; Liu, Y. Dual DNA unwinding activities of the Rothmund-Thomson syndrome protein, RECQ4. *EMBO J.* **2009**, *28*, 568–577.

41. Kamimura, Y.; Masumoto, H.; Sugino, A.; Araki, H. Sld2, which interacts with Dpb11 in Saccharomyces cerevisiae, is required for chromosomal DNA replication. *Mol. Cell. Biol.* **1998**, *18*, 6102–6109.

42. Im, J.S.; Ki, S.H.; Farina, A.; Jung, D.S.; Hurwitz, J.; Lee, J.K. Assembly of the Cdc45-Mcm2-7-GINS complex in human cells requires the Ctf4/And-1, RecQL4, and Mcm10 proteins. *Proc. Natl. Acad. Sci. USA* **2009**, *106*, 15628–15632.

43. Xu, X.; Rochette, P.J.; Feyissa, E.A.; Su, T.V.; Liu, Y. MCM10 mediates RECQ4 association with MCM2-7 helicase complex during DNA replication. *EMBO J.* **2009**, *28*, 3005–3014.

44. Thangavel, S.; Mendoza-Maldonado, R.; Tissino, E.; Sidorova, J.M.; Yin, J.; Wang, W.; Monnat, R.J., Jr.; Falaschi, A.; Vindigni, A. Human RECQ1 and RECQ4 helicases play distinct roles in DNA replication initiation. *Mol. Cell. Biol.* **2010**, *30*, 1382–1396.

45. Im, J.S.; Park, S.Y.; Cho, W.H.; Bae, S.H.; Hurwitz, J.; Lee, J.K. RecQL4 is required for the association of Mcm10 and Ctf4 with replication origins in human cells. *Cell Cycle* **2015**, *14*, 1001–1009.

46. Sangrithi, M.N.; Bernal, J.A.; Madine, M.; Philpott, A.; Lee, J.; Dunphy, W.G.; Venkitaraman, A.R. Initiation of DNA replication requires the RECQL4 protein mutated in Rothmund-Thomson syndrome. *Cell* **2005**, *121*, 887–898.

47. Matsuno, K.; Kumano, M.; Kubota, Y.; Hashimoto, Y.; Takisawa, H. The *N*-terminal noncatalytic region of Xenopus RecQ4 is required for chromatin binding of DNA polymerase α in the initiation of DNA replication. *Mol. Cell. Biol.* **2006**, *26*, 4843–4852.

48. Ichikawa, K.; Noda, T.; Furuichi, Y. Preparation of the gene targeted knockout mice for human premature aging diseases, Werner syndrome, and Rothmund-Thomson syndrome caused by the mutation of DNA helicases. *Nihon Yakurigaku Zasshi* **2002**, *119*, 219–226.

49. Mann, M.B.; Hodges, C.A.; Barnes, E.; Vogel, H.; Hassold, T.J.; Luo, G. Defective sister-chromatid cohesion, aneuploidy and cancer predisposition in a mouse model of type II Rothmund-Thomson syndrome. *Hum. Mol. Genet.* **2005**, *14*, 813–825.

50. Marino, F.; Vindigni, A.; Onesti, S. Bioinformatic analysis of RecQ4 helicases reveals the presence of a RQC domain and a Zn knuckle. *Biophys. Chem.* **2013**, *177–178*, 34–39.

51. Kohzaki, M.; Chiourea, M.; Versini, G.; Adachi, N.; Takeda, S.; Gagos, S.; Halazonetis, T.D. The helicase domain and *C*-terminus of human RecQL4 facilitate replication elongation on DNA templates damaged by ionizing radiation. *Carcinogenesis* **2012**, *33*, 1203–1210.

52. Lucic, B.; Zhang, Y.; King, O.; Mendoza-Maldonado, R.; Berti, M.; Niesen, F.H.; Burgess-Brown, N.A.; Pike, A.C.; Cooper, C.D.; Gileadi, O.; *et al.* A prominent beta-hairpin structure in the winged-helix domain of RECQ1 is required for DNA unwinding and oligomer formation. *Nucleic Acids Res.* **2011**, *39*, 1703–1717.

53. Chi, Z.; Nie, L.; Peng, Z.; Yang, Q.; Yang, K.; Tao, J.; Mi, Y.; Fang, X.; Balajee, A.S.; Zhao, Y. RecQL4 cytoplasmic localization: Implications in mitochondrial DNA oxidative damage repair. *Int. J. Biochem. Cell Biol.* **2012**, *44*, 1942–1951.

54. Croteau, D.L.; Rossi, M.L.; Canugovi, C.; Tian, J.; Sykora, P.; Ramamoorthy, M.; Wang, Z.M.; Singh, D.K.; Akbari, M.; Kasiviswanathan, R.; *et al.* RECQL4 localizes to mitochondria and preserves mitochondrial DNA integrity. *Aging Cell* **2012**, *11*, 456–466.

55. Gupta, S.; De, S.; Srivastava, V.; Hussain, M.; Kumari, J.; Muniyappa, K.; Sengupta, S. RECQL4 and p53 potentiate the activity of polymerase gamma and maintain the integrity of the human mitochondrial genome. *Carcinogenesis* **2014**, *35*, 34–45.

56. Wang, J.T.; Xu, X.; Alontaga, A.Y.; Chen, Y.; Liu, Y. Impaired p32 regulation caused by the lymphoma-prone RECQ4 mutation drives mitochondrial dysfunction. *Cell Rep.* **2014**, *7*, 848–858.

57. Muta, T.; Kang, D.; Kitajima, S.; Fujiwara, T.; Hamasaki, N. p32 protein, a splicing factor 2-associated protein, is localized in mitochondrial matrix and is functionally important in maintaining oxidative phosphorylation. *J. Biol. Chem.* **1997**, *272*, 24363–24370.

58. West, A.P.; Shadel, G.S.; Ghosh, S. Mitochondria in innate immune responses. *Nat. Rev. Immunol.* **2011**, *11*, 389–402.

59. Fogal, V.; Richardson, A.D.; Karmali, P.P.; Scheffler, I.E.; Smith, J.W.; Ruoslahti, E. Mitochondrial p32 protein is a critical regulator of tumor metabolism via maintenance of oxidative phosphorylation. *Mol. Cell. Biol.* **2010**, *30*, 1303–1318.

60. Itahana, K.; Zhang, Y. Mitochondrial p32 is a critical mediator of ARF-induced apoptosis. *Cancer Cell* **2008**, *13*, 542–553.

61. Dhar, S.K.; St Clair, D.K. Nucleophosmin blocks mitochondrial localization of p53 and apoptosis. *J. Biol. Chem.* **2009**, *284*, 16409–16418.

62. Dumas, L.B.; Lussky, J.P.; McFarland, E.J.; Shampay, J. New temperature-sensitive mutants of *Saccharomyces cerevisiae* affecting DNA replication. *Mol. Gen. Genet.* **1982**, *187*, 42–46.

63. Eki, T.; Okumura, K.; Shiratori, A.; Abe, M.; Nogami, M.; Taguchi, H.; Shibata, T.; Murakami, Y.; Hanaoka, F. Assignment of the closest human homologue (DNA2L:KIAA0083) of the yeast DNA2 helicase gene to chromosome band 10q21.3-q22.1. *Genomics* **1996**, *37*, 408–410.

64. Imamura, O.; Campbell, J.L. The human Bloom syndrome gene suppresses the DNA replication and repair defects of yeast DNA2 mutants. *Proc. Natl. Acad. Sci. USA* **2003**, *100*, 8193–8198.

65. Kim, J.H.; Kim, H.D.; Ryu, G.H.; Kim, D.H.; Hurwitz, J.; Seo, Y.S. Isolation of human DNA2 endonuclease and characterization of its enzymatic properties. *Nucleic Acids Res.* **2006**, *34*, 1854–1864.

66. Lee, C.H.; Lee, M.; Kang, H.J.; Kim, D.H.; Kang, Y.H.; Bae, S.H.; Seo, Y.S. The *N*-terminal 45-kDa domain of DNA2 endonuclease/helicase targets the enzyme to secondary structure DNA. *J. Biol. Chem.* **2013**, *288*, 9468–9481.

67. Masuda-Sasa, T.; Imamura, O.; Campbell, J.L. Biochemical analysis of human DNA2. *Nucleic Acids Res.* **2006**, *34*, 1865–1875.

68. Bae, S.H.; Kim, D.W.; Kim, J.; Kim, J.H.; Kim, D.H.; Kim, H.D.; Kang, H.Y.; Seo, Y.S. Coupling of DNA helicase and endonuclease activities of yeast DNA2 facilitates Okazaki fragment processing. *J. Biol. Chem.* **2002**, *277*, 26632–26641.

69. Hu, J.; Sun, L.; Shen, F.; Chen, Y.; Hua, Y.; Liu, Y.; Zhang, M.; Hu, Y.; Wang, Q.; Xu, W.; *et al.* The intra-S phase checkpoint targets DNA2 to prevent stalled replication forks from reversing. *Cell* **2012**, *149*, 1221–1232.

70. Formosa, T.; Nittis, T. DNA2 mutants reveal interactions with DNA polymerase α and Ctf4, a Pol α accessory factor, and show that full DNA2 helicase activity is not essential for growth. *Genetics* **1999**, *151*, 1459–1470.

71. Peng, G.; Dai, H.; Zhang, W.; Hsieh, H.J.; Pan, M.R.; Park, Y.Y.; Tsai, R.Y.; Bedrosian, I.; Lee, J.S.; Ira, G.; *et al.* Human nuclease/helicase DNA2 alleviates replication stress by promoting DNA end resection. *Cancer Res.* **2012**, *72*, 2802–2813.

72. Karanja, K.K.; Cox, S.W.; Duxin, J.P.; Stewart, S.A.; Campbell, J.L. DNA2 and EXO1 in replication-coupled, homology-directed repair and in the interplay between HDR and the FA/BRCA network. *Cell Cycle* **2012**, *11*, 3983–3996.

73. Duxin, J.P.; Dao, B.; Martinsson, P.; Rajala, N.; Guittat, L.; Campbell, J.L.; Spelbrink, J.N.; Stewart, S.A. Human DNA2 is a nuclear and mitochondrial DNA maintenance protein. *Mol. Cell. Biol.* **2009**, *29*, 4274–4282.

74. Nimonkar, A.V.; Genschel, J.; Kinoshita, E.; Polaczek, P.; Campbell, J.L.; Wyman, C.; Modrich, P.; Kowalczykowski, S.C. BLM-DNA2-RPA-MRN and EXO1-BLM-RPA-MRN constitute two DNA end resection machineries for human DNA break repair. *Genes Dev.* **2011**, *25*, 350–362.

75. Daley, J.M.; Chiba, T.; Xue, X.; Niu, H.; Sung, P. Multifaceted role of the Topo IIIα-RMI1-RMI2 complex and DNA2 in the BLM-dependent pathway of DNA break end resection. *Nucleic Acids Res.* **2014**, *42*, 11083–11091.

76. Sturzenegger, A.; Burdova, K.; Kanagaraj, R.; Levikova, M.; Pinto, C.; Cejka, P.; Janscak, P. DNA2 cooperates with the WRN and BLM RecQ helicases to mediate long-range DNA end resection in human cells. *J. Biol. Chem.* **2014**, *289*, 27314–27326.

77. Lin, W.; Sampathi, S.; Dai, H.; Liu, C.; Zhou, M.; Hu, J.; Huang, Q.; Campbell, J.; Shin-Ya, K.; Zheng, L.; *et al.* Mammalian DNA2 helicase/nuclease cleaves G-quadruplex DNA and is required for telomere integrity. *EMBO J.* **2013**, *32*, 1425–1439.

78. Zheng, L.; Zhou, M.; Guo, Z.; Lu, H.; Qian, L.; Dai, H.; Qiu, J.; Yakubovskaya, E.; Bogenhagen, D.F.; Demple, B.; *et al.* Human DNA2 is a mitochondrial nuclease/helicase for efficient processing of DNA replication and repair intermediates. *Mol. Cell* **2008**. *32*, 325–336.

79. Ronchi, D.; Di Fonzo, A.; Lin, W.; Bordoni, A.; Liu, C.; Fassone, E.; Pagliarani, S.; Rizzuti, M.; Zheng, L.; Filosto, M.; *et al.* Mutations in DNA2 link progressive myopathy to mitochondrial DNA instability. *Am. J. Hum. Genet.* **2013**, *92*, 293–300.

80. Foury, F.; Kolodynski, J. PIF mutation blocks recombination between mitochondrial ρ⁺ and ρ⁻ genomes having tandemly arrayed repeat units in Saccharomyces cerevisiae. *Proc. Natl. Acad. Sci. USA* **1983**, *80*, 5345–5349.

81. Mateyak, M.K.; Zakian, V.A. Human PIF helicase is cell cycle regulated and associates with telomerase. *Cell Cycle* **2006**, *5*, 2796–2804.

82. Zhang, D.H.; Zhou, B.; Huang, Y.; Xu, L.X.; Zhou, J.Q. The human PIF1 helicase, a potential Escherichia coli RecD homologue, inhibits telomerase activity. *Nucleic Acids Res.* **2006**, *34*, 1393–1404.

83.   Futami, K.; Shimamoto, A.; Furuichi, Y. Mitochondrial and nuclear localization of human PIF1 helicase. *Biol. Pharm. Bull.* **2007**, *30*, 1685–1692.

84.   Gu, Y.; Masuda, Y.; Kamiya, K. Biochemical analysis of human PIF1 helicase and functions of its *N*-terminal domain. *Nucleic Acids Res.* **2008**, *36*, 6295–6308.

85.   George, T.; Wen, Q.; Griffiths, R.; Ganesh, A.; Meuth, M.; Sanders, C.M. Human PIF1 helicase unwinds synthetic DNA structures resembling stalled DNA replication forks. *Nucleic Acids Res.* **2009**, *37*, 6491–6502.

86.   Sanders, C.M. Human PIF1 helicase is a G-quadruplex DNA-binding protein with G-quadruplex DNA-unwinding activity. *Biochem. J.* **2010**, *430*, 119–128.

87.   Bochman, M.L.; Sabouri, N.; Zakian, V.A. Unwinding the functions of the PIF1 family helicases. *DNA Repair (Amst.)* **2010**, *9*, 237–249.

88.   Gu, Y.; Wang, J.; Li, S.; Kamiya, K.; Chen, X.; Zhou, P. Determination of the biochemical properties of full-length human PIF1 ATPase. *Prion* **2013**, *7*, 341–347.

89.   Duan, X.L.; Liu, N.N.; Yang, Y.T.; Li, H.H.; Li, M.; Dou, S.X.; Xi, X. G-quadruplexes significantly stimulate PIF1 helicase-catalyzed duplex DNA unwinding. *J. Biol. Chem.* **2015**, *290*, 7722–7735.

90.   Hou, X.M.; Wu, W.Q.; Duan, X.L.; Liu, N.N.; Li, H.H.; Fu, J.; Dou, S.X.; Li, M.; Xi, X.G. Molecular mechanism of G-quadruplex unwinding helicase: Sequential and repetitive unfolding of G-quadruplex by PIF1 helicase. *Biochem. J.* **2015**, *466*, 189–199.

91.   Zhou, R.; Zhang, J.; Bochman, M.L.; Zakian, V.A.; Ha, T. Periodic DNA patrolling underlies diverse functions of PIF1 on R-loops and G-rich DNA. *Elife* **2014**, *3*, e02190.

92.   Byrd, A.K.; Raney, K.D. A parallel quadruplex DNA is bound. Tightly but unfolded slowly by PIF1 helicase. *J. Biol. Chem.* **2015**, *290*, 6482–6494.

93.   Gagou, M.E.; Ganesh, A.; Thompson, R.; Phear, G.; Sanders, C.; Meuth, M. Suppression of apoptosis by PIF1 helicase in human tumor cells. *Cancer Res.* **2011**, *71*, 4998–5008.

94.   Gagou, M.E.; Ganesh, A.; Phear, G.; Robinson, D.; Petermann, E.; Cox, A.; Meuth, M. Human PIF1 helicase supports DNA replication and cell growth under oncogenic-stress. *Oncotarget* **2014**, *5*, 11381–11398.

95.   Cheng, X.; Ivessa, A.S. Association of the yeast DNA helicase PIF1p with mitochondrial membranes and mitochondrial DNA. *Eur. J. Cell Biol.* **2010**, *89*, 742–747.

96.   Cheng, X.; Dunaway, S.; Ivessa, A.S. The role of Pif1p, a DNA helicase in *Saccharomyces cerevisiae*, in maintaining mitochondrial DNA. *Mitochondrion* **2007**, *7*, 211–222.

97.   Bharti, S.K.; Sommers, J.A.; Zhou, J.; Kaplan, D.L.; Spelbrink, J.N.; Mergny, J.L.; Brosh, R.M., Jr. DNA sequences proximal to human mitochondrial DNA deletion breakpoints prevalent in human disease form G-quadruplexes, a class of DNA structures inefficiently unwound by the mitochondrial replicative Twinkle helicase. *J. Biol. Chem.* **2014**, *289*, 29975–29993.

98.   Budd, M.E.; Reis, C.C.; Smith, S.; Myung, K.; Campbell, J.L. Evidence suggesting that PIF1 helicase functions in DNA replication with the DNA2 helicase/nuclease and DNA polymerase delta. *Mol. Cell. Biol.* **2006**, *26*, 2490–2500.

99.   Butow, R.A.; Zhu, H.; Perlman, P.; Conrad-Webb, H. The role of a conserved dodecamer sequence in yeast mitochondrial gene expression. *Genome* **1989**, *31*, 757–760.

100. Dmochowska, A.; Kalita, K.; Krawczyk, M.; Golik, P.; Mroczek, K.; Lazowska, J.; Stepien, P.P.; Bartnik, E. A human putative SUV3-like RNA helicase is conserved between Rhodobacter and all eukaryotes. *Acta Biochim. Pol.* **1999**, *46*, 155–162.

101. Chen, P.L.; Chen, C.F.; Chen, Y.; Guo, X.E.; Huang, C.K.; Shew, J.Y.; Reddick, R.L.; Wallace, D.C.; Lee, W.H. Mitochondrial genome instability resulting from SUV3 haploinsufficiency leads to tumorigenesis and shortened lifespan. *Oncogene* **2013**, *32*, 1193–1201.

102. Wang, D.D.; Shu, Z.; Lieser, S.A.; Chen, P.L.; Lee, W.H. Human mitochondrial SUV3 and polynucleotide phosphorylase form a 330-kDa heteropentamer to cooperatively degrade double-stranded RNA with a 3'-to-5' directionality. *J. Biol. Chem.* **2009**, *284*, 20812–20821.

103. Minczuk, M.; Piwowarski, J.; Papworth, M.A.; Awiszus, K.; Schalinski, S.; Dziembowski, A.; Dmochowska, A.; Bartnik, E.; Tokatlidis, K.; Stepien, P.P.; *et al.* Localisation of the human hSUV3p helicase in the mitochondrial matrix and its preferential unwinding of dsDNA. *Nucleic Acids Res.* **2002**, *30*, 5074–5086.

104. Veno, S.T.; Kulikowicz, T.; Pestana, C.; Stepien, P.P.; Stevnsner, T.; Bohr, V.A. The human SUV3 helicase interacts with replication protein A and flap endonuclease 1 in the nucleus. *Biochem. J.* **2011**, *440*, 293–300.

105. Wang, D.D.; Guo, X.E.; Modrek, A.S.; Chen, C.F.; Chen, P.L.; Lee, W.H. Helicase SUV3, polynucleotide phosphorylase, and mitochondrial polyadenylation polymerase form a transient complex to modulate mitochondrial mRNA polyadenylated tail lengths in response to energetic changes. *J. Biol. Chem.* **2014**, *289*, 16727–16735.

106. Khidr, L.; Wu, G.; Davila, A.; Procaccio, V.; Wallace, D.; Lee, W.H. Role of SUV3 helicase in maintaining mitochondrial homeostasis in human cells. *J. Biol. Chem.* **2008**, *283*, 27064–27073.

107. Szczesny, R.J.; Obriot, H.; Paczkowska, A.; Jedrzejczak, R.; Dmochowska, A.; Bartnik, E.; Formstecher, P.; Polakowska, R.; Stepien, P.P. Down-regulation of human RNA/DNA helicase SUV3 induces apoptosis by a caspase- and AIF-dependent pathway. *Biol. Cell* **2007**, *99*, 323–332.

108. Szczesny, R.J.; Borowski, L.S.; Brzezniak, L.K.; Dmochowska, A.; Gewartowski, K.; Bartnik, E.; Stepien, P.P. Human mitochondrial RNA turnover caught in flagranti: Involvement of hSUV3p helicase in RNA surveillance. *Nucleic Acids Res.* **2010**, *38*, 279–298.

109. Pereira, M.; Mason, P.; Szczesny, R.J.; Maddukuri, L.; Dziwura, S.; Jedrzejczak, R.; Paul, E.; Wojcik, A.; Dybczynska, L.; Tudek, B.; *et al.* Interaction of human SUV3 RNA/DNA helicase with BLM helicase: Loss of the *SUV3* gene results in mouse embryonic lethality. *Mech. Ageing Dev.* **2007**, *128*, 609–617.

110. Crawford, D.R.; Wang, Y.; Schools, G.P.; Kochheiser, J.; Davies, K.J. Down-regulation of mammalian mitochondrial RNAs during oxidative stress. *Free Radic. Biol. Med.* **1997**, *22*, 551–559.

111. Desler, C.; Marcker, M.L.; Singh, K.K.; Rasmussen, L.J. The importance of mitochondrial DNA in aging and cancer. *J. Aging Res.* **2011**, *2011*, 407536.

112. Almeida, M. Aging and oxidative stress: A new look at old bone. *IBMS BoneKEy* **2010**, *7*, 340–352.

113. Siitonen, H.A.; Sotkasiira, J.; Biervliet, M.; Benmansour, A.; Capri, Y.; Cormier-Daire, V.; Crandall, B.; Hannula-Jouppi, K.; Hennekam, R.; Herzog, D.; *et al.* The mutation spectrum in RECQL4 diseases. *Eur. J. Hum. Genet.* **2009**, *17*, 151–158.

114. Carew, J.S.; Nawrocki, S.T.; Xu, R.H.; Dunner, K.; McConkey, D.J.; Wierda, W.G.; Keating, M.J.; Huang, P. Increased mitochondrial biogenesis in primary leukemia cells: The role of endogenous nitric oxide and impact on sensitivity to fludarabine. *Leukemia* **2004**, *18*, 1934–1940.

115. Lan, Q.; Lim, U.; Liu, C.S.; Weinstein, S.J.; Chanock, S.; Bonner, M.R.; Virtamo, J.; Albanes, D.; Rothman, N. A prospective study of mitochondrial DNA copy number and risk of non-Hodgkin lymphoma. *Blood* **2008**, *112*, 4247–4249.

116. D'Souza, A.D.; Parikh, N.; Kaech, S.M.; Shadel, G.S. Convergence of multiple signaling pathways is required to coordinately up-regulate mtDNA and mitochondrial biogenesis during T cell activation. *Mitochondrion* **2007**, *7*, 374–385.

117. Jeon, J.P.; Shim, S.M.; Nam, H.Y.; Baik, S.Y.; Kim, J.W.; Han, B.G. Copy number increase of 1p36.33 and mitochondrial genome amplification in Epstein-Barr virus-transformed lymphoblastoid cell lines. *Cancer Genet. Cytogenet.* **2007**, *173*, 122–130.

118. Shapovalov, Y.; Hoffman, D.; Zuch, D.; de Mesy Bentley, K.L.; Eliseev, R.A. Mitochondrial dysfunction in cancer cells due to aberrant mitochondrial replication. *J. Biol. Chem.* **2011**, *286*, 22331–22338.

119. Akiyama, T.; Dass, C.R.; Choong, P.F. Novel therapeutic strategy for osteosarcoma targeting osteoclast differentiation, bone-resorbing activity, and apoptosis pathway. *Mol. Cancer Ther.* **2008**, *7*, 3461–3469.

120. Miyazaki, T.; Mori, S.; Shigemoto, K.; Larsson, N.; Nakamura, T.; Kato, S.; Nakashima, T.; Takayanagi, H.; Tanaka, S. Maintenance of mitochondrial DNA copy number is essential for osteoclast survival. *Arthritis Res. Ther.* **2012**, *14*, 40.

121. Jeng, J.Y.; Yeh, T.S.; Lee, J.W.; Lin, S.H.; Fong, T.H.; Hsieh, R.H. Maintenance of mitochondrial DNA copy number and expression are essential for preservation of mitochondrial function and cell growth. *J. Cell. Biochem.* **2008**, *103*, 347–357.

Treatment Strategies that Enhance the Efficacy and Selectivity of Mitochondria-Targeted Anticancer Agents

Josephine S. Modica-Napolitano [1,*] and Volkmar Weissig [2]

[1] Department of Biology, Merrimack College, North Andover, MA 01845, USA
[2] Department of Pharmaceutical Sciences, Midwestern University, College of Pharmacy, Glendale, AZ 85308, USA; E-Mail: vweiss@midwestern.edu

* Author to whom correspondence should be addressed;
E-Mail: josephine.modicanapolitano@merrimack.edu

Academic Editors: Jaime M. Ross and Giuseppe Coppotelli

Abstract: Nearly a century has passed since Otto Warburg first observed high rates of aerobic glycolysis in a variety of tumor cell types and suggested that this phenomenon might be due to an impaired mitochondrial respiratory capacity in these cells. Subsequently, much has been written about the role of mitochondria in the initiation and/or progression of various forms of cancer, and the possibility of exploiting differences in mitochondrial structure and function between normal and malignant cells as targets for cancer chemotherapy. A number of mitochondria-targeted compounds have shown efficacy in selective cancer cell killing in pre-clinical and early clinical testing, including those that induce mitochondria permeability transition and apoptosis, metabolic inhibitors, and ROS regulators. To date, however, none has exhibited the standards for high selectivity and efficacy and low toxicity necessary to progress beyond phase III clinical trials and be used as a viable, single modality treatment option for human cancers. This review explores alternative treatment strategies that have been shown to enhance the efficacy and selectivity of mitochondria-targeted anticancer agents *in vitro* and *in vivo*, and may yet fulfill the clinical promise of exploiting the mitochondrion as a target for cancer chemotherapy.

Keywords: mitochondria; cancer; drug delivery systems; photodynamic therapy; combination therapy

---

1. Introduction

Despite enormous investments in the areas of basic research and medical science during the past few decades, cancer remains a leading health threat worldwide. Today in the United States alone, it is estimated that one in four adult men and one in five adult women are at risk of dying from cancer [1]. A resurgence of interest in the study of mitochondria has led to the discovery of several notable differences in the structure and function of this organelle between normal and cancer cells, and various attempts have been made to exploit these differences as novel and site specific targets for chemotherapy. Although a number of mitochondria-targeted compounds have shown some efficacy in selective cancer cell killing in pre-clinical and early clinical testing, the success of mitochondria-targeted therapeutic agents as a single modality treatment option for human cancers has been quite limited. This article presents an overview of mitochondria structure and function, especially as it relates to those differences found between normal and cancer cells, and highlights the progress made in exploiting this organelle as a target for chemotherapy. In addition, it summarizes three alternative treatment strategies that enhance the efficacy and selectivity of mitochondria-targeted anticancer agents *in vitro* and *in vivo* and offer the promise of therapeutic benefit. These include: mitochondria-targeted drug delivery systems; photodynamic therapy; and combination chemotherapy.

2. Mitochondria Structure and Function

In living cells, mitochondria are dynamic organelles comprising a network of long, filamentous structures that can be seen extending, contracting, fragmenting and fusing with one another as they move in three dimensions throughout the cytoplasm [2,3]. In electron micrographs of fixed tissue specimens, mitochondria appear as oval shaped particles similar in size to the bacterium *Escherichia coli* (1–2 microns long × 0.5–1.0 microns wide) and bound by two membranes. The outer membrane encloses the entire contents of the organelle. The inner membrane, which folds inward to form cristae, encloses the inner space, or matrix. Interestingly, the surface area of the inner mitochondrial membrane correlates with the degree of metabolic activity of the cell, and can vary considerably from cell type to cell type, or within a given cell depending upon its functional state. Mitochondria contain the enzymes and cofactors involved in a number of important metabolic reactions and pathways, including the tricarboxylic acid (TCA) cycle, oxidative phosphorylation, fatty acid degradation, the urea cycle, and gluconeogenesis. In mammalian cells, the matrix also typically contains up to 10,000 copies of a 16.6 kb closed circular double helical molecule of mitochondrial DNA (mtDNA), which is compacted *in vivo* to form a nucleoprotein complex, or nucleoid [4]. Although representing less than 1% of the total cellular DNA, mtDNA encodes two rRNAs, twenty-two tRNAs and thirteen highly hydrophobic polypeptide subunit components of four different respiratory enzyme Complexes (I, III, IV and V) that are localized to the inner mitochondrial membrane.

Mitochondria are considered the "powerhouse" of eukaryotic cells because of their central role in the process of aerobic metabolism. In carbohydrate metabolism, this begins when pyruvate, the end product of glycolysis, is transported from the cytosol into the mitochondrial matrix to undergo oxidative decarboxylation via the pyruvate dehydrogenase complex. In lipid metabolism, this begins when fatty acids are transported into the mitochondrial matrix to undergo sequential rounds of oxidative decarboxylation via the β-oxidation pathway. In either case, the resultant metabolic product is acetyl coA, which is further oxidized in the mitochondrial matrix via the TCA cycle. The net metabolic yield of the TCA cycle includes two molecules of CO_2, one molecule of GTP (the energetic equivalent of ATP), three molecules of reduced nicotinamide adenine dinucleotide (NADH), and one molecule of reduced flavin adenine dinucleotide ($FADH_2$). NADH and $FADH_2$ go on to serve as respiratory substrates for oxidative phosphorylation, which couples the oxidation of these high-energy electron donors to the synthesis of ATP. In this process, electrons are transferred from NADH and $FADH_2$ to oxygen via four multi-subunit electron transfer complexes located on the inner mitochondrial membrane. Complexes I, III and IV of the mitochondrial electron transfer chain assemble into functional supramolecular complexes, called respirasomes [5]. These three respiratory complexes also serve as proton pumps at which the energy derived from the transfer of electrons down the electron transport chain (ETC) is coupled to the translocation of protons from the matrix space outward to the space between the inner and outer mitochondrial membranes (*i.e.*, inter-membrane space). Under normal physiological conditions, the inner mitochondrial membrane is relatively impermeable to the backflow of protons and an electrochemical gradient is established across the membrane. The energy stored in this proton gradient, the proton-motive force, is then used to drive the synthesis of ATP from ADP and P_i via the inner membrane bound enzyme, mitochondrial ATP sythetase (Complex V). Oxidative phosphorylation supplies the vast majority of ATP produced by a cell under aerobic conditions.

Mitochondria are the main intracellular source of reactive oxygen species (ROS) in most tissues. It has been estimated that under physiological conditions, 1%–2% of the molecular oxygen consumed is converted to ROS molecules as a byproduct of oxidative phosphorylation [6]. ROS production can occur when a small fraction of reducing equivalents from Complex I or Complex III of the mitochondrial electron transport chain "leak" electrons directly to molecular oxygen, generating the superoxide anion O_2^-. Mitochondrial superoxide dismutase converts O_2^- to H_2O_2, which can then acquire an additional electron from a reduced transition metal to generate the highly reactive hydroxyl radical ˙OH. There is increasing evidence that Complex II can also be a major regulator of mitochondrial ROS production under physiological and pathophysiological circumstances [7,8]. ROS play an important role as signaling molecules that mediate changes in cell proliferation, differentiation, and gene transcription [9,10]. Uncontrolled ROS activity, or oxidative stress, can damage intracellular protein and lipid components, and affect the integrity of biological membranes. High levels of ROS can also damage both nuclear and mtDNA. The mitochondrial genome is especially susceptible to ROS damage due to its proximity to the site of ROS production (*i.e.*, the ETC), as well as the fact that it has no introns or protective histones and a limited capacity for DNA repair. Thus, oxidative stress can impair mitochondrial function directly at the level of mitochondrial enzyme complexes, or as a consequence of its genotoxicity to mtDNA. Severe or prolonged oxidative stress can lead to irreversible oxidative damage and cell death [11].

Mitochondria also play a key role in mediating intrinsic apoptosis, an energy dependent cell death pathway regulated by numerous positive and negative signaling factors that exist in dynamic equilibrium [12]. Distally, intrinsic apoptosis can be induced by a variety of physiological or pathological cell stressors, such as toxins, viral infections, hypoxia, hyperthermia, free radicals, and DNA damage. Proximately, the intrinsic pathway is induced by the loss of anti-apoptotic proteins, (e.g., Bcl-2 and Bcl-x) or by activation of pro-apoptotic proteins (e.g., Bax and Bak). Intrinsic apoptosis involves mitochondrial outer membrane permeabilization (MOMP), the critical, irreversible step in the pathway that commits the cell to ultimate destruction. MOMP is followed by the release of cytochrome c and other apoptogenic proteins from the mitochondrial inter-membrane space. Once released into the cytosol, these proteins activate a caspase cascade, which leads to the proteolytic cleavage of intracellular proteins, DNA degradation, formation of apoptotic bodies, and other morphological changes that are considered hallmarks of apoptotic cell death. Both the intrinsic apoptotic pathway and the extrinsic apoptotic pathway, which involves cell membrane receptor-mediated interactions, play significant roles in normal development, tissue remodeling, aging, wound healing, immune response, and maintaining homeostasis in the adult human body.

3. Some Notable Differences between Mitochondria of Cancer Cells and Normal Cells

Nearly a century has passed since Otto Warburg first observed high rates of aerobic glycolysis in a variety of tumor cell types and suggested that this phenomenon might be due to an impaired respiratory capacity in these cells [13]. Warburg's observations prompted many scientists to focus their investigative efforts on the mitochondria of cancer cells in an attempt to understand the underlying basis for the "Warburg Effect", i.e., enhanced glucose uptake, high rate of glycolysis in the presence of sufficient oxygen, and an increase in lactic acid as a byproduct of the glycolytic pathway. It is now known that at least some cancer cells possess a normal capacity for oxidative phosphorylation and can, under certain conditions, generate a majority of their ATP from this process [14–21]. In addition, recent evidence suggests that the enhanced glucose uptake and metabolic shift toward aerobic glycolysis in cancer cells is more likely due to their greater need for glucose metabolites, which serve as precursors for the biosynthesis of nucleic acids, amino acids, and lipids in these rapidly dividing cell populations [22], rather than to any specific impairment in respiratory function. In the years since Warburg's initial observations, however, a number of notable differences between the mitochondria of normal and transformed cells have been identified [23–28]. These include differences in the size, number and shape of the organelle, the rates of protein synthesis and organelle turnover, and the polypeptide and lipid profiles of the inner mitochondrial membrane. Metabolic aberrations specifically associated with mitochondrial bioenergetic function in cancer cells include differences with regard to preference for respiratory substrates, rates of electron and anion transport, calcium uptake and retention, and decreased activities of certain enzymes integral to the process of oxidative phosphorylation, such as cytochrome c oxidase [29,30], adenine nucleotide translocase [31–33], and mitochondrial ATPase [34]. The mitochondrial membrane potential has also been shown to be significantly higher in carcinoma cells than in normal epithelial cells [35–37].

Alterations in mitochondrial genome sequence have also been linked to a variety of cancers [38–40]. Some are germ-line mutations. Among these, a human polymorphic variant in the NADH dehydrogenase 3 (ND3) gene at nt 10,398 (nt G10398A) that alters the structure of Complex I in the mitochondrial ETC was associated with an increased risk for invasive breast cancer in African–American women [38,41], the A12308G mutation in tRNA$^{Leu(CUN)}$ was associated with increased risk of both renal and prostate cancers [42], and a variant in a non-coding region of mtDNA (16189T>C) was associated with increased susceptibility to endometrial cancer [43]. Somatic mutations in the mitochondrial genome are more common and have been observed in a wide variety of cancers, including ovarian, uterine, liver, lung, colon, gastric, brain, bladder, prostate, and breast cancer, melanoma and leukemia [26]. The displacement loop (or D-loop) region, a triple stranded non-coding sequence of mtDNA (np 16024-516) that houses cis regulatory elements required for replication and transcription of the molecule, has been shown to be a mutational "hot spot" in human cancer. However, mutations in genes encoding the polypeptide subunits of enzymes involved in oxidative phosphorylation also occur and can be of functional significance. Some of these are thought to be adaptive mutations that confer a selective advantage under the harsh growth conditions of the tumor microenvironment [40]. Others have been shown to be involved directly in tumor initiation and/or progression. For example, introduction of the pathogenic mtDNA *ATP6* T8993G mutation into the PC3 prostate cancer cell line through cybrid transfer produced tumors in nude mice that were 7-fold greater in size than those produced by wild-type cybrids [39]. Additionally, mutations in the mtDNA gene encoding NADH dehydrogenase subunit 6 (*ND6*) produced a deficiency in respiratory Complex I activity that was associated with an enhanced metastatic potential of tumor cells [44].

In general, tumor cells also exhibit higher levels of ROS than normal cells [9], and oxidative stress has been suggested to underlie the development and/or maintenance of the malignant phenotype. As noted previously, oxidative stress can cause somatic mutations in mtDNA. Evidence suggests that the converse is also true, *i.e.*, certain mutations in mtDNA, especially those in genes encoding ETC enzyme subunits, can cause ROS overproduction. Oncogene activation is also known to enhance the production of mitochondrial ROS, which has been implicated as a mechanism for K-RAS and MYC-mediated cell transformation [45,46]. In tumor cells, oxidative stress activates signaling pathways that promote cell growth and metastasis. One such pathway involves hypoxia-inducible factor (HIF), which regulates the transcription of a large number of genes that facilitate cell survival at low oxygen pressures [47]. Under the hypoxic conditions of tumor cell growth, mitochondria act as O_2 sensors and further enhance ROS generation as an adaptive response [48]. ROS overproduction stabilizes the HIF-α subunit, facilitating its dimerization with the HIF-β subunit. This activates a number of different genes, including those mediating a metabolic shift toward glycolysis, angiogenesis, and metastasis. ROS have also been shown to activate MAP kinase and phosphoinositide 3-kinase pathways, which are important for cell proliferation and survival [9], and to up-regulate the expression of matrix metalloproteinases (MMPs) and Snail proteins, which are involved in epithelial-to-mesenchymal transition and metastasis, respectively [49].

Inhibition of the intrinsic apoptotic pathway is also observed in a number of hematopoietic malignancies and solid tumors, and has been implicated in cancer initiation, progression and metastasis [50,51]. This is thought to occur as a result of dysregulation of mitochondrial outer membrane proteins of the Bcl-2 family, and may involve overexpression or enhanced function of anti-apoptotic proteins, under-expression or loss of function of pro-apoptotic proteins, or a combination of both. For example, malignant chronic lymphocytic leukemia (CLL) cells express high levels of anti-apoptotic Bcl-2 and low levels of pro-apoptotic proteins such as Bax [52]. Interestingly, the progression of CLL is thought to be due to reduced apoptosis rather than increased proliferation *in vivo* [53]. Overexpression of Bcl-2 has also been shown to inhibit apoptosis in prostate [54], lung, colorectal and gastric cancers [55,56], neuroblastoma, glioblastoma, and breast carcinoma cells [57]. An imbalance in the expression of the anti- and pro-apoptotic Bcl-2 family of proteins is thought to stabilize the outer mitochondrial membrane, prevent MOMP and the release of cytochrome c, and ultimately, inhibit programmed cell death. This failure of normal cell turnover contributes to cell accumulation, transformation, and survival under extreme conditions, such as the hypoxic or acidic environments common in tumors. Interestingly, the inhibition of apoptosis that results from dysregulation of Bcl-2 protein expression has also been shown to underlie the development of drug resistance in cancer cells. For example, the overexpression Bcl-XL protects murine pro-lymphocytic cells from a wide variety of apoptotic stimuli and confers a multidrug resistance phenotype [58], and drug-induced apoptosis in B-CLL cells cultured *in vitro* is inversely related to Bcl-2/Bax ratios [52].

4. Mitochondria-Targeted Drugs that Show Selective Cancer Cell Killing

During the past few decades, scientists have been exploring the possibility that certain structural and functional differences that exist between the mitochondria of normal and transformed cells might serve as targets for selective cell killing by novel and site-specific anticancer agents. Recently, the term "mitocan" (an acronym for mitochondria and cancer) has been proposed to classify mitochondria-targeted anticancer agents, especially those that induce mitochondrial destabilization [59]. A number of these compounds have shown efficacy in selective cancer cell killing in pre-clinical and early clinical testing (see Table 1 for a representative sampling).

Table 1. Representative mitochondria-targeted compounds that exhibit selective cancer cell killing.

Class	Compound	Mode of Action	Demonstrated Efficacy	References
OxPhos Inhibitors	Rhodamine 123	ATP Synthase inhibitor	Preclinical (*in vitro*, *in vivo*)	[60–62]
	Dequalinium Chloride	Complex I inhibitor	Preclinical (*in vitro*, *in vivo*)	[63,64]
	AA-1	ATP Synthase inhibitor	Preclinical (*in vitro*, *in vivo*)	[65]
	MKT-077	General inhibition of ETC enzymes	Preclinical (*in vitro*, *in vivo*) / Clinical, Phase I	[66–69]
	Metformin	Complex I inhibitor	Preclinical (*in vitro*, *in vivo*) / Clinical, Phase I	[70–89]
ROS Regulators	Elesclomol	Enhanced ROS production	Preclinical (*in vitro*, *in vivo*) / Clinical, Phase I	[90–92]
	Bezielle	Enhanced ROS production	Preclinical (*in vitro*, *in vivo*) / Clinical, Phase I	[93–99]
Intrinsic Apoptosis Inducers	ABT-737	BH3 mimetic	Preclinical (*in vitro*, *in vivo*)	[100–102]
	ABT-263 (Navitoclax)	BH3 mimetic	Preclinical (*in vitro*, *in vivo*) / Clinical, Phase I/II	[103–105]
	Gossypol	BH3 mimetic	Preclinical (*in vitro*, *in vivo*)	[106,107]
	GX15-070 (Obatoclax)	BH3 mimetic	Preclinical (*in vitro*, *in vivo*)	[108,109]
	HA14-1	BH3 mimetic	Preclinical (*in vitro*, *in vivo*)	[110,111]

Among the earliest known mitochondria-targeted anticancer agents are the delocalized lipophilic cations (DLCs). Due to their lipophilicity and positive charge, these compounds selectively accumulate in the mitochondria of carcinoma cells in response to a higher, negative inside membrane potential (e.g., approximately 160 mV in carcinoma *vs.* 100 mV in control epithelial cells) [36,37]. Several DLCs have exhibited efficacy in carcinoma cell killing *in vitro* and *in vivo* [60–69,112,113], including the class prototype Rhodamine 123 (Rh123), dequalinium chloride (DECA), and the thiopyrylium AA-1. Although all DLCs are taken up into mitochondria by a common mechanism and display dose dependent mitochondrial toxicity, their specific mechanism of action can be quite varied. For example, Rh123 and AA-1 inhibit mitochondrial ATP synthesis at the level of F0F1-ATPase activity [62,65,113], while DECA and certain DLC thiacarbocyanines interfere with NADH-ubiquinone reductase (ETC Complex I) activity [64,112]. Another DLC, the water-soluble rhodacyanine dye analogue MKT-077, was shown to cause a more generalized deleterious effect on respiratory function through membrane perturbation and consequent inhibition of membrane-bound enzymes [67]. MKT-077 was the first DLC with a favorable pharmacological and toxicological profile and showed great promise as a selective anticancer agent in preclinical studies [66]. Phase I trials were undertaken to evaluate the safety and pharmacokinetics of MKT-077, but were halted due to recurrent but reversible renal toxicity in about half of the patients treated [68]. It was determined, however, that it is feasible to target mitochondria with rhodacyanine analogues if drugs with higher therapeutic indices could be developed [69].

More recently, evidence suggests that the widely prescribed anti-diabetic biguanide derivative, metformin, may also be effective in the prevention and treatment of human cancer via inhibition of mitochondrial respiratory function. Retrospective analyses show an association between the use of metformin and diminished cancer risk, progression and mortality in diabetic patients [70–74]. *In vitro* laboratory studies demonstrate that metformin has a direct and selective inhibitory effect on breast, colon, ovary, pancreas, lung, and prostate cancer cell lines [75–79]. In addition, at doses that had no effect on the viability of non-cancer stem cells, metformin inhibited transformation and selectively killed cancer stem cells resistant to chemotherapeutic agents [80]. *In vivo*, metformin inhibits the growth of spontaneous and carcinogen-induced tumors, and impacts tumor growth in mouse xenograft and syngeneic models [81–85]. Furthermore, prospective studies investigating the therapeutic efficacy of metformin use in non-diabetic cancer patients suggest its promise for the chemoprevention of colorectal cancer and treatment of early breast cancer [86–88]. It has been postulated that the therapeutic effects of metformin may be associated with both direct (insulin-independent) and indirect (insulin-dependent) actions of the drug [74]. However, results of a recent study showed that the direct inhibition of cancer cell mitochondrial Complex I by metformin was required to decrease cell proliferation *in vitro* and tumorigenesis *in vivo* [89]. Interestingly, it has been shown that cancer cell lines harboring mutations in mtDNA encoded Complex I subunits or having impaired glucose utilization exhibit enhanced biguanide sensitivity when grown under the low glucose conditions seen in the tumor microenvironment [114]. Metformin is a very safe and well-tolerated drug that is now prescribed to almost 120 million people in the world for the treatment of type II diabetes. Clinical trials using metformin alone and in combination with conventional anticancer agents in non-diabetic patients are ongoing and should clarify its potential use in cancer therapy.

Mitochondria-targeted ROS regulators have also shown efficacy as anticancer agents. Although the generally higher endogenous levels of ROS in tumor *versus* normal cells contribute to the development and/or maintenance of the malignant phenotype, they also render cancer cells more vulnerable to irreversible oxidative damage and consequent cell death. Therefore, pro-oxidant pharmacological agents that either enhance ROS production or inhibit ROS scavenging activity have the potential to increase ROS level beyond the threshold of lethality in cancer cells while leaving normal cells viable [115].

One such compound that targets mitochondria is elesclomol (STA-4783), an investigational, first-in-class small molecule that has been shown to enhance ROS production and induce a transcriptional gene profile characteristic of an oxidative stress response *in vitro*. Interestingly, the antioxidant *N*-acetylcysteine blocks elesclomol induced gene expression and apoptosis, indicating that ROS generation is the primary mechanism of cytotoxicity of the drug [115]. Comparative growth assays using the yeast model *S. cerevisiae* demonstrated that elesclomol interacts with the mitochondrial ETC to generate high levels of ROS and induce apoptosis [90]. In the same study, elesclomol was shown to interact similarly with the ETC in human melanoma cells. Elesclomol was granted fast-track designation by the FDA in 2006 for the treatment of metastatic melanoma. A randomized, double-blind, controlled SYMMETRY study evaluating the combination of paclitaxel and elesclomol in patients with advanced melanoma was stopped after all patients were enrolled because the addition of elesclomol to paclitaxel did not significantly improve progression free survival in unselected patients [91]. Studies are ongoing to determine the effect of elesclomol treatment alone and in combination with paclitaxel in patients with acute myeloid leukemia, and ovarian cancer [92].

Bezielle (BZL101), an aqueous extract from the herb *Scutellaria barbata*, is another ROS regulator that displays selective cytotoxicity against a variety of cancers *in vitro* and *in vivo* [93–95]. Early studies showed that in tumor cells, but not in non-transformed cells, Bezielle induces ROS production and causes severe DNA damage followed by hyperactivation of PARP-1, depletion of the cellular ATP and NAD, inhibition of glycolysis, and cell death [96]. It was later shown that treatment of tumor cells with Bezielle induces progressively higher levels of both mitochondrial superoxide and peroxide type ROS, and that Bezielle inhibits oxidative phosphorylation [97]. In addition, tumor cells lacking functional mitochondria did not generate mitochondrial superoxide and were protected from cell death in the presence of Bezielle, supporting the hypothesis that mitochondria are the primary target of the compound [97]. Bezielle has shown promising efficacy and excellent safety in the early phase clinical trials for advanced breast cancer [98,99].

Mitochondria-targeted compounds that induce outer membrane permeabilization and intrinsic apoptosis in cancer cells also show potential as anti-cancer agents. As previously discussed, BCL-2 family proteins, which share one or more of the four BCL-2 homology domains (BH1–BH4), regulate the intrinsic apoptotic pathway. Anti-apoptotic members of the family (such as BCL-2, BCL-X$_L$, BCL-W and MCL-1), which are overexpressed in many cancers, function by sequestering the pro-apoptotic executioners of the MOMP (such as BAX and BAK). Inhibition of programmed cell death is antagonized by BH3-only proteins, a BCL-2 protein subfamily comprised of only the α-helical BH3 domain. These small proteins interact with anti-apoptotic molecules in their BH3-binding groove, causing the release and activation of BAX/BAK and inducing apoptosis [116]. Certain small molecules mimic the effect of BH3-only proteins. Among these BH3 mimetics, the synthetically derived ABT-737 has been shown to induce BAX/BAK-dependent apoptosis in a variety of cancer cell lines *in vitro*, and to display antitumor effects as a single agent *in vivo* [100–102]. Navitoclax (ABT-263), a potent, orally bioavailable analog of ABT-737 with similar biological activity, was shown to elicit complete tumor regression in small cell lung cancer (SCLC) and acute lymphoblastic leukemia xenograft models [103]. A phase I clinical study investigating the single-agent activity of navitoclax in the treatment of recurrent SCLC yielded encouraging preliminary safety and efficacy data [104]. However, in a subsequent phase II study navitoclax treatment induced only a low positive response and was limited by a dose-dependent and clinically significant thrombocytopenia [105]. Since both ABT-737 and navitoclax have been shown to potentiate the efficacy of standard cytotoxic agents against a variety of cancers [103,117–121], combinatorial regimens may ultimately prove a more promising therapeutic strategy for these compounds. Pre-clinical and clinical studies have shown that several other BH3 mimetics, such as the natural polyphenolic compound gossypol, and the synthetic compounds GX15-070 (obatoclax) and HA14-1 (ethyl 2-amino-6-bromo-4-(1-cyano-2-ethoxy-2-oxoethyl)-4*H*-chromene-3-carboxylate), also demonstrate anti-cancer activity, supporting the therapeutic potential of this class of mitochondria-targeted agents in the treatment of human cancer [106–111].

5. Alternative Treatment Strategies that Enhance the Efficacy and Selectivity of Mitochondria-Targeted Anticancer Agents

The fact that several mitochondria-targeted compounds have exhibited potent cancer cell killing in pre-clinical and early clinical studies is encouraging, and further research and testing of these compounds as viable, single modality treatment options for human cancers is warranted. However, the current limitations of this approach suggest the need also to explore the use of alternative treatment strategies in an effort to improve the efficacy and selectivity of these anticancer agents. Presented below (and summarized in Table 2) are three treatment strategies that have been shown *in vitro* and *in vivo* to enhance the selective cancer cell killing of several compounds known to have direct or indirect effects on mitochondrial function. It is proposed that by expanding the application of these strategies to include additional mitochondria-targeted compounds already known to exhibit significant preclinical and clinical anticancer activity as single agents (e.g., oxidative phosphorylation inhibitors, ROS regulators, and apoptosis inducers), the therapeutic efficacy of these compounds might also be improved.

Table 2. Treatment strategies that have been shown to enhance the efficacy and selectivity of anticancer agents.

Strategy	Carrier/Class	Anticancer Agent	References
Mitochondria-Targeted Drug Delivery Systems	TPP+-conjugated molecules	Vitamin E succinate	[122,123]
		Coenzyme Q	[124]
	DQAsomes	Paclitaxel	[125–127]
		Curcumin	[128]
		Resveratrol	[129]
	STPP+ liposomes	Paclitaxel	[130,131]
		Doxorubicin	[132]
	Mito-targeted nanontubes	Platinum (IV)	[133]
Photodynamic Therapy	Cationic photosensitizers	EDKC	[134]
		Rh123	[135]
		MKT-077	[136]
	Non-cationic photosensitizers	Pba	[137–143]
		BBr2	[144]
Combination Chemotherapy	Inhibitors of glycolysis and oxidative phosphorylation	2-DG plus metformin	[145,146]
	Inhibitors of two or more mitochondrial target sites	AZT plus MKT-077	[147]

5.1. Mitochondria-Targeted Drug Delivery Systems

Over the past several decades, attempts have been made to develop mitochondriotropic drug delivery systems for a variety of therapeutic purposes. One early strategy employed mitochondrial protein-import machinery to deliver macromolecules to mitochondria. For example, a mitochondrial signal sequence was used to direct green fluorescent protein to mitochondria to allow the visualization of mitochondria within living cells [148]. Another strategy employed conjugation with well-established mitochondriotropic cations, such as triphenylphosphonium (TPP$^+$) to successfully target low-molecular weight molecules to mammalian mitochondria. These molecules rapidly permeate lipid bilayers and, in response to the plasma and mitochondrial membrane potentials (negative inside), accumulate several hundredfold inside the organelle. One study demonstrated that significant doses of the TPP-conjugated antioxidants coenzyme Q or vitamin E could be fed safely to mice over long periods, and achieve steady-state distributions within the heart, brain, liver, and muscle [149]. These results showed that mitochondria-targeted bioactive molecules can be administered orally, leading to their accumulation at potentially therapeutic concentrations in those tissues most affected by mitochondrial dysfunction. More recently, mitochondria-targeted, TPP-conjugated vitamin E succinate has been shown to act preferentially on cancer cells, suppressing mitochondrial function and mtDNA transcription and blocking proliferation at low concentrations [122], and inducing apoptosis at higher concentrations [123]. In another study, Mito-Q (coenzyme-Q conjugated to an alkyl triphenylphosphonium cation) and Mito-CP (a 5-membered nitroxide, CP, conjugated to a TPP cation) potently inhibited the proliferation of breast cancer cells (MCF-7 and MDA-MB-231) [124] and human colon cancer cells (HCT-116) [45], further demonstrating the anticancer potential of TPP-conjugated molecules.

A quantitative structure activity relationship (QSAR) model was developed to facilitate guided synthesis and selection of optimal mitochondriotropic structures [150]. In theory, any compound that acts on mitochondria can be chemically modified to become mitochondriotropic. However, there are limitations to this strategy. First, not all potentially therapeutic compounds with molecular targets at or inside mammalian mitochondria find their way to mitochondria once inside a cell. This is because the intracellular distribution of a low-molecular weight compound is strongly affected not only by its own physico-chemical properties, but also by the cytoskeletal network, dissolved macromolecules, and dispersed organelles. Furthermore, any chemical modification that renders a compound mitochondriotropic may adversely affect its inherent pharmacological activity. In contrast, pharmaceutical nanocarriers offer an alternative approach to improve the intracellular disposition of potentially therapeutic compounds. The benefit of this strategy is that all chemistry can be carried out on the components of the nanocarrier, leaving the pharmacological profile of the compound unaltered [151]. Furthermore, nanocarrier delivery can overcome several limitations for the therapeutic use of free compounds, such as lack of water solubility, non-specific biodistribution and targeting, and low therapeutic indices.

The idea that nanocarriers could serve as effective mitochondria-targeted drug delivery systems arose in the late 1990s with the accidental discovery of the vesicle-forming capacity of dequalinium chloride, a cationic bolaamphiphile comprising two quinaldinium rings linked by ten methylene groups [152]. The compound was found to self-assemble into liposome-like vesicles, called DQAsomes (DeQAlinium-based lipoSOMES), and to have a strong affinity for mitochondria [153,154]. Follow-up studies confirmed the suitability of DQAsomes for the delivery of bioactive compounds to mitochondria, and DQAsomes are now considered the prototype for all vesicular mitochondria-specific nanocarriers [155]. *In vitro* and *in vivo* studies have shown that DQAsomal preparations of the anticancer agent paclitaxel increase the solubility of the drug by a factor of 3000, and enhance its efficiency in triggering apoptosis by direct action on mitochondria [125–127]. More recently, DQAsomes have been used for the pulmonary delivery of curcumin [128], a potent antioxidant with anti-inflammatory and potential anticancer properties. Due to its water-insolubility, however, curcumin's bioavailability following oral administration is extremely low. Curcumin encapsulated into DQAsomes displays enhanced antioxidant activity in comparison to the free compound.

Interestingly, a mitochondria-targeting drug delivery system in which dequalinium chloride has been covalently linked to the hydrophilic distal end of polyethylene glycol-distearoylphosphatidylethanolamine (DQA-PEG(2000)-DSPE) has also been prepared [129]. These nanocarriers were used to deliver resveratrol to mitochondria in human lung adenocarcinoma A549 cells, resistant A549/cDDP cells, A549 and A549/cDDP tumor spheroids as well as the xenografted resistant A549/cDDP cancers in nude mice. Results demonstrated that the mitochondrial targeting of resveratrol induced apoptosis in both non-resistant and resistant cancer cells by dissipating the mitochondria membrane potential, releasing cytochrome c and increasing the activities of caspase 9 and 3 [129]. DQAsomes have also been used to deliver an artificial mini-mitochondrial genome construct encoding Green Fluorescence Protein (GFP) to the mitochondrial compartment of a mouse macrophage cell line resulting in the expression of GFP mRNA and protein [156]. Though the transfection efficiency for GFP was very low this work constitutes the very first reported successful transgene expression inside mitochondria within living mammalian cells.

Conventional liposomes are another type of pharmaceutical nanocarrier that can also be rendered mitochondria-specific via the surface attachment of known mitochondriotropic residues, such as the cation TPP [157–160]. Preparation of liposomes in the presence of hydrophilic molecules, which have been artificially hydrophobized via linkage to fatty acid or phospholipid derivatives, results in the covalent "anchoring" of the hydrophilic moiety to the liposomal surface [161,162]. In 2005, TPP cations were conjugated to stearyl residues (yielding stearyl-TPP, or STPP), and STPP-bearing liposomes were first shown to exhibit *in vitro* mitochondriotropism [157]. The same group later demonstrated that surface modification of nanocarriers with mitochondriotropic TPP cations facilitates the efficient subcellular delivery of a model compound, ceramide, to mitochondria of mammalian cells and improves its cytotoxic and pro-apoptotic activities *in vitro* and *in vivo* [158]. More recently, STPP liposomes have been used as nanocarriers to enhance the efficacy of mitochondria-targeted anticancer agents. For example, paclitaxel loaded STPP liposomes were shown to co-localize with mitochondria and to significantly increase cytotoxicity by paclitaxel in a drug resistant ovarian carcinoma cell line [130]. The improvement in cytotoxicity was found to result from the increased accumulation of paclitaxel in mitochondria, as well as from the specific toxicity of STPP towards the resistant cell line. Mechanistic studies revealed that the cytotoxicity of STPP was associated with a decrease in mitochondrial membrane potential and other hallmarks related to caspase-independent cell death. Interestingly, mitochondriotropic STPP liposomes can be made to exhibit even greater cancer cell specificity with the addition of another ligand, folic acid. Cancer cell-specific targeting via surface modification with these dual ligands has been shown to enhance the cellular and mitochondrial delivery of doxorubicin in KB cells, and produce a synergistic effect on ROS production and cytotoxicity in this tumor cell line [132].

The preparation of TPP-surface modified liposomes utilizing an alternative hydrophobic anchor for TPP cations has also been described. For example, a d-alpha-tocopheryl polyethylene glycol 1000 succinate-triphenylphosphine conjugate (TPGS1000-TPP) was synthesized as the mitochondrial targeting molecule and incorporated into the membranes of paclitaxel-loaded liposomes [131]. The paclitaxel loaded TPGS1000-TPP conjugated liposomes were shown to selectively accumulate in the mitochondria. This targeted delivery of paclitaxel caused the release of cytochrome c, initiated a cascade of caspase 9 and 3 reactions, and enhanced apoptosis by activating pro-apoptotic pathways and inhibiting anti-apoptotic pathways. In comparison with taxol and regular paclitaxel liposomes, the mitochondria targeted paclitaxel liposomes exhibited the strongest anticancer efficacy against drug resistant lung cancer cells *in vitro* and in a nude mouse xenograft model *in vivo*, suggesting a potential therapeutic treatment for drug-resistant lung cancer.

A number of other TPP^+ modified nanocarriers have shown promise as effective mitochondrial specific drug delivery systems. One novel mitochondriotropic nanocarrier based on an oligolysine scaffold with the addition of two triphenylphosphonium cations per oligomer, and another based on a 5 poly(amidoamine) dendrimer conjugated with TPP^+, were shown to be efficiently taken up by cells and display a high degree of mitochondrial specificity [163,164]. A TPP-conjugated, mitochondria-targeted nano delivery system for coenzyme Q10 (CoQ10) has also been shown to reach mitochondria and to deliver CoQ10 in adequate quantities [165]. The multifunctional nanocarrier is composed of poly(ethylene glycol), polycaprolactone and triphenylphosphonium bromide and was synthesized using a combination of click chemistry with ring-opening polymerization followed by self-assembly into nanosized micelles. A potential disadvantage of this system, however, is the localization of the mitochondrial targeting moiety, which is seated between the two polymers, *i.e.*, between the poly(ethylene glycol) and polycaprolactone units. In a different approach, TPP^+ was linked to the PEG side of a PLGA-PEG-based block copolymer, thereby enhancing the availability of the targeting moiety for any potential interaction with mitochondrial membranes [166]. In a follow-up study, Zinc phtalocyanine (ZnPc) was encapsulated inside PLGA-b-PEG-TPP polymer nanoparticles. By targeting ZnPc to the mitochondria, singlet oxygen was locally produced inside the mitochondria to effectively initiate apoptosis [167]. Interestingly, TPP-conjugated poly(ethylene imine) hyperbranched polymer nanoassemblies were also shown to successfully deliver doxorubicin to the mitochondria of human prostate carcinomas cells and cause rapid and severe cytotoxicity within few hours of incubation, even at sub-micromolar incubation concentrations [168].

The mitochondrial cationic dye, rhodamine-110, has also been used for rendering carbon nanotubes (CNTs) mitochondriotropic. In one study, multi-walled carbon nanotubes (MWCNTs) were functionalized with either mitochondrial-targeting fluorescent rhodamine-110 (MWCNT-Rho) or non-targeting fluorescein (MWCNT-Fluo) as a control [133]. Results demonstrated that MWCNT-Rho co-localized well with mitochondria (*ca.* 80% co-localization) in contrast to MWCNT-Fluo, which showed poor association with mitochondria (*ca.* 21% co-localization). In addition, platinum (IV), a prodrug of cis-platin, displayed significantly enhanced cytotoxicity towards several cancer cell lines when incorporated into mitochondria-targeted carbon nanotubes in comparison to non-targeted formulations [133]. MWCNTs have also been functionalized with peptides having a mitochondria-targeted peptide sequence (MTS). The association of such MWCNT-MTS conjugates with mitochondria inside murine macrophages and HeLa cells has been confirmed by wide-field epifluorescence microscopy, confocal laser scanning microscopy and transmission electron microscopy (TEM). The localization of the MTS-MWCNT conjugates with mitochondria was further confirmed by analyzing the isolated organelles using TEM [169]. The use of nanoparticles for the delivery of small molecule anticancer agents has thus shown past success and holds much promise for further development and therapeutic application.

5.2. Photodynamic Therapy

Photodynamic therapy (PDT) involves the use of a photoreactive drug, or photosensitizer, that is selectively taken up or retained by target cells or tissues. Upon administration of light of a specific wavelength, the photosensitizer becomes activated from a ground state to an excited state. As the photosensitizer returns to the ground state, the energy is transferred to molecular oxygen, thus generating ROS and inducing cellular toxicity in the particular areas of tissue that have been exposed to light [170]. There has been considerable interest in PDT as a treatment modality for a variety of cancers [170,171]. Photofrin, which was first used in PDT in 1993 for the prophylactic treatment of bladder cancer, is the most common photosensitizer in clinical use today. However, a number of other photosensitizers have been approved for clinical use or have undergone clinical testing to treat cancers of the head and neck, brain, lung, pancreas, intraperitoneal cavity, breast, prostate and skin. The selectivity of a photosensitizer and its site of action within a cell contribute to the efficacy of PDT. Evidence suggests that subcellular localization is more important than photochemical reactivity in terms of overall cell killing, and that mitochondrial localization represents a highly desirable property for the development of highly specific and efficient photosensitizers for photodynamic therapy applications [172].

Cationic photosensitizers are particularly promising as potential PDT agents. Like other DLCs, these compounds are concentrated by cells and into mitochondria in response to negative-inside transmembrane potentials, and are thus selectively accumulated in the mitochondria of carcinoma cells. In combination with localized photoirradiation, the cationic photosensitizer can be converted to a reactive and highly toxic species, thus enhancing its selectivity for and toxicity to carcinoma cells, and providing a means of highly specific tumor cell killing without injury to normal cells. Several cationic photosensitizers have shown promise for use in PDT. For example, selective photoxicity of carcinomas *in vitro* and *in vivo* has been observed for a series of triarylmethane derivatives [173] and the kryptocyanine EDKC [134]. Both Rh123 and the chalcogenapyrylium dye 8b have been evaluated as photosensitizers for the photochemotherapy of malignant gliomas [135,174]. In another study, photoactivation of the selective anticancer agent MKT-077 was shown to enhance its mitochondrial toxicity [136]. As expected, the mechanisms of mitochondrial toxicity exhibited by these compounds are varied, and range from specific inhibition of mitochondrial enzymes to non-specific perturbation of mitochondrial function due to singlet oxygen production.

Non-cationic photosensitizers that target mitochondria have also shown promise for use in PDT. Pheophorbide a (Pba), is a chlorophyll breakdown product isolated from silkworm excreta and the Chinese medicinal herb, Scutellaria barbata [137,175]. Because Pba absorbs light at longer wavelengths than the first-generation photosensitizer photofrin, tissue penetration is enhanced. Pba has been shown to accumulate in mitochondria and cause apoptosis in a variety of cancer cells, including leukemia, and uterine, breast, pancreatic, colon and hepatocellular carcinoma [137–143]. *In vivo* animal studies have supported the efficacy of Pba-PDT in preventing tumor cell growth. [139,143]. In addition, the tetra-aryl brominated porphyrin and the corresponding diaryl derivative are also promising sensitizers with good photodynamic properties that have the ability to accumulate in mitochondria and induce cell death in human melanoma and colorectal adenocarcinoma *in vitro* and *in vivo* [144]. These results have positive implications for the use of mitochondria-targeted PDT compounds in cancer therapy.

5.3. Combination Chemotherapy

As noted previously, the two major pathways for cellular ATP production are glycolysis and mitochondrial oxidative phosphorylation. The high rate of aerobic glycolysis in cancer cells makes them particularly vulnerable to chemotherapeutic agents that inhibit glycolytic enzymes. For example, 2-deoxy-D-glucose (2DG), 3-bromopyruvate (3-BrPA), and lonidamine, which inhibit the hexokinase (HK) catalyzed first step in glycolysis, each have demonstrated significant anticancer activity against a variety of cell types *in vitro* and *in vivo* [176–181]. Unfortunately, the therapeutic efficacy of these compounds as single agents appears to be quite limited. Perhaps this is due to the fact that many cancer cells have functionally competent mitochondria and can overcome inhibition of the glycolytic pathway by increasing mitochondrial ATP production.

Recent evidence suggests that combination chemotherapy, simultaneously aimed at both glycolytic and mitochondrial pathways for ATP production, can be a more effective chemotherapeutic approach for the selective cytotoxicity of cancer cells. In one study [145], the *in vitro* antitumor activity 2DG alone was found insufficient to promote tumor cell death in human breast cancer and osteosarcoma cell lines, reflecting its limited efficacy in clinical trials. However, the combination of 2DG and metformin led to significant cell death associated with a decrease in cellular ATP. Gene expression analysis and functional assays revealed that metformin compromised OXPHOS. Furthermore, forced energy restoration with methyl pyruvate reversed the cell death induced by 2DG and metformin, suggesting a critical role of energetic deprivation in the underlying mechanism of cell death. The combination of 2DG and metformin also inhibited tumor growth and metastasis in mouse xenograft tumor models [145]. In another study, the combination of 2DG and metformin was shown to inhibit both mitochondrial respiration and glycolysis in prostate cancer cells leading to a severe depletion in cellular ATP. This combination of drugs induced a 96% inhibition of cell viability in LNCaP prostate cancer cells, a cytotoxic effect that was much greater than that induced by treatment with either drug alone. In contrast, only a moderate effect by the combination of 2DG and metformin on cell viability was observed in normal prostate epithelial cells [146].

The selective tumor cell killing by mitochondria-targeted DLCs can also be enhanced by combination with anticancer agents having alternative mitochondria target sites. For example, 3-azido deoxythymidine (AZT) as a single agent was found to induce a dose-dependent inhibition of cell growth of several human carcinoma cells, yet cause no significant effect on the growth of control epithelial cells [147]. Combination treatment employing a constant concentration of a delocalized lipophilic cation (dequalinium chloride or MKT-077) plus varying concentrations of AZT enhanced the AZT-induced cytotoxicity of carcinoma cells up to four-fold. The drug combination of constant DLC and varying AZT had no significant effect on the growth of control cells. Furthermore, clonogenic assays demonstrated up to 20-fold enhancement of selective carcinoma cell killing by combination *vs.* single agent treatment, depending on the specific drug combination and concentrations used. It was hypothesized that the efficacy of the AZT/DLC drug combination in carcinoma cell killing may be based on a dual selectivity involving inhibition of mitochondrial energy metabolism and inhibition of DNA synthesis due to limited deoxythymidine monophosphate availability [147].

Although limited in scope and number, the results of these drug combination studies are encouraging. More importantly, they suggest that additional studies should be undertaken to assess the anticancer activity of novel combinations of metabolic inhibitors targeting both major pathways of ATP production, and of novel combinations of compounds that target different sites in mitochondria.

6. Summary and Concluding Remarks

A persistent challenge in cancer therapy is to find ways to improve the efficacy and selectivity of a therapeutic compound while minimizing its systemic toxicity and treatment-limiting side effects. The central role that mitochondria play in the life and death of a cell, together with the many differences found to exist between the mitochondria of normal and transformed cells, make them prime targets for anticancer agents. However, despite the fact that a number of mitochondria-targeted compounds have exhibited potent and selective cancer cell killing in preclinical and early clinical testing, currently none has achieved the standards for high selectivity and efficacy and low toxicity necessary to progress beyond phase III clinical trials and to be used as a viable, single modality treatment option for human cancers. The limitations of this approach suggest the need to explore the use of alternative treatment strategies to enhance the efficacy and selectivity of mitochondria-targeted anticancer agents. Mitochondria-targeted drug delivery systems, photodynamic therapy, and combination chemotherapy are three strategies that have been shown to enhance the efficacy and selectivity of certain mitochondria-targeted anticancer agents *in vitro* and *in vivo*. These strategies enhance the effects of potential therapeutic agents either by delivering them directly to the site of action (mitochondria-targeted drug delivery systems), or by increasing their potency once they have reached their target site (PDT, combination chemotherapy). It is proposed that by expanding the application of these strategies to include additional mitochondria-targeted compounds that have already demonstrated significant preclinical and clinical anticancer activity as single agents, including but not limited to those summarized in this review, the therapeutic efficacy of these compounds might also be improved. New and ongoing research in this area is warranted, and may yet fulfill the clinical promise of exploiting the mitochondrion as a target for cancer chemotherapy.

Author Contributions

This review was a joint effort between Josephine S. Modica-Napolitano and Volkmar Weissig. Both contributed to the development, research and writing of the article.

References

1. American Cancer Society. Lifetime Risk of Developing or Dying from Cancer. Available online: http://www.cancer.org/cancer/cancerbasics/lifetime-probability-of-developing-or-dying-from-cancer (accessed on 18 June 2015).

2. Chen, H.; Chan, D.C. Emerging functions of mammalian mitochondrial fusion and fission. *Hum. Mol. Genet.* **2005**, *14*, R283–R289.

3. Mishra, P.; Chan, D.C. Mitochondrial dynamics and inheritance during cell division, development and disease. *Nat. Rev. Mol. Cell Biol.* **2014**, *15*, 634–646.

4. Kukat C.; Larsson, N.G. mtDNA makes a U-turn for the mitochondrial nucleoid. *Trends Cell Biol.* **2013**, *23*, 457–463.

5. Shagger, H.; Pfeiffer, K. Supercomplexes in the respiratory chains of yeast and mammalian mitochondria. *EMBO J.* **2000**, *19*, 1777–1783.

6. Ott, M.; Gogvadze, V.; Orrenius, S.; Zhivotovsky, B. Mitochondria, oxidative stress and cell death. *Apoptosis* **2007**, *12*, 913–922.

7. Quinlan, C.L.; Orr, A.L.; Perevoshchikova, I.V.; Treberg, J.R.; Ackrell, B.A.; Brand, M.D. Mitochondrial Complex II can generate reactive oxygen species at high rates in both the forward and reverse reactions. *J. Biol. Chem.* **2012**, *287,* 27255–27264.

8. Drose, S. Differential effects of Complex II on mitochondrial ROS production and their relation to cardioprotective pre- and post-conditioning. *Biochim. Biophys. Acta* **2013**, *1827*, 578–587.

9. Weinberg, F.; Chandel, N.S. Reactive oxygen species-dependent signaling regulates cancer. *Cell. Mol. Life Sci.* **2009**, *66*, 3663–3673.

10. Kamata, H.; Hirata, H. Redox regulation of cellular signalling. *Cell Signal.* **1999**, *11*, 1–14.

11. Lee, Y.J.; Shacter, E. Oxidative stress inhibits apoptosis in human lymphoma cells. *J. Biol. Chem.* **1999**, *274*, 19792–19798.

12. Elmore, S. Apoptosis: A review of programmed cell death. *Toxicol. Pathol.* **2007**, *35*, 495–516.

13. Warburg, O.; Dickens, F. *The Metabolism of Tumors*; Arnold Constable: London, UK, 1930.

14. Fan, J.; Kamphorst, J.J.; Mathew, R.; Chung, M.K.; White, E.; Shlomi, T.; Rabinowitz, J.D. Glutamine-driven oxidative phosphorylation is a major ATP source in transformed mammalian cells in both normoxia and hypoxia. *Mol. Syst. Biol.* **2013**, *9*, 712.

15. Tan, A.S.; Baty, J.W.; Dong, L.F.; Bezawork-Geleta, A.; Endaya, B.; Goodwin, J.; Bajzikova, M.; Kovarova, J.; Peterka, M.; Yan, B.; *et al.* Mitochondrial genome acquisition restores respiratory function and tumorigenic potential of cancer cells without mitochondrial DNA. *Cell Metab.* **2015**, *21*, 81–94.

16. LeBleu, V.S.; O'Connell, J.T.; Gonzalez Herrera, K.N.; Wikman-Kocher, H.; Pantel, K.; Haigis, M.C.; de Carvalho, F.M.; Damascena, A.; Domingos Chinen, L.T.; Rocha, R.M.; *et al.* PGC-1 mediates mitochondrial biogenesis and oxidative phosphorylation to promote metastasis. *Nat. Cell Biol.* **2014**, *16*, 992–1015.

17. Viale, A.; Pettazzoni, P.; Lyssiotis, C.A.; Ying, H.; Sánchez, N.; Marchesini, M.; Carugo, A.; Green, T.; Seth, S.; Giuliani, V.; *et al.* Oncogene ablation-resistant pancreatic cancer cells depend on mitochondrial function. *Nature* **2014**, *514*, 628–632.

18. Lu, C.L.; Qin, L.; Liu, H.C.; Candas, D.; Fan, M.; Li, J.J. Tumor cells switch to mitochondrial oxidative phosphorylation under radiation via mTOR-mediated hexokinase II inhibition—A Warburg-reversing effect. *PLoS ONE* **2015**, *10*, e0121046.

19. Guppy, M.; Leedman, P.; Zu, X.L.; Russell, V. Contribution by different fuels and metabolic pathways to the total ATP turnover of proliferating MCF-7 breast cancer cells. *Biochem. J.* **2002**, *364*, 309–315.

20. Lagadinou, E.D.; Sach, A.; Callahan, K.; Rossi, R.M.; Neering, S.J.; Minhajuddin, M.; Ashton, J.M.; Pei, S.; Grose, V.; O'Dwyer, K.M.; *et al.* Bcl-2 inhibition targets oxidative phosphorylation and selectively eradicates quiescent human leukemia stem cells. *Cell Stem Cell* **2013**, *12*, 329–341.

21. Vlashi, E.; Lagadec, C.; Vergnes, L.; Matsutani, T.; Masui, K.; Poulou, M.; Popescu, R.; Della Donna, L.; Evers, P.; Dekmezian, C.; *et al.* Metabolic state of glioma stem cells and nontumorigenic cells. *Proc. Natl. Acad. Sci. USA* **2011**, *108*, 16062–16067.

22. Vander Heiden, M.G.; Lunt, S.Y.; Dayton, T.L.; Fiske, B.P.; Israelsen, W.J.; Mattaini, K.R.; Vokes, N.I.; Stephanopoulos, G.; Cantley, L.C.; Metallo, C.M.; *et al.* Metabolic pathway alterations that support cell proliferation. *Cold Spring Harb. Symp. Quant. Biol.* **2011**, *76*, 325–334.

23. Pedersen, P.L. Tumor mitochondria and the bioenergetics of cancer cells. *Prog. Exp. Tumor Res.* **1978**, *22*, 190–274.

24. Modica-Napolitano, J.S.; Singh, K.K. Mitochondria as targets for detection and treatment of cancer. *Expert Rev. Mol. Med.* **2002**, *4*, 1–19.

25. Modica-Napolitano, J.S.; Singh, K.K. Mitochondrial dysfunction in cancer. *Mitochondrion* **2004**, *4*, 755–762.

26. Modica-Napolitano, J.S.; Kulawiec, M.; Singh, K.K. Mitochondria and human cancer. *Curr. Mol. Med.* **2007**, *7*, 121–31.

27. Kroemer, G. Mitochondria in cancer. *Oncogene* **2006**, *25*, 4630–4632.

28. Fogg, V.C.; Lanning, N.J.; MacKeigan, J.P. Mitochondria in cancer: At the crossroads of life and death. *Chin. J. Cancer* **2011**, *30*, 526–539.

29. Modica-Napolitano, J.S.; Touma, S.E. Functional differences in mitochondrial enzymes from normal epithelial and carcinoma cells. In *Mitochondrial Dysfunction in Pathogenesis*; Keystone Symposia: Silverthorne, CO, USA, 2000.

30. Sun, A.S.; Sepkowitz, K.; Geller, S.A. A study of some mitochondrial and peroxisomal enzymes in human colonic adenocarcinoma. *Lab. Investig.* **1981**, *44*, 13–17.

31. Chan, S.H.; Barbour, R.L. Adenine nucleotide transport in hepatoma mitochondria. Characterization of factors influencing the kinetics of ADP and ATP uptake. *Biochim. Biophys. Acta* **1983**, *723*, 104–113.

32. Sul, H.S.; Shrago, E.; Goldfarb, S.; Rose, F. Comparison of the adenine nucleotide translocase in hepatomas and rat liver mitochondria. *Biochim. Biophys. Acta* **1979**, *551*, 148–155.

33. Woldegiorgis, G.; Shrago, E. Adenine nucleotide translocase activity and sensitivity to inhibitors in hepatomas. Comparison of the ADP/ATP carrier in mitochondria and in a purified reconstituted liposome system. *J. Biol. Chem.* **1985**, *260*, 7585–7590.

34. Pedersen, P.L.; Morris, H.P. Uncoupler-stimulated adenosine triphosphatase activity. Deficiency in intact mitochondria from Morris hepatomas and ascites tumor cells. *J. Biol. Chem.* **1974**, *249*, 3327–3334.

35. Johnson, L.V.; Walsh, M.L.; Bockus, B.J.; Chen, L.B. Monitoring of relative mitochondrial membrane potential in living cells by fluorescence microscopy. *J. Cell Biol.* **1981**, *88*, 526–535.

36. Davis, S.; Weiss, M.J.; Wong, J.R.; Lampidis, T.J.; Chen, L.B. Mitochondrial and plasma membrane potentials cause unusual accumulation and retention of rhodamine 123 by human breast adenocarcinoma-derived MCF-7 cells. *J. Biol. Chem.* **1985**, *260*, 13844–13850.

37. Modica-Napolitano, J.S.; Aprille, J.R. Basis for the selective cytotoxicity of rhodamine 123. *Cancer Res.* **1987**, *47*, 4361–4365.

38. Canter, J.A.; Kallianpur, A.R.; Parl, F.F.; Millikan, R.C. Mitochondrial DNA G10398A polymorphism and invasive breast cancer in African–American women. *Cancer Res.* **2005**, *65*, 8028–8033.

39. Petros, J.A.; Baumann, A.K.; Ruiz-Pesini, E.; Amin, M.B.; Sun, C.Q.; Hall, J.; Lim, S.; Issa, M.M.; Flanders, W.D.; Hosseini, S.H.; *et al.* mtDNA mutations increase tumorigenicity in prostate cancer. *Proc. Natl. Acad. Sci. USA* **2005**, *102*, 719–724.

40. Brandon, M.; Baldi, P.; Wallace, D.C.; Mitochondrial mutations in cancer. *Oncogene* **2006**, *25*, 4647–4662.

41. Kulawiec, M.; Owens, K.M.; Singh, K.K. mtDNA G10398A variant in African–American women with breast cancer provides resistance to apoptosis and promotes metastasis in mice. *J. Hum. Genet.* **2009**, *54*, 647–654.

42. Booker, L.M.; Habermacher, G.M.; Jessie, B.C.; Sun, Q.C.; Baumann, A.K.; Amin, M.; Lim, S.D.; Fernandez-Golarz, C.; Lyles, R.H.; Brown, M.D.; *et al.* North American white mitochondrial haplogroups in prostate and renal cancer. *J. Urol.* **2006**, *175*, 468–472.

43. Liu, V.W.; Wang, Y.; Yang, H.J.; Tsang, P.C.; Ng, T.Y.; Wong, L.C.; Nagley, P.; Ngan, H.Y. Mitochondrial DNA variant 16189T>C is associated with susceptibility to endometrial cancer. *Hum. Mutat.* **2003**, *22*, 173–174.

44. Ishikawa, K.; Takenaga, K.; Akimoto, M.; Koshikawa, N.; Yamaguchi, A.; Imanishi, H.; Nakada, K.; Honma, Y.; Hayashi, J. ROS-generating mitochondrial DNA mutations can regulate tumor cell metastasis. *Science* **2008**, *320*, 661–664.

45. Weinberg, F.; Hamanaka, R.; Wheaton, W.W.; Weinberg, S.; Joseph, J.; Lopez, M.; Kalyanaraman, B.; Mutlu, G.M.; Budinger, G.R.; Chandel, N.S. Mitochondrial metabolism and ROS generation are essential for Kras-mediated tumorigenicity. *Proc. Natl. Acad. Sci. USA* **2010**, *107*, 8788–8793.

46. Vafa, O.; Wade, M.; Kern, S.; Beeche, M.; Pandita, T.K.; Hampton, G.M.; Wahl, G.M. c-Myc can induce DNA damage, increase reactive oxygen species, and mitigate p53 function: A mechanism for oncogene-induced genetic instability. *Mol. Cell* **2002**, *9*, 1031–1044.

47. Fruehauf, J.P.; Meyskens, F.L., Jr. Reactive oxygen species: A breath of life or death? *Clin. Cancer Res.* **2007**, *13*, 789–794.

48. Guzy, R.D.; Schumacker, P.T. Oxygen sensing by mitochondria at Complex III: The paradox of increased reactive oxygen species during hypoxia. *Exp. Physiol.* **2006**, *91*, 807–819.

49. Cannito, S.; Novo, E.; di Bonzo, L.V.; Busletta, C.; Colombatto, S.; Parola, M. Epithelial-mesenchymal transition: From molecular mechanisms, redox regulation to implications in human health and disease. *Antioxid. Redox Signal.* **2010**, *12*, 1383–1430.

50. Reed, J.C. Dysregulation of apoptosis in cancer. *J. Clin. Oncol.* **1999**, *17*, 2941–2953.

51. Wong, R. Apoptosis in cancer: From pathogenesis to treatment. *J. Exp. Clin. Cancer Res.* **2011**, *30*, 87.

52. Pepper, C.; Hoy, T.; Bentley, D.P. Bcl-2/Bax ratios in chronic lymphocytic leukaemia and their correlation with *in vitro* apoptosis and clinical resistance. *Br. J. Cancer* **1997**, *76*, 935–938.

53. Goolsby, C; Paniagua, M.; Tallman, M.; Gartenhaus, R.B. Bcl-2 regulatory pathway is functional in chronic lymphocytic leukaemia. *Cytom. Part B Clin. Cytom.* **2005**, *63*, 36–46.

54. Raffo, A.J.; Perlman, H.; Chen, M.W.; Day, M.L.; Streitman, J.S.; Buttyan, R. Overexpression of Bcl-2 protects prostate cancer cells from apoptosis *in vitro* and confers resistance to androgen depletion *in vivo*. *Cancer Res.* **1995**, *55*, 4438–4445.

55. Kitada, S.; Pedersen, I.M.; Schimmer, A.D.; Reed, J.C. Dysregulation of apoptosis genes in hematopoietic malignancies. *Oncogene* **2002**, *21*, 3459–3474.

56. Kirkin, V.; Joos, S.; Zornig, M. The role of Bcl-2 family members in tumorigenesis. *Biochim. Biophys. Acta* **2004**, *1644*, 229–249.

57. Fulda, S.; Meyer, E.; Debatin, K.M. Inhibition of TRAIL-induced apoptosis by Bcl-2 overexpression. *Oncogene* **2000**, *21*, 2283–2294.

58. Minn, A.J.; Rudin, C.M.; Boise, L.H.; Thompson, C.B. Expression of Bcl-XL can confer a multidrug resistance phenotype. *Blood* **1995**, *86*, 1903–1910.

59. Neuzil, J.; Dong, L.F.; Rohlena, J.; Truksa, J.; Ralph, S.J. Classification of mitocans, anti-cancer drugs acting on mitochondria. *Mitochondrion* **2013**, *13*, 199–208.

60. Bernal, S.D.; Lampidis, T.J.; Summerhayes, I.C.; Chen, L.B. Rhodamine-123 selectively reduces clonal growth of carcinoma cells *in vitro*. *Science* **1982**, *218*, 1117–1119.

61. Bernal, S.D.; Lampidis, T.J.; McIsaac, R.M.; Chen, L.B. Anticarcinoma activity *in vivo* of rhodamine 123, a mitochondrial-specific dye. *Science* **1983**, *222*, 169–172.

62. Modica-Napolitano, J.S.; Weiss, M.J.; Chen, L.B.; Aprille, J.R. Rhodamine 123 inhibits bioenergetic function in isolated rat liver mitochondria. *Biochem. Biophys. Res. Commun.* **1984**, *118*, 717–723.

63. Bleday, R.; Weiss, M.J.; Salem, R.R.; Wilson, R.E.; Chen, L.B.; Steele, G., Jr. Inhibition of rat colon tumor isograft growth with dequalinium chloride. *Arch. Surg.* **1986**, *121*, 1272–1275.

64. Weiss, M.J.; Wong, J.R.; Ha, C.S.; Bleday, R.; Salem, R.R.; Steele, G.D., Jr.; Chen, L.B. Dequalinium, a topical antimicrobial agent, displays anticarcinoma activity based on selective mitochondrial accumulation. *Proc. Natl. Acad. Sci. USA* **1987**, *84*, 5444–5448.

65. Sun, X.; Wong, J.R.; Song, K.; Hu, J.; Garlid, K.D.; Chen, L.B. AA1, a newly synthesized monovalent lipophilic cation, expresses potent *in vivo* antitumor activity. *Cancer Res.* **1994**, *54*, 1465–1471.

66. Koya, K.; Li, Y.; Wang, H.; Ukai, T.; Tatsuta, N.; Kawakami, M.; Shishido, T.; Chen, L.B. MKT-077, a novel rhodacyanine dye in clinical trials, exhibits anticarcinoma activity in preclinical studies based on selective mitochondrial accumulation. *Cancer Res.* **1996**, *56*, 538–543.

67. Modica-Napolitano, J.S.; Koya, K.; Weisberg, E.; Brunelli, B.T.; Li, Y.; Chen, L.B. Selective damage to carcinoma mitochondria by the rhodacyanine MKT-077. *Cancer Res.* **1996**, *56*, 544–550.

68. Britten, C.D.; Rowinsky, E.K.; Baker, S.D.; Weiss, G.R.; Smith, L.; Stephenson, J.; Rothenberg, M.; Smetzer, L.; Cramer, J.; Collins, W.; *et al.* A phase I and pharmacokinetic study of the mitochondrial-specific rhodacyanine dye analog MKT 077. *Clin. Cancer Res.* **2000**, *6*, 42–49.

69. Propper, D.J.; Braybrooke, J.P.; Taylor, D.J.; Lodi, R.; Styles, P.; Cramer, J.A.; Collins, W.C.J.; Levitt, N.C.; Talbot, D.C.; Ganesan, T.S.; *et al.* Phase I trial of the selective mitochondrial toxin MKT 077 in chemo-resistant solid tumours. *Ann. Oncol.* **1999**, *10*, 923–927.

70. Evans, J.M.; Donnelly, L.A.; Emslie-Smith, A.M.; Alessi, D.R.; Morris, A.D. Metformin and reduced risk of cancer in diabetic patients. *BMJ* **2005**, *330*, 1304–1305.

71. Libby, G.; Donnelly, L.A.; Donnan, P.T.; Alessi, D.R.; Morris, A.D.; Evans, J.M. New users of metformin are at low risk of incident cancer: A cohort study among people with type 2 diabetes. *Diabetes Care* **2009**, *32*, 1620–1625.

72. Murtola, T.J.; Tammela, T.L.; Lahtela, J.; Auvinen, A. Antidiabetic medication and prostate cancer risk: A population-based case-control study. *Am. J. Epidemiol.* **2008**, *168*, 925–931.

73. Jiralerspong, S.; Angulo, A.M.; Hung, M.C. Expanding the arsenal: Metformin for the treatment of triple-negative breast cancer? *Cell Cycle* **2009**, *8*, 2681.

74. Dowling, R.J.; Niraula, S.; Stambolic, V.; Goodwin, P.J. Metformin in cancer: Translational challenges. *J. Mol. Endocrinol.* **2012**, *48*, R31–R43.

75. Ben Sahra, I.; Laurent, K.; Loubat, A.; Giorgetti-Peraldi, S.; Colosetti, P; Auberger, P.; Tanti, J.F.; Le Marchand-Brustel, Y.; Bost, F. The antidiabetic drug metformin exerts an antitumoral effect *in vitro* and *in vivo* through a decrease of cyclin D1 level. *Oncogene* **2008**, *27*, 3576–3586.

76. Zakikhani, M.; Dowling, R.; Fantus, I.G.; Sonenberg, N.; Pollak, M. Metformin is an AMP kinase-dependent growth inhibitor for breast cancer cells. *Cancer Res.* **2006**, *66*, 10269–10273.

77. Gotlieb, W.H.; Saumet, J.; Beauchamp, M.C.; Gu, J.; Lau, S.; Pollak, M.N.; Bruchim, I. *In vitro* metformin antineoplastic activity in epithelial ovarian cancer. *Gynecol. Oncol.* **2008**, *110*, 246–250.

78. Wang, L.W.; Li, Z.S.; Zou, D.W.; Jin, Z.D.; Gao, J.; Xu, G.M. Metformin induces apoptosis of pancreatic cancer cells. *World J. Gastroenterol.* **2008**, *14*, 7192–7198.

79. Buzzai, M.; Jones, R.G.; Amaravadi, R.K.; Lum, J.J.; DeBerardinis, R.J.; Zhao, F.; Viollet, B.; Thompson, C.B. Systemic treatment with the antidiabetic drug metformin selectively impairs p53-deficient tumor cell growth. *Cancer Res.* **2007**, *67*, 6745–6752.

80. Hirsch, H.A.; Iliopoulos, D.; Tsichlis, P.N.; Struhl, K. Metformin selectively targets cancer stem cells, and acts together with chemotherapy to block tumor growth and prolong remission. *Cancer Res.* **2009**, *69*, 507–511.

81. Anisimov, V.N.; Berstein, L.M.; Egormin, P.A.; Piskunova, T.S.; Popovich, I.G.; Zabezhinski, M.A.; Kovalenko, I.G.; Poroshina, T.E.; Semenchenko, A.V.; Provinciali, M.; *et al.* 2005 Effect of metformin on life span and on the development of spontaneous mammary tumors in HER-2/neu transgenic mice. *Exp. Gerontol.* **2005**, *40*, 685–693.

82. Huang, X.; Wullschleger, S.; Shpiro, N.; McGuire, V.A.; Sakamoto, K.; Woods, Y.L.; McBurnie, W.; Fleming, S.; Alessi, D.R. Important role of the LKB1–AMPK pathway in suppressing tumorigenesis in PTEN-deficient mice. *Biochem. J.* **2008**, *412*, 211–221.

83. Memmott, R.M.; Mercado, J.R.; Maier, C.R.; Kawabata, S.; Fox, S.D.; Dennis, P.A. Metformin prevents tobacco carcinogen–induced lung tumorigenesis. *Cancer Prev. Res.* **2010**, *3*, 1066–1076.

84. Algire, C.; Zakikhani, M.; Blouin, M.J.; Shuai, J.H.; Pollak, M. 2008 Metformin attenuates the stimulatory effect of a high-energy diet on *in vivo* LLC1 carcinoma growth. *Endocr. Relat. Cancer* **2008**, *15*, 833–839.

85. Phoenix, K.N.; Vumbaca, F.; Fox, M.M.; Evans, R.; Claffey, K.P. Dietary energy availability affects primary and metastatic breast cancer and metformin efficacy. *Breast Cancer Res. Treat.* **2010**, *123*, 333–344.

86. Hosono, K.; Endo, H.; Takahashi, H.; Sugiyama, M.; Sakai, E.; Uchiyama, T.; Suzuki, K.; Iida, H.; Sakamoto, Y.; Yoneda, K.; *et al.* Metformin suppresses colorectal aberrant crypt foci in a short-term clinical trial. *Cancer Prev. Res.* **2010**, *3*, 1077–1083.

87. Niraula, S.; Dowling, R.J.; Ennis, M.; Chang, M.C.; Done, S.J.; Hood, N.; Escallon, J.; Leong, W.L.; McCready, D.R.; Reedijk, M.; *et al.* Metformin in early breast cancer: A prospective window of opportunity neoadjuvant study. *Breast Cancer Res. Treat.* **2012**, *135*, 821–830.

88. Hadad, S.; Iwamoto, T.; Jordan, L.; Purdie, C.; Bray, S.; Baker, L.; Jellema, G.; Deharo, S.; Hardie, D.G.; Pusztai, L.; *et al.* 2011 Evidence for biological effects of metformin in operable breast cancer: A pre-operative, window-of-opportunity, randomized trial. *Breast Cancer Res. Treat.* **2011**, *128*, 783–794.

89. Wheaton, W.W.; Weinberg, S.E.; Hamanaka, R.B.; Soberanes, S.; Sullivan, L.B.; Anso, E.; Glasauer, A.; Dufour, E.; Mutlu, G.M.; Budigner, G.R.S.; *et al.* Metformin inhibits mitochondrial Complex I of cancer cells to reduce tumorigenesis. *eLife* **2014**, *3*, e02242.

90. Blackman, R.K.; Cheung-Ong, K.; Gebbia, M.; Proia, D.A.; He, S.; Kepros, J.; Jonneaux, A.; Marchetti, P.; Kluza, J.; Rao, P.E.; *et al.* Mitochondrial electron transport is the cellular target of the oncology drug elesclomol. *PLoS ONE* **2012**, *7*, e29798.

91. O'Day, S.J.; Eggermont, A.M.; Chiarion-Sileni, V.; Kefford, R.; Grob, J.J.; Mortier, L.; Robert, C.; Schachter, J.; Testori, A.; Mackiewicz, J.; *et al.* Final results of phase III SYMMETRY study: Randomized, double-blind trial of elesclomol plus paclitaxel *versus* paclitaxel alone as treatment for chemotherapy-naive patients with advanced melanoma. *J. Clin. Oncol.* **2013**, *31*, 1211–1218.

92. ClinicalTrials.gov. Available online: https://clinicaltrials.gov/ct2/results?term=elesclomol&Search= Search (accessed on 19 May 2015).

93. Dai, Z.J.; Wang, X.J.; Li, Z.F.; Ji, Z.Z.; Ren, H.T.; Tang, W.; Liu, X.X.; Kang, H.F.; Guan, H.T.; Song, L.Q. *Scutellaria barbate* extract induces apoptosis of hepatoma H22 cells via the mitochondrial pathway involving caspase-3. *World J. Gastroenterol.* **2008**, *14*, 7321–7328.

94. Kim, E.K.; Kwon, K.B.; Han, M.J.; Song, M.Y.; Lee, J.H.; Ko, Y.S.; Shin, B.C.; Yu, J.; Lee, Y.R.; Ryu, D.G.; *et al.* Induction of G1 arrest and apoptosis by *Scutellaria barbata* in the human promyelocytic leukemia HL-60 cell line. *Int. J. Mol. Med.* **2007**, *20*, 123–128.

95. Marconett, C.N.; Morgenstern, T.J.; san Roman, A.K.; Sundar, S.N.; Singhal, A.K.; Firestone, G.L. BZL101, a phytochemical extract from the *Scutellaria barbata* plant, disrupts proliferation of human breast and prostate cancer cells through distinct mechanisms dependent on the cancer cell phenotype. *Cancer Biol. Ther.* **2010**, *10*, 397–405.

96. Fong, S.; Shoemaker, M.; Cadaoas, J.; Lo, A.; Liao, W.; Tagliaferri, M.; Cohen, I.; Shtivelman, E. Molecular mechanisms underlying selective cytotoxic activity of BZL101, an extract of *Scutellaria barbata*, towards breast cancer cells. *Cancer Biol. Ther.* **2008**, *7*, 577–586.

97. Chen, V.; Staub, R.E.; Fong, S.; Tagliaferri, M.; Cohen, I.; Shtivelman, E. Bezielle selectively targets mitochondria of cancer cells to inhibit glycolysis and OXPHOS. *PLoS ONE* **2012**, *7*, e30300.

98. Rugo, H.; Shtivelman, E.; Perez, A.; Vogel, C.; Franco, S.; Chiu, E.T.; Melisko, M.; Tagliaferri, M.; Cohen, I.; Shoemaker, M.; *et al.* Phase I trial and antitumor effects of BZL101 for patients with advanced breast cancer. *Breast Cancer Res. Treat.* **2007**, *105*, 17–28.

99. Perez, A.T.; Arun, B.; Tripathy, D.; Tagliaferri, M.A.; Shaw, H.S.; Kimmick, G.G.; Cohen, I.; Shtivelman, E.; Caygill, K.A.; Grady, D.; *et al.* A phase 1B dose escalation trial of *Scutellaria barbata* (BZL101) for patients with metastatic breast cancer. *Breast Cancer Res. Treat.* **2010**, *120*, 111–118.

100. Oltersdorf, T.; Elmore, S.W.; Shoemaker, A.R.; Armstrong, R.C.; Augeri, D.J.; Belli, B.A.; Bruncko, M.; Deckwerth, T.L.; Dinges, J.; Hajduk, P.J.; *et al.* An inhibitor of Bcl-2 family proteins induces regression of solid tumours. *Nature* **2005**, *435*, 677–681.

101. Konopleva, M.; Contractor, R.; Tsao, T.; Samudio, I.; Ruvolo, P.P.; Kitada, S.; Deng, X.; Zhai, D.; Shi, Y.X.; Sneed, T.; *et al.* Mechanisms of apoptosis sensitivity and resistance to the BH3 mimetic ABT-737 in acute myeloid leukemia. *Cancer Cell* **2006**, *10*, 375–388.

102. Hann, C.L.; Daniel, V.C.; Sugar, E.A.; Dobromilskaya, I.; Murphy, S.C.; Cope, L.; Lin, X.; Hierman, J.S.; Wilburn, D.L.; Neil Watkins, D.; *et al.* Therapeutic efficacy of ABT-737, a selective inhibitor of Bcl-2, in small cell lung cancer. *Cancer Res.* **2008**, *68*, 2321–2328.

103. Tse, C.; Shoemaker, A.R.; Adickes, J.; Anderson, M.G.; Chen, J.; Jin, S.; Johnson, E.F.; Marsh, K.C.; Mitten, M.J.; Nimmer, P.; *et al.* ABT-263: A potent and orally bioavailable Bcl-2 family inhibitor. *Cancer Res.* **2008**, *68*, 3421–3428.

104. Gandhi, L.; Camidge, D.R.; de Oliveira, M.R.; Bonomi, P.; Gandara, D.; Khaira, D.; Hann, C.L.; McKeegan, E.M.; Litvinovich, E.; Hemken, P.M.; *et al.* Phase I study of navitoclax (ABT-263), a novel Bcl-2 family inhibitor, in patients with small-cell lung cancer and other solid tumors. *J. Clin. Oncol.* **2011**, *29*, 909–916.

105. Rudin, C.M.; Hann, C.L.; Garon, E.B.; de Oliveira, M.R.; Bonomi, P.D.; Camidge, D.R.; Chu, Q.; Giaccone, G.; Khaira, D.; Ramalingam, S.S.; *et al.* Phase II study of single-agent navitoclax (ABT-263) and biomarker correlates in patients with relapsed small cell lung cancer. *Clin. Cancer Res.* **2012**, *18*, 3163–3169.

106. Sadahira, K.; Sagawa, M.; Nakazato, T.; Uchida, H.; Ikeda, Y.; Okamoto, S.; Nakajima, H.; Kizaki, M. Gossypol induces apoptosis in multiple myeloma cells by inhibition of interleukin-6 signaling and Bcl-2/Mcl-1 pathway. *Int. J. Oncol.* **2014**, *45*, 2278–2286.

107. Kline, M.P.; Rajkumar, S.V.; Timm, M.M.; Kimlinger, T.K.; Haug, J.L.; Lust, J.A.; Greipp, P.R.; Kumar, S. *R*-(−)-gossypol (AT-101) activates programmed cell death in multiple myeloma cells. *Exp. Hematol.* **2008**, *36*, 568–576.

108. Konopleva, M.; Watt, J.; Contractor, R.; Tsao, T.; Harris, D.; Estrov, Z.; Bornmann, W.; Kantarjian, H.; Viallet, J.; Samudio, I.; *et al.* Mechanisms of antileukemic activity of the novel BH3 mimetic GX15–070 (obatoclax). *Cancer Res.* **2008**, *68*, 3413–3420.

109. Nguyen, M.; Marcellus, R.C.; Roulston, A.; Watson, M.; Serfass, L.; Madiraju, S.R.M.; Goulet, D.; Viallet, J.; Bélec, L.; Billot, X.; *et al.* Small molecule obatoclax (GX15–070) antagonizes MCL-1 and overcomes MCL-1-mediated resistance to apoptosis. *Proc. Natl. Acad. Sci. USA* **2007**, *104*, 19512–19517.

110. Heikaus, S.; van den Berg, L.; Kempf, T.; Mahotka, C.; Gabbert, H.E.; Ramp, U. HA14–1 is able to reconstitute the impaired mitochondrial pathway of apoptosis in renal cell carcinoma cell lines. *Cell Oncol.* **2008**, *30*, 419–433.

111. Rehman, K.; Tariq, M.; Akash, M.S.; Gillani, Z.; Qazi, M.H. Effect of HA14–1 on apoptosis-regulating proteins in HeLa cells. *Chem. Biol. Drug Des.* **2014**, *83*, 317–323.

112. Anderson, W.M.; Wood, J.M.; Anderson, A.C. Inhibition of mitochondrial and Paracoccus denitrificans NADH-ubiquinone reductase by oxacarbocyanine dyes. A structure-activity study. *Biochem. Pharmacol.* **1993**, *45*, 691–696.

113. Rideout, D.; Bustamante, A.; Patel, J. Mechanism of inhibition of FaDu hypopharyngeal carcinoma cell growth by tetraphenylphosphonium chloride. *Int. J. Cancer* **1994**, *57*, 247–253.

114. Birsoy, K.; Possemato, R.; Lorbeer, F.K.; Bayraktar, E.C.; Thiru, P.; Yucel, B.; Wang, T.; Chen, W.W.; Clish, C.B.; Sabatini, D.M. Metabolic determinants of cancer cell sensitivity to glucose limitation and biguanides. *Nature* **2014**, *508*, 108–112.

115. Kong, Q.; Beel, J.A.; Lillehei, K.O. A threshold concept for cancer therapy. *Med. Hypotheses* **2000**, *55*, 29–35.

116. Billard, C. BH3 mimetics: Status of the field and new developments. *Mol. Cancer Ther.* **2013**, *12*, 1691–1700.

117. Shoemaker, A.R.; Oleksijew, A.; Bauch, J.; Belli, B.A.; Borre, T.; Bruncko, M.; Deckwirth, T.; Frost, D.J.; Jarvis, K.; Joseph, M.K.; *et al.* A small-molecule inhibitor of Bcl-X$_L$ potentiates the activity of cytotoxic drugs *in vitro* and *in vivo*. *Cancer Res.* **2006**, *66*, 8731–8739.

118. Hikita, H.; Takehara, T.; Shimizu, S.; Kodama, T.; Shigekawa, M.; Iwase, K.; Hosui, A.; Miyagi, T.; Tatsumi, T.; Ishida, H.; *et al.* The Bcl-xL inhibitor, ABT-737, efficiently induces apoptosis and suppresses growth of hepatoma cells in combination with sorafenib. *Hepatology* **2010**, *52*, 1310–1321.

119. Jain, H.V.; Meyer-Hermann, M. The molecular basis of synergism between carboplatin and ABT-737 therapy targeting ovarian carcinomas. *Cancer Res.* **2011**, *71*, 705–715.

120. Zall, H.; Weber, A.; Besch, R.; Zantl, N.; Hacker, G. Chemotherapeutic drugs sensitize human renal cell carcinoma cells to ABT-737 by a mechanism involving the Noxa-dependent inactivation of Mcl-1 or A1. *Mol. Cancer* **2010**, *9*, 164.

121. Tan, N.; Malek, M.; Zha, J.; Yue, P.; Kassees, R.; Berry, L.; Fairbrother, W.J.; Sampath, D.; Belmont, L.D. Navitoclax enhances the efficacy of taxanes in non-small cell lung cancer models. *Clin. Cancer Res.* **2011**, *17*, 1394–1404.

122. Truksa, J.; Dong, L.F.; Rohlena, J.; Stursa, J.; Vondrusova, M.; Goodwin, J.; Nguyen, M.; Kluckova, K.; Rychtarcikova, Z.; Lettlova, S.; *et al.* Mitochondrially targeted vitamin E succinate modulates expression of mitochondrial DNA transcripts and mitochondrial biogenesis. *Antiox. Redox Signal.* **2015**, *22*, 883–900.

123. Dong, L.F.; Jameson, V.J.A.; Tilly, D.; Cerny, J.; Mahdavian, E.; Marín-Hernandez, A.; Hernandez-Esquivel, L.; Rodríguez-Enríquez, S.; Stursa, J.; Witting, P.K.; *et al.* Mitochondrial targeting of vitamin E succinate enhances its pro-apoptotic and anti-cancer activity via mitochondrial Complex II. *J. Biol. Chem.* **2011**, *286*, 3717–3728.

124. Rao, V.A.; Klein, S.R.; Bonar, S.J.; Zielonka, J.; Mizuno, N.; Dickey, J.S.; Keller, P.W.; Joseph, J.; Kalyanaraman, B.; Shacter, E. The antioxidant transcription factor Nrf2 negatively regulates autophagy and growth arrest induced by the anticancer redox agent mitoquinone. *J. Biol. Chem.* **2010**, *285*, 34447–34459.

125. D'Souza, G.G.M.; Cheng, S.M.; Boddapati, S.V.; Horobin, R.W.; Weissig, V. Nanocarrier-assisted sub-cellular targeting to the site of mitochondria improves the pro-apoptotic activity of paclitaxel. *J. Drug Target.* **2008**, *16*, 578–585.

126. Paliwal, R.; Rai, S.; Vaidya, B.; Gupta, P.N.; Mahor, S.; Khatri, K.; Goyal, A.K.; Rawat, A.; Vyas, S.P. Cell-selective mitochondrial targeting: Progress in mitochondrial medicine. *Curr. Drug Deliv.* **2007**, *4*, 211–224.

127. Biswas, S.; Dodwadkar, N.S.; Deshpande, P.P.; Torchilin, V.P. Liposomes loaded with paclitaxel and modified with novel triphenylphosphonium-PEG-PE conjugate possess low toxicity, target mitochondria and demonstrate enhanced antitumor effects *in vitro* and *in vivo*. *J. Control. Release* **2012**, *159*, 393–402.

128. Zupancic, S.; Kocbek, P.; Zariwala, M.G.; Renshaw, D.; Gul, M.O.; Elsaid, Z.; Taylor, K.M.; Somavarapu, S. Design and development of novel mitochondrial targeted nanocarriers, DQAsomes for curcumin inhalation. *Mol. Pharm.* **2014**, *11*, 2334–2345.

129. Wang, X.X.; Li, Y.B.; Yao, H.J.; Ju, R.J.; Zhang, Y.; Li, R.J.; Yu, Y.; Zhang, L.; Lu, W.L. The use of mitochondrial targeting resveratrol liposomes modified with a dequalinium polyethylene glycol-distearoylphosphatidyl ethanolamine conjugate to induce apoptosis in resistant lung cancer cells. *Biomaterials* **2011**, *32*, 5673–5687.

130. Solomon, M.A.; Shah, A.A.; D'Souza, G.G. *In vitro* assessment of the utility of stearyl triphenyl phosphonium modified liposomes in overcoming the resistance of ovarian carcinoma Ovcar-3 cells to paclitaxel. *Mitochondrion* **2013**, *13*, 464–472.

131. Zhou. J.; Zhao, W.Y.; Ma, X.; Ju, R.J.; Li, X.Y.; Li, N.; Sun, M.G.; Shi, J.F.; Zhnag, C.X.; Lu, W.L. The anticancer efficacy of paclitaxel liposomes modified with mitochondrial targeting conjugate in resistant lung cancer. *Biomaterials* **2013**, *34*, 3626–3638.

132. Malhi, S.S.; Budhiraja, A.; Arora, S.; Chaudhari, K.R.; Nepali, K.; Kumar, R.; Sohi, H.; Murthy, R.S. Intracellular delivery of redox cycler-doxorubicin to the mitochondria of cancer cell by folate receptor targeted mitocancerotropic liposomes. *Int. J. Pharm.* **2012**, *432*, 63–74.

133. Yoong, S.L.; Wong, B.S.; Zhou, Q.L.; Chin, C.F.; Li, J.; Venkatesan, T.; Ho, H.K.; Yu, V.; Ang, W.H.; Pastorin, G. Enhanced cytotoxicity to cancer cells by mitochondria-targeting MWCNTs containing platinum(IV) prodrug of cisplatin. *Biomaterials* **2014**, *35*, 748–759.

134. Ara, G.; Aprille, J.R.; Malis, C.D.; Kane, S.B.; Cincotta, L.; Foley, J.; Bonventre, J.V.; Oseroff, A.R. Mechanisms of mitochondrial photosensitization by the cationic dye, *N*,*N*'-bis(2-ethyl-l,3-dioxylene)kryptocyanine (EDKC): Preferential inactivation of Complex I in the electron transport chain. *Cancer Res.* **1987**, *47*, 6580–6585.

135. Powers, S.K.; Pribil, S.; Gillespie, G.Y.; Watkins, P.J. Laser photochemotherapy of rhodamine-123 sensitized human glioma cells *in vitro*. *J. Neurosurg.* **1986**, *64*, 918–923.

136. Modica-Napolitano, J.S.; Brunelli, B.T.; Koya, K.; Chen, L.B. Photoactivation enhances the mitochondrial toxicity of the cationic rhodacyanine MKT-077. *Cancer Res.* **1998**, *58*, 71–75.

137. Chan, J.Y.; Tang, P.M.; Hon, P.M.; Au, S.W.; Tsui, S.K.; Waye, M.M.; Kong, S.K.; Mak, T.C.; Fung, K.P. Pheophorbide *a*, a major antitumor component purified from *Scutellaria barbata*, induces apoptosis in human hepatocellular carcinoma cells. *Planta Med.* **2006**, *72*, 28–33.

138. Li, W.T.; Tsao, H.W.; Chen, Y.Y.; Cheng, S.W.; Hsu, Y.C. A study on the photodynamic properties of chlorophyll derivatives using human hepatocellular carcinoma cells. *Photochem. Photobiol. Sci.* **2007**, *6*, 1341–1348.

139. Hajri, A.; Coffy, S.; Vallat, F.; Evrard, S.; Marescaux, J.; Aprahamian, M. Human pancreatic carcinoma cells are sensitive to photodynamic therapy *in vitro* and *in vivo*. *Br. J. Surg.* **1999**, *86*, 899–906.

140. Hibasami, H.; Kyohkon, M.; Ohwaki, S.; Katsuzaki, H.; Imai, K.; Nakagawa, M.; Ishi, Y.; Komiya, T. Pheophorbide *a*, a moiety of chlorophyll *a*, induces apoptosis in human lymphoid leukemia molt 4B cells. *Int. J. Mol. Med.* **2000**, *6*, 277–279.

141. Tang, P.M.; Liu, X.Z.; Zhang, D.M.; Fong, W.P.; Fung, K.P. Pheophorbide *a* based photodynamic therapy induces apoptosis via mitochondrial-mediated pathway in human uterine carcinosarcoma. *Cancer Biol. Ther.* **2009**, *8*, 533–539.

142. Hoi, S.W.; Wong, H.M.; Chan, J.Y.; Yue, G.G.; Tse, G.M.; Law, B.K.; Fong, W.P.; Fung, K.P. Photodynamic therapy of Pheophorbide *a* inhibits the proliferation of human breast tumour via both caspase-dependent and -independent apoptotic pathways in *in vitro* and *in vivo* models. *Phytother. Res.* **2012**, *26*, 734–742.

143. Hajri, A.; Wack, S.; Meyer, C.; Smith, M.K.; Leberquier, C.; Kedinger, M.; Aprahamian, M. *In vitro* and *in vivo* efficacy of Photofrin® and pheophorbide *a*, a bacteriochlorin, in photodynamic therapy of colonic cancer cells. *Photochem. Photobiol.* **2002**, *75*, 140–148.

144. Laranjo, M.; Serra, A.C.; Abrantes, M.; Piñeiro, M.; Gonçalves, A.C.; Casalta-Lopes, J.; Carvalho, L.; Sarmento-Ribeiro, A.B.; Rocha-Gonsalves, A.; Botelho, F. 2-Bromo-5-hydroxyphenylporphyrins for photodynamic therapy: Photosensitization efficiency, subcellular localization and *in vivo* studies. *Photodiagn. Photodyn. Ther.* **2013**, *10*, 51–61.

145. Cheong, J.H.; Park, E.S.; Liang, J.; Dennison, J.B.; Tsavachidou, D.; Nguyen-Charles, C.; Cheng, K.W.; Hall, H.; Zhang, D.; Lu, Y.; *et al.* Dual inhibition of tumor energy pathway by 2-deoxyglucose and metformin is effective against a broad spectrum of preclinical cancer models. *Mol. Cancer Ther.* **2011**, *10*, 2350–2362.

146. Ben Sahra, I.; Laurent, K.; Giuliano, S.; Larbret, F.; Ponzio, G.; Gounon, P.; Le Marchand-Brustel, Y.; Giorgetti-Peraldi, S.; Cormont, M.; Bertolotto, C.; *et al.* Targeting cancer cell metabolism: The combination of metformin and 2-deoxyglucose induces p53-dependent apoptosis in prostate cancer cells. *Cancer Res.* **2010**, *70*, 2465–2475.

147. Modica-Napolitano, J.S.; Nalbandian, R.; Kidd, M.E.; Nalbandian, A.; Nguyen, C.C. The selective *in vitro* cytotoxicity of carcinoma cells by AZT is enhanced by concurrent treatment with delocalized lipophilic cations. *Cancer Lett.* **2003**, *19*, 859–868.

148. Westermann, B.; Neupert, W. Mitochondria-targeted green fluorescent proteins: Convenient tools for the study of organelle biogenesis in *Saccharomyces cerevisiae. Yeast* **2000**, *16*, 1421–1427.

149. Smith, R.A.; Porteous, C.M.; Gane, A.M.; Murphy, M.P. Delivery of bioactive molecules to mitochondria *in vivo. Proc. Natl. Acad. Sci. USA* **2003**, *100*, 5407–5412.

150. Horobin, R.W.; Trapp, S.; Weissig, V. Mitochondriotropics: A review of their mode of action, and their applications for drug and DNA delivery to mammalian mitochondria. *J. Control. Release* **2007**, *121*, 125–136.

151. D'Souza, G.G.M.; Weissig, V. An introduction to subcellular and nanomedicine: Current trends and future developments. In *Organelle-Specific Pharmaceutical Nanotechnology*; John Wiley & Sons, Inc.: Hoboken, NJ, USA, 2010; pp. 1–13.

152. Weissig, V.; Lasch, J.; Erdos, G.; Meyer, H.W.; Rowe, T.C.; Hughes, J. DQAsomes: A novel potential drug and gene delivery system made from dequalinium. *Pharm. Res.* **1998**, *15*, 334–337.

153. Weissig, V.; Torchilin, V.P. Towards mitochondrial gene therapy: DQAsomes as a strategy. *J. Drug Target.* **2001**, *9*, 1–13.

154. Weissig, V.; Torchilin, V.P. Cationic bolasomes with delocalized charge centers as mitochondria-specific DNA delivery systems. *Adv. Drug Deliv. Rev.* **2001**, *49*, 127–149.

155. Weissig, V. DQAsomes as the prototype of mitochondria-targeted pharmaceutical nanocarriers: Preparation, characterization, and use. *Methods Mol. Biol.* **2015**, *1265*, 1–11.

156. Lyrawati, D.; Trounson, A.; Cram, D. Expression of GFP in the mitochondrial compartment using DQAsome-mediated delivery of an artificial mini-mitochondrial genome. *Pharm. Res.* **2011**, *28*, 2848–2862.

157. Boddapati, S.V.; Tongcharoensirikul, P.; Hanson, R.N.; D'Souza, G.G.; Torchilin, V.P.; Weissig, V. Mitochondriotropic liposomes. *J. Liposome Res.* **2005**, *15*, 49–58.

158. Boddapati, S.V.; D'Souza, G.G.; Erdogan, S.; Torchilin, V.P.; Weissig, V. Organelle-targeted nanocarriers: Specific delivery of liposomal ceramide to mitochondria enhances its cytotoxicity *in vitro* and *in vivo. Nano Lett.* **2008**, *8*, 2559–2263.

159. Boddapati, S.V.; D'Souza, G.G.; Weissig, V. Liposomes for drug delivery to mitochondria. *Methods Mol. Biol.* **2010**, *605*, 295–303.

160. Weissig, V.; Boddapati, S.V.; Cheng, S.M.; D'Souza, G.G. Liposomes and liposome-like vesicles for drug and DNA delivery to mitochondria. *J. Liposome Res.* **2006**, *16*, 249–264.

161. Weissig, V.; Lasch, J.; Klibanov, A.L.; Torchilin, V.P. A new hydrophobic anchor for the attachment of proteins to liposomal membranes. *FEBS Lett.* **1986**, *202*, 86–90.

162. Weissig, V., Lasch, J.; Gregoriadis, G. Covalent coupling of sugars to liposomes. *Biochim. Biophys. Acta* **1989**, *1003*, 54–57.

163. Theodossiou, T.A.; Sideratou, Z.; Tsiourvas, D.; Paleos, C.M. A novel mitotropic oligolysine nanocarrier: Targeted delivery of covalently bound D-Luciferin to cell mitochondria. *Mitochondrion* **2011**, *11*, 982–986.

164. Biswas, S.; Dodwadkar, N.S.; Piroyan, A.; Torchilin, V.P. Surface conjugation of triphenylphosphonium to target poly(amidoamine) dendrimers to mitochondria. *Biomaterials* **2012**, *33*, 4773–4782.

165. Sharma, A.; Soliman, G.M.; Al-Hajaj, N.; Sharma, R.; Maysinger, D.; Kakkar, A. Design and evaluation of multifunctional nanocarriers for selective delivery of coenzyme Q10 to mitochondria. *Biomacromolecules* **2012**, *13*, 239–252.

166. Marrache, S.; Dhar, S. Engineering of blended nanoparticle platform for delivery of mitochondria-acting therapeutics. *Proc. Natl. Acad. Sci. USA* **2012**, *109*, 16288–16293.

167. Pathak, R.K.; Kolishetti, N.; Dhar, S. Targeted nanoparticles in mitochondrial medicine. *Wiley Interdiscip. Rev. Nanomed. Nanobiotechnol.* **2015**, *7*, 315–329.

168. Theodossiou, T.A.; Sideratou, Z.; Katsarou, M.E.; Tsiourvas, D. Mitochondrial delivery of doxorubicin by triphenylphosphonium-functionalized hyperbranched nanocarriers results in rapid and severe cytotoxicity. *Pharm. Res.* **2013**, *30*, 2832–2842.

169. Battigelli, A.; Russier, J.; Venturelli, E.; Fabbro, C.; Petronilli, V.; Bernardi, P.; Da Ros, T.; Prato, M.; Bianco, A. Peptide-based carbon nanotubes for mitochondrial targeting. *Nanoscale* **2013**, *5*, 9110–9117.

170. Dougherty, T.J.; Gomer, C.J.; Henderson, B.W.; Jori, G.; Kessel, D.; Korbelik, M.; Moan, J.; Peng, Q. Photodynamic therapy. *J. Natl. Cancer Inst.* **1998**, *90*, 889–905.

171. Dolmans, D.E.; Fukumura, D.; Jain, R.K. Photodynamic therapy for cancer. *Nat. Rev. Cancer* **2003**, *3*, 380–387.

172. Oliveira, C.S.; Turchiello, R.; Kowaltowski, A.J.; Indig, G.L.; Baptista, M.S. Major determinants of photoinduced cell death: Subcellular localization versus photosensitization efficiency. *Free Radic. Biol. Med.* **2011**, *51*, 824–833.

173. Modica-Napolitano, J.S.: Joyal, J.L.; Ara, G.; Oseroff, A.R.; Aprille, J.R. Mitochondrial toxicity of cationic photosensitizers for photochemotherapy. *Cancer Res.* **1990**, *50*, 7876–7881.

174. Powers, S.K.; Walstad, D.L.; Brown, J.T.; Detty, M.; Watkins, P.J. Photosensitization of human glioma cells by chalcogenapyrylium dyes. *J. Neurooncol.* **1989**, *7*, 179–188.

175. Park, Y.J.; Lee, W.Y.; Hahn, B.S.; Han, M.J.; Yang, W.I.; Kim, B.S. Chlorophyll derivatives—A new photosensitizer for photodynamic therapy of cancer in mice. *Yonsei Med. J.* **1989**, *30*, 212–218.

176. Zhang, X.D.; Deslandes, E.; Villedieu, M.; Poulain, L.; Duval, M.; Gauduchon, P.; Scwartz, L.; Icard, P. Effect of 2-deoxy-D-glucose on various malignant cell lines *in vitro*. *Anticancer Res.* **2006**, *26*, 3561–3566.

177. Zhang, D.; Li, J.; Wang, F.; Hu, J.; Wang, S.; Sun, Y. 2-Deoxy-D-glucose targeting of glucose metabolism in cancer cells as a potential therapy. *Cancer Lett.* **2014**, *355*,176–183.

178. Ko, Y.H.; Pedersen, P.L.; Geschwind, J.F. Glucose catabolism in the rabbit VX2 tumor model for liver cancer: Characterization and targeting hexokinase. *Cancer Lett.* **2001**, *173*, 83–91.

179. Pedersen, P.L. 3-Bromopyruvate (3BP) a fast acting, promising, powerful, specific, and effective "small molecule" anti-cancer agent taken from labside to bedside: Introduction to a special issue. *J. Bioenerg. Biomembr.* **2012**, *44*, 1–6.

180. Oudard, S.; Poirson, F.; Miccoli, L.; Bourgeois, Y.; Vassault, A.; Poisson, M.; Magdelénat, H.; Dutrillaux, B.; Poupon, M.F. Mitochondria-bound hexokinase as target for therapy of malignant gliomas. *Int. J. Cancer* **1995**, *62*, 216–222.

181. Pulselli, R.; Amadio, L.; Fanciulli, M.; Floridi, A. Effect of lonidamine on the mitochondrial potential *in situ* in Ehrlich ascites tumor cells. *Anticancer Res.* **1996**, *16*, 419–423.

8

Thyroid Hormone Mediated Modulation of Energy Expenditure

Janina A. Vaitkus, Jared S. Farrar and Francesco S. Celi *

Division of Endocrinology and Metabolism, Department of Internal Medicine,
Virginia Commonwealth University School of Medicine, Richmond, VA 23298, USA;
E-Mails: vaitkusj@vcu.edu (J.A.V.); farrarj@vcu.edu (J.S.F.)

* Author to whom correspondence should be addressed; E-Mail: fsceli@vcu.edu

Academic Editors: Jaime M. Ross and Giuseppe Coppotelli

Abstract: Thyroid hormone (TH) has diverse effects on mitochondria and energy expenditure (EE), generating great interest and research effort into understanding and harnessing these actions for the amelioration and treatment of metabolic disorders, such as obesity and diabetes. Direct effects on ATP utilization are a result of TH's actions on metabolic cycles and increased cell membrane ion permeability. However, the majority of TH induced EE is thought to be a result of indirect effects, which, in turn, increase capacity for EE. This review discusses the direct actions of TH on EE, and places special emphasis on the indirect actions of TH, which include mitochondrial biogenesis and reduced metabolic efficiency through mitochondrial uncoupling mechanisms. TH analogs and the metabolic actions of T2 are also discussed in the context of targeted modulation of EE. Finally, clinical correlates of TH actions on metabolism are briefly presented.

Keywords: thyroid hormone; mitochondria; uncoupling mechanisms; mitochondrial biogenesis; metabolism; energy expenditure; thyroid hormone receptors

1. Introduction

The maintenance of life is dependent on the metabolism of substrates in the form of carbohydrates, fats, and proteins to provide energy, and in the form of ATP to assure cell integrity and functions. Although in humans the day-to-day variations in energy flux are dramatic, over time, the dynamic equilibrium between energy intake (EI) and energy expenditure (EE) is remarkable. Indeed, a small but sustained imbalance between EE and EI can lead to dramatic and severe clinical presentations, such as obesity or cachexia, both of which represent life-limiting conditions [1,2]. A variety of biochemical pathways are involved in energy metabolism, but in its broadest sense, the common requirement is chemical energy. Basal EE, otherwise defined as resting energy expenditure (REE), is the energy required to maintain basic cell and organ functions. Total EE (TEE) is defined as REE plus the energy consumed during activity (activity EE (AEE)) and diet-induced thermogenesis (DIT), the energy used to metabolize substrates above and beyond the requirements of intestinal tract mobility and absorption [3]. It is important to note that TEE is not static, as REE, AEE, and DIT are all variable and modifiable by a variety of factors. While there are several modulators of REE, and therefore overall EE, the focus of this review will be on thyroid hormone (TH) and its mechanisms of action, particularly on mitochondria. Following the complex integration of various afferent metabolic signals to the hypothalamus [4], TH releasing hormone (TRH) prompts the pituitary gland to secrete thyroid-stimulating hormone (TSH), which in turn activates the thyroid gland to produce and secrete TH [5]. In humans, this is mostly in the form of tetraiodothyronine (also referred to as thyroxine, T4), and to some degree, triiodothyronine (T3) [5]. T4 is then converted into T3 by deiodinase enzymes [5,6], which allow for time- and tissue-specific pre-receptor modulation of the hormonal signal. Most T4 and T3 are bound to thyroxine binding globulin (TBG) and other carriers in circulation, and only unbound or "free" TH exerts biological effects [7]. For the purposes of this review, TH will refer to T3 and T4, while other forms, referred to as TH analogs and "non-classical" THs, will be discussed later.

The critical role of TH in EE modulation has been known for more than a century, starting with the groundbreaking work of Magnus-Levy in 1895 (summarized in [8]). However, each specific mechanism, and in particular their regulatory systems, have yet to be fully elucidated. This review will discuss the developments in knowledge in this area, specifically regarding TH's role in modulating EE.

2. Direct Effects

Direct effects refer to TH actions that inherently cause an increase in ATP utilization. In general, these actions can be further classified into those that are related to metabolic cycles, and those that are related to ion leaks.

2.1. Metabolic Cycles

Metabolic cycles, also referred to as substrate or futile cycles, are the combination of two or more reactions which act in a cyclical manner; for a two reaction cycle, the reactions operate in reverse under the control of separate enzymes [9]. In the process of these reactions occurring, ATP is utilized, yet no product is consumed due to the cyclical nature of the products and reactants (hence the designation as a *futile cycle*). Examples of these cycles on the enzymatic level include hexokinase/glucose-6-phosphatase, phosphofructokinase/fructose 1,6-diphosphatase [9], and pyruvate kinase/malic enzyme [10]. Broadly then, futile cycles include such processes as glycolysis/gluconeogenesis, lipolysis (also referred to as fatty acid oxidation)/lipogenesis, and protein turnover, among others [9,11,12]. TH action promotes substrate cycling (reviewed by [9–11,13]). Interestingly, Grant and colleagues demonstrated that this increase in cycling results in a reduction in reactive oxygen species (ROS) formation in states of over nutrition [13]. Therefore, TH, by promoting "futile" cycles, plays an important role as an antioxidant in addition to increasing EE. With respect to TEE, however, the EE fraction affected by TH action on metabolic cycles is low compared to other mechanisms discussed later in this review [14,15].

2.2. Ion Leaks

A similar yet distinct target of TH activity is an increase in ion leakage, resulting from TH-induced increased cellular membrane permeability to ions. Consequently, a new ion gradient is established, and cells act to re-establish the desired ion concentrations across the membrane of interest at the cost of increased ATP utilization. Two of the most widely studied and understood ion leaks which are induced by TH and lead to futile ion cycling are the Na^+/K^+ ATPase and the sarco/endoplasmic reticulum Ca^{2+} ATPase (SERCA) (see Figure 1, orange components). TH action increases both Na^+ influx and K^+ efflux into/out of cell plasma membranes, which not only results in increased Na^+/K^+ ATPase activity [16], but also increased expression and insertion of these Na^+/K^+ ATPases into the plasma membrane [17–20]. While not as widely discussed, the Ca^{2+} ATPase on the plasma membrane of erythrocytes has also demonstrated regulation and activity modulation by TH [21], supporting the notion that TH exerts non-genomic effects [22] aside from its well-documented transcriptional action (which will be discussed later). TH also mediates leakage of Ca^{2+} from the sarcoplasmic/endoplasmic reticulum (SR/ER) into the cytosol [11], and induces increased expression of ryanodine receptors, which in turn further increase Ca^{2+} efflux out of the SR/ER into the cytosol [23]. Since Ca^{2+} is an extremely important signaling ion and second messenger used by cells, its leakage has the potential to undermine cell survival. In order to restore homeostasis, the cell compensates by increasing Ca^{2+} influx back into the SR/ER via TH-induced expression of SERCA [6,9,24]. Similar to metabolic cycles described above, futile ion cycling has been estimated to play a less substantial role in TH-dependent increases in EE [14,18].

3. Indirect Effects

While direct effects have been demonstrated to be important in TH-induced EE, the majority of the thermogenesis induced by TH can be attributed to indirect effects [9]. Indirect effects result in an increased capacity for EE through non-genomic pathways and mitochondrial biogenesis, and also a reduction in metabolic efficiency at the stage of ATP production, by activating uncoupling mechanisms.

3.1. Non-Genomic Pathways

TH participates in diverse non-genomic actions which can be initiated at the plasma membrane, in the cytoplasm, or in the mitochondria [7]. These recently discovered non-genomic actions of TH are important for the coordination of normal growth and metabolism, and include regulation of ion channels and oxidative phosphorylation [25]. The principal mediators of non-genomic TH actions on metabolism are the protein kinase signaling cascades [26]. A few examples of non-genomic TH actions are reported below, with comprehensive reviews available elsewhere [6,27]. In an example of plasma membrane TH signaling, T3 binding to the plasma membrane integrin αVβ3 was found to activate the phosphatidylinositol-4,5-

bisphosphate 3-kinase (PI3K) pathway, leading to thyroid hormone receptor-α1 (TRα1) receptor shuttling from the cytoplasm to the nucleus (see Figure 1, pink components) and induction of hypoxia-inducible factor 1-α (*HIF1α*) gene expression [28]. Non-genomic TH actions on the cardiovascular system also involve protein-kinase-dependent signaling cascades, which include protein kinase A (PKA), protein kinase C (PKC), PI3K, and mitogen-activated protein kinase (MAPK), with changes in ion channel and pump activities [29]. Other non-genomic actions of TH have been linked to AMP-activated protein kinase (AMPK) and Akt/protein kinase B [30–32]. T3 and T2 activate AMPK, a particularly important energy sensor in the cell, resulting in increased fatty acid oxidation, mitochondrial biogenesis, and glucose transporter type 4 (GLUT4) translocation [33–35]. Collectively, the non-genomic effects of TH on ion channels and protein kinase signaling cascades may account for a significant component of TH-mediated EE.

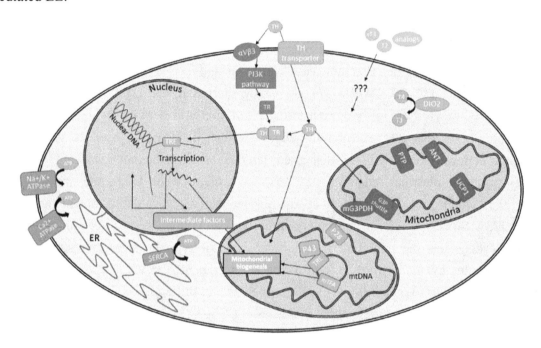

Figure 1. Summary of the mechanisms by which thyroid hormone (TH) modulates energy expenditure (EE) on the cellular level. Orange: Ion leaks. Pink: Non-genomic pathways. Green: Mitochondrial biogenesis resulting from nuclear, intermediate, and mitochondrial-specific pathways. Purple: Uncoupling mechanisms. Yellow: rT3, T2, TH analogs. Blue: TH, ATP, and intermediate steps in TH metabolism and signaling.

3.2. Mitochondrial Biogenesis

Of the roughly 1500 mitochondrial genes, the vast majority are housed within the nuclear genome, while the remainder are in the mitochondrial genome [36,37]. In 1992, Wiesner and colleagues demonstrated that the mechanisms of regulation for these two genomes are distinct [38]. TH exerts some of its thermogenic effects by stimulating mitochondrial biogenesis, which has substantial EE implications. Of note, the elevated oxidative capacity due to an increase in the number of mitochondria is not synonymous with an increase in baseline EE, but rather reflects the potential for expansion of respiration in response to an increased demand (such as muscle contraction or adaptive thermogenic response activation) [39].

TH-dependent mitochondrial biogenesis occurs via three mechanisms discussed below: (1) action on nuclear TH receptors; (2) activation of mitochondrial transcription; and (3) expression and activation of intermediate factors that span both the nucleus and the mitochondria (see Figure 1, green components).

3.2.1. Nuclear

In mammals, two genes, *c-ErbAα* and *c-ErbAβ*, lead to the production of TH receptors (TRs) (reviewed in [40]). TRα1, TRα2, and TRα3 are the protein products of *c-ErbAα*, yet only the TRα1 isoform binds TH and is functionally relevant [41]. TRβ1 and TRβ2, both of which bind TH, are the products of *c-ErbAβ* [42]. TR isoforms are tissue specific, developmentally regulated, and may have distinct functions [43]. All functional TR isoforms contain multiple functional domains, which include a DNA-binding domain (DBD) and a carboxyl-terminal ligand-binding domain (LBD) [7]. The DBD is highly conserved and interacts with specific DNA segments known as TH response elements, or TREs [7]. Thus, TRs are nuclear receptors which modulate gene expression specifically and locally through binding of circulating TH. TRs can exist as monomers, homodimers, and heterodimers; as heterodimers, they can interact with retinoid X receptor (RXR) or retinoic acid receptor (RAR) [44,45]. Through their LBD, TR can also interact with coactivators and corepressors, further modulating TH activity in a tissue specific manner [46]. TH nuclear actions modulate the activities of other transcription factors and coactivators (see Section 3.2.3 below) which are important in metabolic control and the regulation of mitochondrial DNA replication and transcription [47–49]. TH also promotes mitochondrial biogenesis through the induction of nuclear encoded mitochondrial genes such as cytochrome c, cytochrome c oxidase subunit IV, and cytochrome c subunit VIIIa [50]. Other TR interacting proteins and TR functions are reviewed extensively elsewhere [6].

3.2.2. Mitochondrial

In addition to the effects described above, TH exerts actions in/on mitochondria [51]. Aside from the nuclear genomic-based pathway of mitochondrial biogenesis, TH also induces mitochondrial genome transcription [25]. TH promotes mitochondrial genome transcription via two distinct mechanisms: directly by binding within the mitochondria to activate transcription machinery, and indirectly by binding to TR nuclear receptors which induce the expression of intermediate factors, which then go on to mitochondria and induce mitochondrial genome-specific gene expression (reviewed by [25] and discussed further in Section 3.2.3 below).

It is important to recognize that direct TH action on mitochondria is not sufficient *per se* to promote mitochondrial biogenesis, since the vast majority of the mitochondrial proteome is encoded by and regulated within the cell's nuclear genome and cytoplasm [36,37]. Still, there is evidence of direct TH action on the mitochondrial genome. Truncated forms of TRα1, p43 (mitochondrial matrix T3-binding protein) and p28 (inner mitochondrial membrane T3 binding protein), have been isolated in the mitochondrial matrix and inner mitochondrial membrane, respectively [52]. This was a novel and exciting finding, since prior to this discovery there was no knowledge of a non-nuclear TR. Subsequently, Casas and colleagues [53] demonstrated that p43 is indeed restricted to the mitochondria, and that it has similar ligand binding affinity to TRα1, indicating that p43 is the receptor which drives TH mediated transcription of the mitochondrial genome [54,55]. p43 translocates into the mitochondria via fusion to a cytosolic protein [56], and once within the mitochondrial matrix, TH binding to p43 results in p43 interaction with the mitochondrial genome via TREs located in the D loop of the heavy strand [6] to initiate transcription. This mechanism explains the observation of an increased mRNA/rRNA ratio within the mitochondria after exposure to TH [57].

3.2.3. Intermediate Factors

TH also induces mitochondrial biogenesis by bridging nuclear and mitochondrial transcription. This "bridge" is formed by a TH-dependent increase in nuclear expression of a variety of intermediate factors, which can then act on the nucleus, generating a positive feedback loop to either induce nuclear transcription, or to act on the mitochondria to induce mitochondrial transcription [25]. In an extensive review on this topic, Weitzel and Iwen distinguish two distinct classes of intermediate factors: Transcription factors and coactivators [25]. The expression of mitochondrial transcription factor A (mTFA, also referred to as TFAM) is directly regulated by TH, and modulates *in vivo* mitochondrial transcription [58]. Nuclear respiratory factors 1 and 2 (NRF1, NRF2) are transcription factors with multifaceted actions leading to stimulation of mitochondrial biogenesis ([25], and [59] for extensive review). While these intermediate factors function as transcription factors, others function as coactivators of transcription. An example of this class is represented by steroid hormone receptor coactivator 1 (SRC-1), whose action as a coactivator of TH modulates white and brown adipose tissue (BAT) energy balance [60]. Peroxisome proliferator-activated receptor gamma coactivator-1 (PGC-1, both α and β isoforms) are also transcriptionally regulated by TH [25,61] and play a pivotal role in the oxidative capacity of skeletal muscle and BAT (see below). For many metabolism-related genes which are regulated by TH, a putative TRE has yet to be found, further supporting a role for intermediate factors in TH metabolic control [48].

3.3. Uncoupling Mechanisms within the Mitochondria

While mitochondrial biogenesis increases the capacity for EE, uncoupling mechanisms manipulate and decrease the efficiency of ATP production within the cell, thereby increasing EE. TH has been demonstrated to play a role in these mechanisms (see Figure 1, purple components), as discussed below.

3.3.1. Uncoupling Proteins

Non-shivering thermogenesis consists of the direct conversion of chemical energy into heat, allowing for a rapid and efficient adaptation to changes in environmental temperature. This ultimately contributed to the evolutionary success of mammals, as it expands the ability to survive in hostile climates [62]. The biochemical hallmark of non-shivering thermogenesis is represented by uncoupling oxidative phosphorylation in the mitochondria, particularly in brown adipose tissue (BAT) [63]. This is accomplished by uncoupling protein-1 (UCP1), which renders the inner membrane of the mitochondria permeable to electrons [64]. This allows for the dissipation of chemical energy as heat, shunting the production of ATP away from the respiration complexes and therefore increasing

EE. TH plays an important role in modulating this process. UCP1 transcription is positively regulated by a TRE [65], which therefore implicates TH in this energy-expending activity. Interestingly, in BAT, the intracellular concentration of T3 is relatively independent from the circulating levels of TH, and it is regulated by type 2 deiodinase (DIO2) [66]. DIO2 is driven by the β-adrenergic cyclic AMP (cAMP) signaling cascade [67], which promotes an increase in intracellular conversion of the prohormone T4 into T3, the ligand for the TH receptor. This signal pathway ultimately assures a time- and tissue-specific modulation of TH action relatively independent of circulating TH levels [66], with obvious effects on EE [68].

In addition to UCP1, which is the hallmark of brown adipose tissue transcriptome signature, other structurally-related proteins with putative uncoupling properties have been described in other tissues. UCP2 and UCP3 are the most well studied and their transcription is induced by TH [69,70]. UCP3, which is predominantly expressed in skeletal muscle, has been associated with TH-induced modulation of REE [71] and fatty acid peroxide-induced mitochondrial uncoupling [72]. Additional actions of uncoupling proteins are reviewed elsewhere [9,73].

3.3.2. PCG-1α

While TH action directly stimulates EE in the mitochondria by promoting the uncoupling of substrate oxidation from ADP phosphorylation, TH also augments the overall capacity for non-shivering thermogenesis and therefore EE by positively regulating the transcription of PGC-1α, the master regulator of brown and "beige" adipocyte differentiation and mitochondria proliferation [74]. PGC-1α is also an important modulator of EE in muscle, where it promotes the switch from glycolytic function toward oxidative metabolism [75]. Interestingly, PGC-1α also plays a role in modulating the relative ratio between the transcriptionally active isoform of the TH receptor (TRα1) and the "inactive" TRα2 isoform devoid of the ligand binding domain, thereby generating a sort of intracellular negative feedback [76].

3.3.3. Mitochondrial Permeability Transition Pore

Mitochondrial uncoupling by T3 is driven by gating of the mitochondrial permeability transition pore (PTP) [77]. Previous studies have shown that mitochondrial PTP opening is exquisitely sensitive to mitochondrial Ca^{2+} [78], which is classically increased in states of cell stress [79]. Prolonged opening of the PTP results in mitochondrial depolarization and swelling, and if PTP conductance is sufficiently elevated, mitochondrial rupture will ensue with release of pro-apoptotic proteins and programmed cell death [80]. Interestingly, in addition to its historic role in apoptosis, recent evidence has emerged to implicate PTP in TH-mediated EE. Yehuda-Shnaidman *et al.* found that mitochondrial uncoupling by T3 required activation of the endoplasmic reticulum inositol 1,4,5-triphosphate receptor 1 (IP(3)R1), suggesting an upstream role for IP(3)R1 in the action of T3 on EE [77]. This study indicated a novel target for TH-dependent mitochondrial EE and the potential for targeting future TH analogs to this pathway. While much research is still necessary in this area, it is possible that IP(3)R1 may result in increased PTP opening, uncoupling, and therefore EE. For a more extensive discussion of the mitochondrial PTP and its role in TH induced EE, please see a recent review by Yehuda-Shnaidman and colleagues [9].

3.3.4. ANT

The mitochondrial adenosine diphosphate/adenosine triphosphate (ADP/ATP) translocase, or ANT, forms a gated pore in the inner mitochondrial membrane, allowing ADP to flow into the mitochondrial matrix and ATP in the opposite direction towards the cytoplasm [81]. ANT serves an important role in oxidative phosphorylation by controlling the flow of ADP substrate into the mitochondria, which is subsequently phosphorylated to ATP. As an important regulator of mitochondrial EE, ANT and cytosolic and mitochondrial ADP/ATP ratios were an early focus of studies into TH stimulated EE [82,83]. Indeed, in 1985, Seitz and colleagues demonstrated that T3 could rapidly increase mitochondrial respiration, ATP regeneration, and the activity of ANT in rat liver [82]. T3 stimulation of ANT was later confirmed and more expansively studied in rat liver mitochondrial isolates [84]. Mowbray and colleagues proposed a model in which T3 caused covalent modification of ANT, promoting a conformation with elevated ADP and cation flux [85]. This study directly linked T3 to mitochondrial uncoupling and provided evidence for the role of TH in shunting substrate towards heat generation in the mitochondria instead of ATP production. Brand *et al.* later demonstrated that basal proton conductance in the mitochondria of mice lacking ANT1 was half that of wild-type controls; firmly establishing the role of ANT in mitochondrial basal uncoupling [86] and therefore EE. Finally, ANT may serve an important role in long-term adaptive thermogenesis. In their study, Ukropec *et al.* found that mice lacking UCP1 were able to induce ANT1/2 and other proteins to compensate for long-term cold exposure [87]. Taken together, these data suggest an important role for ANT in the uncoupling of mitochondrial respiration.

3.3.5. Glycerol-3-Phosphate Shuttle

In order for the electron transport chain to produce ATP, reducing equivalents must also be present in the inner mitochondrial matrix, in addition to ADP as described above. Two mechanisms that allow for this are the malate-aspartate shuttle and the glycerol-3-phosphate (G3P) shuttle [11]. These shuttles differ in the resultant nucleotides which they provide to the electron transport chain within the mitochondria; the malate-aspartate shuttle provides NADH, while the G3P shuttle provides $FADH_2$ [9]. This seemingly minute difference has substantial implications with respect to energy balance, as subsequent oxidative phosphorylation of NADH results in the synthesis of 3 ATP, compared with only 2 ATP for a $FADH_2$ molecule (reviewed in [9]). In this sense, the G3P shuttle is less metabolically efficient, and therefore, if its action is upregulated, it can function as an energy dissipation mechanism. Indeed, TH regulates the G3P shuttle at the level of FADH-dependent mitochondrial glycerol-3-phosphate dehydrogenase (mG3PDH) [9]. mG3PDH is located on the outer side of the mitochondrial inner membrane and allows for the conversion of G3P into dihydroxyacetone phosphate (DHAP) [88]. In this conversion, $FADH_2$ is formed and shuttled into complex II of the electron transport chain. Silva and colleagues studied a transgenic *mG3PDH−/−* mouse model and found significantly higher levels of TH ([89], and reviewed in [11]). This evidence suggests a clear role for TH in thermogenesis created by the G3P shuttle. However, total oxygen consumption was not reduced as drastically as expected (only a 7%–10% reduction in the transgenic *mG3PDH−/−* mouse compared to controls) [89].

This suggests that compensatory mechanisms exist to lessen the reduction in EE when mG3PDH is not present.

4. TH Analogs and Non-Classical THs

4.1. TH Analogs

The diverse effects of TH on metabolism prompted researchers to study its use as a potential therapeutic for obesity and dyslipidemia. However, supra-physiologic TH levels cause a toxic state, and their systemic effects such as tachycardia, bone loss, muscle wasting, and neuropsychiatric disturbances prevent therapeutic use [90]. For these reasons, supplementing TH in euthyroid individuals for the treatment of obesity was abandoned. A logical development from research on TH actions has been the isolation and synthesis of TH derivatives with favorable side effect profiles, or "ideal" target-tissue distribution, to exploit beneficial metabolic effects while minimizing toxicity and systemic adverse effects. Newer TH derivatives have been developed with tissue and TRβ specificity (reviewed in [91,92]) (see Figure 1, yellow components). By focusing on TRβ selectivity, the adverse cardiac effects of TH have been reduced due to the low expression of TRβ receptors in the heart [93]. Tissue specificity has focused on the actions of TH in the liver, in part because synthetic TH derivatives could be made with high first-pass metabolism in the liver and greatly lowered serum concentrations [92]. The synthetic TH analog GC-1 (sobetirome) has been shown to prevent or reduce hepatosteatosis in a rat model [94] and can reduce serum triglyceride and cholesterol levels without significant side-effects on heart rate [95]. Additionally, GC-1 has been shown to increase EE and prevent fat accumulation in female rats [96].

4.2. Non-Classical THs

In addition to the "classic" THs T4 and T3, other naturally occurring "non-classical" THs may have physiological actions or be exploited therapeutically in the modulation of EE (see Figure 1, yellow components). The mechanisms of action of non-classical THs, which include 3,3′,5′-triiodothyronine (rT3), thyronamines (TAMs), and 3,5-diiodothyronine (T2) have been recently reviewed in detail elsewhere [8,97–99]. In this review, we will briefly discuss the metabolic actions of T2. T2 is found at picomolar serum concentrations in humans [100], and at similar concentrations, T2 is able to stimulate oxygen consumption in the isolated perfused livers of hypothyroid rats [101]. T2 has also been shown to directly and rapidly stimulate mitochondrial activity [102] and elevate resting EE in rats [103]. Subsequently, it was demonstrated that T2 can prevent high fat diet-induced hepatosteatosis and obesity in rats by stimulating mitochondrial uncoupling and decreasing ATP synthesis [104,105]. Furthermore, T2 can treat obesity and hepatosteatosis [106] and prevent high fat diet-induced insulin resistance in rats [107]. Finally, recent experimental evidence indicates that T2 is able to activate BAT-dependent thermogenesis and enhance mitochondrial respiration in hypothyroid rats [108]. In an attempt towards translating experimental findings to humans, Antonelli et al. administered T2 to healthy, euthyroid subjects and monitored changes in body weight, resting metabolic rate (RMR) and thyroid function [109]. Compared to baseline, T2-treated subjects had a significant elevation in RMR, reduced body weight, and normal thyroid and cardiac function, while no changes in any of these metrics were observed in the placebo group. Within the limitation of a very small proof-of-concept trial, this study further supports the potential of T2 to therapeutically increase RMR and reduce body weight.

5. Clinical Correlates

The recent discovery of naturally occurring mutations in the *TRα* gene [110] has provided the opportunity to assess *in vivo* the differential effects of TH signaling by comparing and contrasting the effects of TH receptor α and β mutations on energy metabolism. The human phenotype of resistance to TH (RTH) secondary to mutations in the *TRβ* gene is commonly characterized by a combination of hyper- and hypothyroid hormonal signaling at different end-organ tissues, with an overall increase in EE [111]. Conversely, the recently described syndrome of RTH secondary to *TRα* mutations is characterized by increased adiposity and decreased EE [112], in keeping with the predominance of *TRα* in high energy demanding tissues such as myocardium. Interestingly, while both isoforms are present in BAT [113], *TRβ* is the prevalent isoform, playing a critical role in the adaptive thermogenic response [114]. The data therefore strongly suggest that the modulatory activity of lipolysis and EE by *TRα* is primarily due to indirect effects, rather than direct action on the mitochondria. Interestingly, an association between polymorphisms in the *TRα* locus and increased body mass index has been reported, supporting the role of this isoform in energy metabolism [115]. From a clinical standpoint, these findings suggest that the development of a receptor isoform or tissue-specific TH agonist may represent a viable strategy to modulate end-organ targets or pathways with precision, without generating undesirable side effects.

6. Conclusions and Final Remarks

TH has pleiotropic effects on mitochondria and energy expenditure. The modulation of TH's actions is critical in the delivery of time and tissue specific signaling. The effects of TH in increasing energy expenditure via modulation of the adaptive thermogenesis response, coupled with the ability of increasing respiratory capacity by regulating mitochondrial biogenesis, are augmented by the increase in TH's non-mitochondrial effects on futile cycles and ion transport. Finally, the opportunity to selectively modulate TH effects represents a promising therapeutic target for the amelioration of a wide range of metabolic disorders.

Acknowledgments

The authors are grateful to Bin Ni, Ph.D. for his comments and constructive criticisms.

Author Contributions

Janina A. Vaitkus performed the primary literature search, wrote the first draft of the manuscript, and contributed to the subsequent revisions; Jared S. Farrar contributed to the primary literature search and to revisions; Francesco S. Celi designed the structure of the manuscript, supervised the literature search, and contributed to the subsequent revisions.

References

1. Rosen, E.D.; Spiegelman, B.M. Adipocytes as regulators of energy balance and glucose homeostasis. *Nature* **2006**, *444*, 847–853.

2. De Vos-Geelen, J.; Fearon, K.C.; Schols, A.M. The energy balance in cancer cachexia revisited. *Curr. Opin. Clin. Nutr. Metab. Care* **2014**, *17*, 509–514.

3. Haugen, H.A.; Chan, L.N.; Li, F. Indirect calorimetry: A practical guide for clinicians. *Nutr. Clin. Pract.* **2007**, *22*, 377–388.

4. Sotelo-Rivera, I.; Jaimes-Hoy, L.; Cote-Velez, A.; Espinoza-Ayala, C.; Charli, J.L.; Joseph-Bravo, P. An acute injection of corticosterone increases thyrotrophin-releasing hormone expression in the paraventricular nucleus of the hypothalamus but interferes with the rapid hypothalamus pituitary thyroid axis response to cold in male rats. *J. Neuroendocrinol.* **2014**, *26*, 861–869.

5. Medici, M.; Visser, W.E.; Visser, T.J.; Peeters, R.P. Genetic determination of the hypothalamic-pituitary-thyroid axis: Where do we stand? *Endocr. Rev.* **2015**, *36*, 214–244.

6. Cheng, S.Y.; Leonard, J.L.; Davis, P.J. Molecular aspects of thyroid hormone actions. *Endocr. Rev.* **2010**, *31*, 139–170.

7. Cioffi, F.; Senese, R.; Lanni, A.; Goglia, F. Thyroid hormones and mitochondria: With a brief look at derivatives and analogues. *Mol. Cell. Endocrinol.* **2013**, *379*, 51–61.

8. Goglia, F. The effects of 3,5-diiodothyronine on energy balance. *Front. Physiol.* **2014**, *5*, doi:10.3389/fphys.2014.00528.

9. Yehuda-Shnaidman, E.; Kalderon, B.; Bar-Tana, J. Thyroid hormone, thyromimetics, and metabolic efficiency. *Endocr. Rev.* **2014**, *35*, 35–58.

10. Petersen, K.F.; Cline, G.W.; Blair, J.B.; Shulman, G.I. Substrate cycling between pyruvate and oxaloacetate in awake normal and 3,3′-5-triiodo-L-thyronine-treated rats. *Am. J. Physiol.* **1994**, *267*, E273–E277.

11. Silva, J.E. Thermogenic mechanisms and their hormonal regulation. *Physiol. Rev.* **2006**, *86*, 435–464.

12. Newsholme, E.A.; Parry-Billings, M. Some evidence for the existence of substrate cycles and their utility *in vivo. Biochem. J.* **1992**, *285*, 340–341.

13. Grant, N. The role of triiodothyronine-induced substrate cycles in the hepatic response to overnutrition: Thyroid hormone as an antioxidant. *Med. Hypotheses.* **2007**, *68*, 641–649.

14. Freake, H.C.; Oppenheimer, J.H. Thermogenesis and thyroid function. *Annu. Rev. Nutr.* **1995**, *15*, 263–291.

15. Oppenheimer, J.H.; Schwartz, H.L.; Lane, J.T.; Thompson, M.P. Functional relationship of thyroid hormone-induced lipogenesis, lipolysis, and thermogenesis in the rat. *J. Clin. Investig.* **1991**, *87*, 125–132.

16. Haber, R.S.; Ismail-Beigi, F.; Loeb, J.N. Time course of Na, K transport and other metabolic responses to thyroid hormone in clone 9 cells. *Endocrinology* **1988**, *123*, 238–247.

17. Lei, J.; Nowbar, S.; Mariash, C.N.; Ingbar, D.H. Thyroid hormone stimulates Na-K-ATPase activity and its plasma membrane insertion in rat alveolar epithelial cells. *Am. J. Physiol. Lung Cell. Mol. Physiol.* **2003**, *285*, L762–L772.

18. Lei, J.; Mariash, C.N.; Ingbar, D.H. 3,3′,5-triiodo-L-thyronine up-regulation of Na, K-ATPase activity and cell surface expression in alveolar epithelial cells is src kinase- and phosphoinositide 3-kinase-dependent. *J. Biol. Chem.* **2004**, *279*, 47589–47600.

19. Gick, G.G.; Ismail-Beigi, F.; Edelman, I.S. Thyroidal regulation of rat renal and hepatic Na, K-ATPase gene expression. *J. Biol. Chem.* **1988**, *263*, 16610–16618.

20. Gick, G.G.; Ismail-Beigi, F. Thyroid hormone induction of Na^+-K^+-ATPase and its mrnas in a rat liver cell line. *Am. J. Physiol.* **1990**, *258*, C544–C551.

21. Segal, J.; Hardiman, J.; Ingbar, S.H. Stimulation of calcium-atpase activity by 3,5,3′-*tri*-iodothyronine in rat thymocyte plasma membranes. A possible role in the modulation of cellular calcium concentration. *Biochem. J.* **1989**, *261*, 749–754.

22. Vicinanza, R.; Coppotelli, G.; Malacrino, C.; Nardo, T.; Buchetti, B.; Lenti, L.; Celi, F.S.; Scarpa, S. Oxidized low-density lipoproteins impair endothelial function by inhibiting non-genomic action of thyroid hormone-mediated nitric oxide production in human endothelial cells. *Thyroid* **2013**, *23*, 231–238.

23. Jiang, M.; Xu, A.; Tokmakejian, S.; Narayanan, N. Thyroid hormone-induced overexpression of functional ryanodine receptors in the rabbit heart. *Am. J. Physiol. Heart Circ. Physiol.* **2000**, *278*, H1429–H1438.

24. Kahaly, G.J.; Dillmann, W.H. Thyroid hormone action in the heart. *Endocr. Rev.* **2005**, *26*, 704–728.

25. Weitzel, J.M.; Iwen, K.A. Coordination of mitochondrial biogenesis by thyroid hormone. *Mol. Cell. Endocrinol.* **2011**, *342*, 1–7.

26. Bassett, J.H.; Harvey, C.B.; Williams, G.R. Mechanisms of thyroid hormone receptor-specific nuclear and extra nuclear actions. *Mol. Cell. Endocrinol.* **2003**, *213*, 1–11.

27. Moeller, L.C.; Broecker-Preuss, M. Transcriptional regulation by nonclassical action of thyroid hormone. *Thyroid Res.* **2011**, *4* (Suppl. 1), doi: 10.1186/1756-6614-4-S1-S6.

28. Lin, H.Y.; Sun, M.; Tang, H.Y.; Lin, C.; Luidens, M.K.; Mousa, S.A.; Incerpi, S.; Drusano, G.L.; Davis, F.B.; Davis, P.J. L-thyroxine *vs.* 3,5,3′-triiodo-L-thyronine and cell proliferation: Activation of mitogen-activated protein kinase and phosphatidylinositol 3-kinase. *Am. J. Physiol. Cell Physiol.* **2009**, *296*, C980–C991.

29. Axelband, F.; Dias, J.; Ferrao, F.M.; Einicker-Lamas, M. Nongenomic signaling pathways triggered by thyroid hormones and their metabolite 3-iodothyronamine on the cardiovascular system. *J. Cell. Physiol.* **2011**, *226*, 21–28.

30. Irrcher, I.; Walkinshaw, D.R.; Sheehan, T.E.; Hood, D.A. Thyroid hormone (T3) rapidly activates p38 and ampk in skeletal muscle *in vivo*. *J. Appl. Physiol.* **2008**, *104*, 178–185.

31. Moeller, L.C.; Dumitrescu, A.M.; Refetoff, S. Cytosolic action of thyroid hormone leads to induction of hypoxia-inducible factor-1 α and glycolytic genes. *Mol. Endocrinol.* **2005**, *19*, 2955–2963.

32. De Lange, P.; Senese, R.; Cioffi, F.; Moreno, M.; Lombardi, A.; Silvestri, E.; Goglia, F.; Lanni, A. Rapid activation by 3,5,3'-L-triiodothyronine of adenosine 5'-monophosphate-activated protein kinase/acetyl-coenzyme a carboxylase and akt/protein kinase b signaling pathways: Relation to changes in fuel metabolism and myosin heavy-chain protein content in rat gastrocnemius muscle *in vivo*. *Endocrinology* **2008**, *149*, 6462–6470.

33. Canto, C.; Auwerx, J. Amp-activated protein kinase and its downstream transcriptional pathways. *Cell. Mol. Life Sci.* **2010**, *67*, 3407–3423.

34. Krueger, J.J.; Ning, X.H.; Argo, B.M.; Hyyti, O.; Portman, M.A. Triidothyronine and epinephrine rapidly modify myocardial substrate selection: A 13C isotopomer analysis. *Am. J. Physiol. Endocrinol. Metab.* **2001**, *281*, E983–E990.

35. Lombardi, A.; de Lange, P.; Silvestri, E.; Busiello, R.A.; Lanni, A.; Goglia, F.; Moreno, M. 3,5-Diiodo-L-thyronine rapidly enhances mitochondrial fatty acid oxidation rate and thermogenesis in rat skeletal muscle: AMP-activated protein kinase involvement. *Am. J. Physiol. Endocrinol. Metab.* **2009**, *296*, E497–E502.

36. Anderson, S.; Bankier, A.T.; Barrell, B.G.; de Bruijn, M.H.; Coulson, A.R.; Drouin, J.; Eperon, I.C.; Nierlich, D.P.; Roe, B.A.; Sanger, F.; *et al.* Sequence and organization of the human mitochondrial genome. *Nature* **1981**, *290*, 457–465.

37. Lopez, M.F.; Kristal, B.S.; Chernokalskaya, E.; Lazarev, A.; Shestopalov, A.I.; Bogdanova, A.; Robinson, M. High-throughput profiling of the mitochondrial proteome using affinity fractionation and automation. *Electrophoresis* **2000**, *21*, 3427–3440.

38. Wiesner, R.J.; Kurowski, T.T.; Zak, R. Regulation by thyroid hormone of nuclear and mitochondrial genes encoding subunits of cytochrome-c oxidase in rat liver and skeletal muscle. *Mol. Endocrinol.* **1992**, *6*, 1458–1467.

39. Holloszy, J.O. Skeletal muscle "mitochondrial deficiency" does not mediate insulin resistance. *Am. J. Clin. Nutr.* **2009**, *89*, 463S–466S.

40. Lazar, M.A. Thyroid hormone receptors: Multiple forms, multiple possibilities. *Endocr. Rev.* **1993**, *14*, 184–193.

41. Mitsuhashi, T.; Tennyson, G.E.; Nikodem, V.M. Alternative splicing generates messages encoding rat c-erbA proteins that do not bind thyroid hormone. *Proc. Natl. Acad. Sci. USA* **1988**, *85*, 5804–5808.

42. Williams, G.R. Cloning and characterization of two novel thyroid hormone receptor β isoforms. *Mol. Cell. Biol.* **2000**, *20*, 8329–8342.

43. Cioffi, F.; Lanni, A.; Goglia, F. Thyroid hormones, mitochondrial bioenergetics and lipid handling. *Curr. Opin. Endocrinol. Diabetes Obes.* **2010**, *17*, 402–407.

44. Kakizawa, T.; Miyamoto, T.; Kaneko, A.; Yajima, H.; Ichikawa, K.; Hashizume, K. Ligand-dependent heterodimerization of thyroid hormone receptor and retinoid x receptor. *J. Biol. Chem.* **1997**, *272*, 23799–23804.

45. Lee, S.; Privalsky, M.L. Heterodimers of retinoic acid receptors and thyroid hormone receptors display unique combinatorial regulatory properties. *Mol. Endocrinol.* **2005**, *19*, 863–878.

46. Crunkhorn, S.; Patti, M.E. Links between thyroid hormone action, oxidative metabolism, and diabetes risk? *Thyroid* **2008**, *18*, 227–237.

47. McClure, T.D.; Young, M.E.; Taegtmeyer, H.; Ning, X.H.; Buroker, N.E.; Lopez-Guisa, J.; Portman, M.A. Thyroid hormone interacts with PPARα and PGC-1 during mitochondrial maturation in sheep heart. *Am. J. Physiol. Heart Circ. Physiol.* **2005**, *289*, H2258–H2264.

48. Weitzel, J.M.; Hamann, S.; Jauk, M.; Lacey, M.; Filbry, A.; Radtke, C.; Iwen, K.A.; Kutz, S.; Harneit, A.; Lizardi, P.M.; *et al.* Hepatic gene expression patterns in thyroid hormone-treated hypothyroid rats. *J. Mol. Endocrinol.* **2003**, *31*, 291–303.

49. Weitzel, J.M.; Iwen, K.A.; Seitz, H.J. Regulation of mitochondrial biogenesis by thyroid hormone. *Exp. Physiol.* **2003**, *88*, 121–128.

50. Lee, J.Y.; Takahashi, N.; Yasubuchi, M.; Kim, Y.I.; Hashizaki, H.; Kim, M.J.; Sakamoto, T.; Goto, T.; Kawada, T. Triiodothyronine induces UPC-1 expression and mitochondrial biogenesis in human adipocytes. *Am. J. Physiol. Cell Physiol.* **2012**, *302*, C463–C472.

51. Psarra, A.M.; Solakidi, S.; Sekeris, C.E. The mitochondrion as a primary site of action of steroid and thyroid hormones: Presence and action of steroid and thyroid hormone receptors in mitochondria of animal cells. *Mol. Cell. Endocrinol.* **2006**, *246*, 21–33.

52. Wrutniak, C.; Cassar-Malek, I.; Marchal, S.; Rascle, A.; Heusser, S.; Keller, J.M.; Flechon, J.; Dauca, M.; Samarut, J.; Ghysdael, J.; *et al.* A 43-kDa protein related to c-ERb A α1 is located in the mitochondrial matrix of rat liver. *J. Biol. Chem.* **1995**, *270*, 16347–16354.

53. Casas, F.; Rochard, P.; Rodier, A.; Cassar-Malek, I.; Marchal-Victorion, S.; Wiesner, R.J.; Cabello, G.; Wrutniak, C. A variant form of the nuclear triiodothyronine receptor c-ERb A α1 plays a direct role in regulation of mitochondrial rna synthesis. *Mol. Cell. Biol.* **1999**, *19*, 7913–7924.

54. Casas, F.; Pessemesse, L.; Grandemange, S.; Seyer, P.; Baris, O.; Gueguen, N.; Ramonatxo, C.; Perrin, F.; Fouret, G.; Lepourry, L.; *et al.* Overexpression of the mitochondrial T3 receptor induces skeletal muscle atrophy during aging. *PLoS ONE* **2009**, *4*, e5631.

55. Pessemesse, L.; Lepourry, L.; Bouton, K.; Levin, J.; Cabello, G.; Wrutniak-Cabello, C.; Casas, F. p28, a truncated form of TRα1 regulates mitochondrial physiology. *FEBS Lett.* **2014**, *588*, 4037–4043.

56. Carazo, A.; Levin, J.; Casas, F.; Seyer, P.; Grandemange, S.; Busson, M.; Pessemesse, L.; Wrutniak-Cabello, C.; Cabello, G. Protein sequences involved in the mitochondrial import of the 3,5,3'-L-triiodothyronine receptor p43. *J. Cell. Physiol.* **2012**, *227*, 3768–3777.

57. Enriquez, J.A.; Fernandez-Silva, P.; Garrido-Perez, N.; Lopez-Perez, M.J.; Perez-Martos, A.; Montoya, J. Direct regulation of mitochondrial rna synthesis by thyroid hormone. *Mol. Cell. Biol.* **1999**, *19*, 657–670.

58. Garstka, H.L.; Facke, M.; Escribano, J.R.; Wiesner, R.J. Stoichiometry of mitochondrial transcripts and regulation of gene expression by mitochondrial transcription factor A. *Biochem. Biophys. Res. Commun.* **1994**, *200*, 619–626.

59. Scarpulla, R.C. Transcriptional paradigms in mammalian mitochondrial biogenesis and function. *Physiol. Rev.* **2008**, *88*, 611–638.

60. Picard, F.; Gehin, M.; Annicotte, J.; Rocchi, S.; Champy, M.F.; O'Malley, B.W.; Chambon, P.; Auwerx, J. SRC-1 and TIF-2 control energy balance between white and brown adipose tissues. *Cell* **2002**, *111*, 931–941.

61. Wu, Z.; Puigserver, P.; Andersson, U.; Zhang, C.; Adelmant, G.; Mootha, V.; Troy, A.; Cinti, S.; Lowell, B.; Scarpulla, R.C.; *et al.* Mechanisms controlling mitochondrial biogenesis and respiration through the thermogenic coactivator PGC-1. *Cell* **1999**, *98*, 115–124.

62. Oelkrug, R.; Polymeropoulos, E.T.; Jastroch, M. Brown adipose tissue: Physiological function and evolutionary significance. *J. Comp. Physiol.* **2015**, 1–20.

63. Cannon, B.; Hedin, A.; Nedergaard, J. Exclusive occurrence of thermogenin antigen in brown adipose tissue. *FEBS Lett.* **1982**, *150*, 129–132.

64. Lowell, B.B.; Spiegelman, B.M. Towards a molecular understanding of adaptive thermogenesis. *Nature* **2000**, *404*, 652–660.

65. Rabelo, R.; Schifman, A.; Rubio, A.; Sheng, X.; Silva, J.E. Delineation of thyroid hormone-responsive sequences within a critical enhancer in the rat uncoupling protein gene. *Endocrinology* **1995**, *136*, 1003–1013.

66. Silva, J.E.; Larsen, P.R. Adrenergic activation of triiodothyronine production in brown adipose tissue. *Nature* **1983**, *305*, 712–713.

67. Canettieri, G.; Celi, F.S.; Baccheschi, G.; Salvatori, L.; Andreoli, M.; Centanni, M. Isolation of human type 2 deiodinase gene promoter and characterization of a functional cyclic adenosine monophosphate response element. *Endocrinology* **2000**, *141*, 1804–1813.

68. Celi, F.S. Brown adipose tissue—When it pays to be inefficient. *N. Engl. J. Med.* **2009**, *360*, 1553–1556.

69. Larkin, S.; Mull, E.; Miao, W.; Pittner, R.; Albrandt, K.; Moore, C.; Young, A.; Denaro, M.; Beaumont, K. Regulation of the third member of the uncoupling protein family, UCP3, by cold and thyroid hormone. *Biochem. Biophys. Res. Commun.* **1997**, *240*, 222–227.

70. Masaki, T.; Yoshimatsu, H.; Kakuma, T.; Hidaka, S.; Kurokawa, M.; Sakata, T. Enhanced expression of uncoupling protein 2 gene in rat white adipose tissue and skeletal muscle following chronic treatment with thyroid hormone. *FEBS Lett.* **1997**, *418*, 323–326.

71. De Lange, P.; Lanni, A.; Beneduce, L.; Moreno, M.; Lombardi, A.; Silvestri, E.; Goglia, F. Uncoupling protein-3 is a molecular determinant for the regulation of resting metabolic rate by thyroid hormone. *Endocrinology* **2001**, *142*, 3414–3420.

72. Lombardi, A.; Busiello, R.A.; Napolitano, L.; Cioffi, F.; Moreno, M.; de Lange, P.; Silvestri, E.; Lanni, A.; Goglia, F. UCP3 translocates lipid hydroperoxide and mediates lipid hydroperoxide-dependent mitochondrial uncoupling. *J. Biol. Chem.* **2010**, *285*, 16599–16605.

73. Lanni, A.; Moreno, M.; Lombardi, A.; Goglia, F. Thyroid hormone and uncoupling proteins. *FEBS Lett.* **2003**, *543*, 5–10.

74. Wulf, A.; Harneit, A.; Kroger, M.; Kebenko, M.; Wetzel, M.G.; Weitzel, J.M. T3-mediated expression of PGC-1α via a far upstream located thyroid hormone response element. *Mol. Cell. Endocrinol.* **2008**, *287*, 90–95.

75. Rodgers, J.T.; Lerin, C.; Gerhart-Hines, Z.; Puigserver, P. Metabolic adaptations through the PGC-1α and sirt1 pathways. *FEBS Lett.* **2008**, *582*, 46–53.

76. Thijssen-Timmer, D.C.; Schiphorst, M.P.; Kwakkel, J.; Emter, R.; Kralli, A.; Wiersinga, W.M.; Bakker, O. PGC-1α regulates the isoform mrna ratio of the alternatively spliced thyroid hormone receptor α transcript. *J. Mol. Endocrinol.* **2006**, *37*, 251–257.

77. Yehuda-Shnaidman, E.; Kalderon, B.; Azazmeh, N.; Bar-Tana, J. Gating of the mitochondrial permeability transition pore by thyroid hormone. *FASEB J.* **2010**, *24*, 93–104.

78. Bernardi, P. Mitochondrial transport of cations: Channels, exchangers, and permeability transition. *Physiol. Rev.* **1999**, *79*, 1127–1155.

79. Rasola, A.; Bernardi, P. Mitochondrial permeability transition in Ca^{2+}-dependent apoptosis and necrosis. *Cell Calcium* **2011**, *50*, 222–233.

80. Crompton, M. The mitochondrial permeability transition pore and its role in cell death. *Biochem. J.* **1999**, *341*, 233–249.

81. Neckelmann, N.; Li, K.; Wade, R.P.; Shuster, R.; Wallace, D.C. cDNA sequence of a human skeletal muscle ADP/ATP translocator: Lack of a leader peptide, divergence from a fibroblast translocator cDNA, and coevolution with mitochondrial DNA genes. *Proc. Natl. Acad. Sci. USA* **1987**, *84*, 7580–7584.

82. Seitz, H.J.; Muller, M.J.; Soboll, S. Rapid thyroid-hormone effect on mitochondrial and cytosolic ATP/ADP ratios in the intact liver cell. *Biochem. J.* **1985**, *227*, 149–153.

83. Seitz, H.J.; Tiedgen, M.; Tarnowski, W. Regulation of hepatic phosphoenolpyruvate carboxykinase (GTP). Role of dietary proteins and amino acids *in vivo* and in the isolated perfused rat liver. *Biochim. Biophys. Acta* **1980**, *632*, 473–482.

84. Verhoeven, A.J.; Kamer, P.; Groen, A.K.; Tager, J.M. Effects of thyroid hormone on mitochondrial oxidative phosphorylation. *Biochem. J.* **1985**, *226*, 183–192.

85. Mowbray, J.; Hardy, D.L. Direct thyroid hormone signalling via ADP-ribosylation controls mitochondrial nucleotide transport and membrane leakiness by changing the conformation of the adenine nucleotide transporter. *FEBS Lett.* **1996**, *394*, 61–65.

86. Brand, M.D.; Pakay, J.L.; Ocloo, A.; Kokoszka, J.; Wallace, D.C.; Brookes, P.S.; Cornwall, E.J. The basal proton conductance of mitochondria depends on adenine nucleotide translocase content. *Biochem. J.* **2005**, *392*, 353–362.

87. Ukropec, J.; Anunciado, R.P.; Ravussin, Y.; Hulver, M.W.; Kozak, L.P. UCP1-independent thermogenesis in white adipose tissue of cold-acclimated $Ucp1^{-/-}$ mice. *J. Biol. Chem.* **2006**, *281*, 31894–31908.

88. Hagopian, K.; Ramsey, J.J.; Weindruch, R. Enzymes of glycerol and glyceraldehyde metabolism in mouse liver: Effects of caloric restriction and age on activities. *Biosci. Rep.* **2008**, *28*, 107–115.

89. Alfadda, A.; DosSantos, R.A.; Stepanyan, Z.; Marrif, H.; Silva, J.E. Mice with deletion of the mitochondrial glycerol-3-phosphate dehydrogenase gene exhibit a thrifty phenotype: Effect of gender. *Am. J. Physiol. Regul. Integr. Comp. Physiol.* **2004**, *287*, R147–R156.

90. Burch, H.B.; Wartofsky, L. Life-threatening thyrotoxicosis. Thyroid storm. *Endocrinol. Metab. Clin. N. Am.* **1993**, *22*, 263–277.

91. Moreno, M.; de Lange, P.; Lombardi, A.; Silvestri, E.; Lanni, A.; Goglia, F. Metabolic effects of thyroid hormone derivatives. *Thyroid* **2008**, *18*, 239–253.

92. Baxter, J.D.; Webb, P. Thyroid hormone mimetics: Potential applications in atherosclerosis, obesity and type 2 diabetes. *Nat. Rev. Drug Discov.* **2009**, *8*, 308–320.

93. Grover, G.J.; Mellstrom, K.; Ye, L.; Malm, J.; Li, Y.L.; Bladh, L.G.; Sleph, P.G.; Smith, M.A.; George, R.; Vennstrom, B.; *et al.* Selective thyroid hormone receptor-β activation: A strateg−y for reduction of weight, cholesterol, and lipoprotein (a) with reduced cardiovascular liability. *Proc. Natl. Acad. Sci. USA* **2003**, *100*, 10067–10072.

94. Perra, A.; Simbula, G.; Simbula, M.; Pibiri, M.; Kowalik, M.A.; Sulas, P.; Cocco, M.T.; Ledda-Columbano, G.M.; Columbano, A. Thyroid hormone (T3) and TRβ agonist GC-1 inhibit/reverse nonalcoholic fatty liver in rats. *FASEB J.* **2008**, *22*, 2981–2989.

95. Trost, S.U.; Swanson, E.; Gloss, B.; Wang-Iverson, D.B.; Zhang, H.; Volodarsky, T.; Grover, G.J.; Baxter, J.D.; Chiellini, G.; Scanlan, T.S.; *et al.* The thyroid hormone receptor-β selective agonist GC-1 differentially affects plasma lipids and cardiac activity. *Endocrinology* **2000**, *141*, 3057–3064.

96. Villicev, C.M.; Freitas, F.R.; Aoki, M.S.; Taffarel, C.; Scanlan, T.S.; Moriscot, A.S.; Ribeiro, M.O.; Bianco, A.C.; Gouveia, C.H. Thyroid hormone receptor β-specific agonist GC-1 increases energy expenditure and prevents fat-mass accumulation in rats. *J. Endocrinol.* **2007**, *193*, 21–29.

97. Coppola, M.; Glinni, D.; Moreno, M.; Cioffi, F.; Silvestri, E.; Goglia, F. Thyroid hormone analogues and derivatives: Actions in fatty liver. *World J. Hepatol.* **2014**, *6*, 114–129.

98. Senese, R.; Cioffi, F.; de Lange, P.; Goglia, F.; Lanni, A. Thyroid: Biological actions of "nonclassical" thyroid hormones. *J. Endocrinol.* **2014**, *221*, R1–R12.

99. Piehl, S.; Hoefig, C.S.; Scanlan, T.S.; Kohrle, J. Thyronamines—Past, present, and future. *Endocr. Rev.* **2011**, *32*, 64–80.

100. Pinna, G.; Meinhold, H.; Hiedra, L.; Thoma, R.; Hoell, T.; Graf, K.J.; Stoltenburg-Didinger, G.; Eravci, M.; Prengel, H.; Brodel, O.; *et al.* Elevated 3,5-diiodothyronine concentrations in the sera of patients with nonthyroidal illnesses and brain tumors. *J. Clin. Endocrinol. Metab.* **1997**, *82*, 1535–1542.

101. Horst, C.; Rokos, H.; Seitz, H.J. Rapid stimulation of hepatic oxygen consumption by 3,5-*di*-iodo-L-thyronine. *Biochem. J.* **1989**, *261*, 945–950.

102. Lombardi, A.; Lanni, A.; Moreno, M.; Brand, M.D.; Goglia, F. Effect of 3,5-*di*-iodo-L-thyronine on the mitochondrial energy-transduction apparatus. *Biochem. J.* **1998**, *330*, 521–526.

103. Moreno, M.; Lanni, A.; Lombardi, A.; Goglia, F. How the thyroid controls metabolism in the rat: Different roles for triiodothyronine and diiodothyronines. *J. Physiol.* **1997**, *505*, 529–538.

104. Lanni, A.; Moreno, M.; Lombardi, A.; de Lange, P.; Silvestri, E.; Ragni, M.; Farina, P.; Baccari, G.C.; Fallahi, P.; Antonelli, A.; *et al.* 3,5-Diiodo-L-thyronine powerfully reduces adiposity in rats by increasing the burning of fats. *FASEB J.* **2005**, *19*, 1552–1554.

105. Grasselli, E.; Canesi, L.; Voci, A.; de Matteis, R.; Demori, I.; Fugassa, E.; Vergani, L. Effects of 3,5-diiodo-L-thyronine administration on the liver of high fat diet-fed rats. *Exp. Biol. Med.* **2008**, *233*, 549–557.

106. Mollica, M.P.; Lionetti, L.; Moreno, M.; Lombardi, A.; de Lange, P.; Antonelli, A.; Lanni, A.; Cavaliere, G.; Barletta, A.; Goglia, F. 3,5-Diiodo-L-thyronine, by modulating mitochondrial functions, reverses hepatic fat accumulation in rats fed a high-fat diet. *J. Hepatol.* **2009**, *51*, 363–370.

107. Moreno, M.; Silvestri, E.; de Matteis, R.; de Lange, P.; Lombardi, A.; Glinni, D.; Senese, R.; Cioffi, F.; Salzano, A.M.; Scaloni, A.; *et al.* 3,5-Diiodo-L-thyronine prevents high-fat-diet-induced insulin resistance in rat skeletal muscle through metabolic and structural adaptations. *FASEB J.* **2011**, *25*, 3312–3324.

108. Lombardi, A.; Senese, R.; de Matteis, R.; Busiello, R.A.; Cioffi, F.; Goglia, F.; Lanni, A. 3,5-Diiodo-L-thyronine activates brown adipose tissue thermogenesis in hypothyroid rats. *PLoS ONE* **2015**, *10*, e0116498.

109. Antonelli, A.; Fallahi, P.; Ferrari, S.M.; di Domenicantonio, A.; Moreno, M.; Lanni, A.; Goglia, F. 3,5-Diiodo-L-thyronine increases resting metabolic rate and reduces body weight without undesirable side effects. *J. Biol. Regul. Homeost. Agents* **2011**, *25*, 655–660.

110. Bochukova, E.; Schoenmakers, N.; Agostini, M.; Schoenmakers, E.; Rajanayagam, O.; Keogh, J.M.; Henning, E.; Reinemund, J.; Gevers, E.; Sarri, M.; *et al.* A mutation in the thyroid hormone receptor α gene. *N. Engl. J. Med.* **2012**, *366*, 243–249.

111. Moran, C.; Schoenmakers, N.; Agostini, M.; Schoenmakers, E.; Offiah, A.; Kydd, A.; Kahaly, G.; Mohr-Kahaly, S.; Rajanayagam, O.; Lyons, G.; *et al.* An adult female with resistance to thyroid hormone mediated by defective thyroid hormone receptor α. *J. Clin. Endocrinol. Metab.* **2013**, *98*, 4254–4261.

112. Mitchell, C.S.; Savage, D.B.; Dufour, S.; Schoenmakers, N.; Murgatroyd, P.; Befroy, D.; Halsall, D.; Northcott, S.; Raymond-Barker, P.; Curran, S.; *et al.* Resistance to thyroid hormone is associated with raised energy expenditure, muscle mitochondrial uncoupling, and hyperphagia. *J. Clin. Investig.* **2010**, *120*, 1345–1354.

113. Tuca, A.; Giralt, M.; Villarroya, F.; Vinas, O.; Mampel, T.; Iglesias, R. Ontogeny of thyroid hormone receptors and c-erbA expression during brown adipose tissue development: Evidence of fetal acquisition of the mature thyroid status. *Endocrinology* **1993**, *132*, 1913–1920.

114. Martinez de Mena, R.; Scanlan, T.S.; Obregon, M.J. The T3 receptor β isoform regulates UCP1 and D2 deiodinase in rat brown adipocytes. *Endocrinology* **2010**, *151*, 5074–5083.

115. Fernandez-Real, J.M.; Corella, D.; Goumidi, L.; Mercader, J.M.; Valdes, S.; Rojo Martinez, G.; Ortega, F.; Martinez-Larrad, M.T.; Gomez-Zumaquero, J.M.; Salas-Salvado, J.; *et al.* Thyroid hormone receptor α gene variants increase the risk of developing obesity and show gene-diet interactions. *Int. J. Obes.* **2013**, *37*, 1499–1505.

9

Mitochondria as Key Targets of Cardioprotection in Cardiac Ischemic Disease: Role of Thyroid Hormone Triiodothyronine

Francesca Forini [1,*], Giuseppina Nicolini [1,2] and Giorgio Iervasi [1]

[1] CNR Institute of Clinical Physiology, Via G. Moruzzi 1, Pisa 56124, Italy;
E-Mails: nicolini@ifc.cnr.it (G.N.); iervasi@ifc.cnr.it (G.I.)

[2] Tuscany Region G. Monasterio Foundation, Via G. Moruzzi 1, Pisa 56124, Italy

* Author to whom correspondence should be addressed; E-Mail: simona@ifc.cnr.it

Academic Editors: Jaime M. Ross and Giuseppe Coppotelli

Abstract: Ischemic heart disease is the major cause of mortality and morbidity worldwide. Early reperfusion after acute myocardial ischemia has reduced short-term mortality, but it is also responsible for additional myocardial damage, which in the long run favors adverse cardiac remodeling and heart failure evolution. A growing body of experimental and clinical evidence show that the mitochondrion is an essential end effector of ischemia/reperfusion injury and a major trigger of cell death in the acute ischemic phase (up to 48–72 h after the insult), the subacute phase (from 72 h to 7–10 days) and chronic stage (from 10–14 days to one month after the insult). As such, in recent years scientific efforts have focused on mitochondria as a target for cardioprotective strategies in ischemic heart disease and cardiomyopathy. The present review discusses recent advances in this field, with special emphasis on the emerging role of the biologically active thyroid hormone triiodothyronine (T3).

Keywords: cardiac ischemia/reperfusion injury; low T3 syndrome; mitochondrial dysfunction; cardioprotection

1. Introduction

Acute myocardial infarction (AMI) leading to ischemic heart disease is a major debilitating disease and important cause of death worldwide [1]. Deprivation of oxygen and nutrients following coronary occlusion is the primary cause of damage to the myocardium and its severity depends on the extent and duration of artery obstruction. Although timely, reperfusion effectively reduces short-term mortality, the reperfusion process itself yields additional injury, including cardiomyocyte dysfunction and death, which in the long run prompts adverse cardiac remodeling [1–3]. As a consequence, prevention or limitation of cardiac damage in the early stages of reperfusion is a crucial step in ameliorating patient prognosis.

Multiple lines of evidence show that mitochondrial functional impairments are critical determinants for myocyte loss during the acute ischemic stage, as well as for the progressive decline of surviving myocytes during the subacute and chronic stages [3–6]. Therefore, mitochondrial dysfunction is considered to be one of the major mechanisms in the pathogenesis of ischemia/reperfusion injury (IRI) and cardiomyopathy.

In spite of promising mitochondria-targeted therapeutic strategies emerging from experimental studies, very few have successfully completed clinical trials. As such, the mitochondrion is a potential untapped target for new therapies. Although ischemic pre-conditioning is a potent protective strategy first reported many decades ago [7], its utility in myocardial ischemia (MI) patients with an abrupt onset of disease undermines implementation of preconditioning in the clinical settings. Therefore, most modern approaches focus on the application of pharmacological or ischemic post-conditioning maneuvers to combat reperfusion injury and adverse cardiac remodeling [8].

Along this line, a growing body of clinical and experimental evidence shows that thyroid hormone (TH) supplementation may offer a novel option for cardiac diseases [9–12]. Indeed, 3,5,3'-triiodothyronine (T3), the biologically active form of TH, significantly declines after AMI both in animal models and in patients [13–15], with "low-T3 Syndrome" (low-T3S) being a strong independent prognostic predictor of death and major adverse cardiac events [16]. Consistently, treatment for low-T3S exerts cardioprotective effects in both humans and animal models [17–20].

Since the mitochondrion is a common effector of cardioprotective strategy and a main target of TH action [21–23], this review has a dual purpose: (1) to summarize the mitochondria-targeted noxious pathways and protective signaling that could be exploited to improve post-ischemic cardiac recovery and (2) to integrate classic and novel TH actions in a unified, mitochondria-centered picture that highlights how the crosstalk of TH with those molecular networks favors post-ischemic cardiomyocytes' survival.

2. Triggers of Mitochondrial-Dependent Cardiomyocyte Death in Ischemia/Reperfusion

2.1. Mitochondrial Dysfunction in Ischemia/Reperfusion

A wide spectrum of metabolic and ionic derangements occur in ischemia/reperfusion (I/R), culminating in mitochondrial impairment. Oxygen deprivation during ischemia arrests oxidative phosphorylation, decreasing intracellular ATP and favoring anaerobic glycolysis. The accumulation of lactic acid decreases the intracellular pH. As a consequence, the Na^+/H^+ antiporter is activated in an attempt to restore the pH. The resulting accumulation of cytosolic sodium reverses the direction of the Na^+/Ca^{2+} exchanger, leading to an increase in intracellular Ca^{2+} levels. The mitochondria act as a buffer for intracellular calcium, which ultimately causes calcium overload in the mitochondria [24,25]. This leads to an increase in ROS production from mitochondrial electron transfer complexes I and III, which consequently causes a decrease in anti-oxidant defenses [26–28]. The increased oxygen tension at the onset of reperfusion results in a greater burst of oxidative stress [29], which worsens mitochondrial dysfunction and alters membrane properties [5,30–32]. Damage to the mitochondrial outer membrane along with activation of the proapoptotic BCL-2 proteins leads to mitochondrial outer membrane permeabilization, release of cytochrome c, caspase activation, and apoptosis [33]. Massive oxidative stress can lead to a sudden increase in inner mitochondrial membrane permeability that is attributable to the opening of the so-called permeability transition pore (PTP). Opening of the PTP (PTPO) is accompanied by release of ROS and calcium [34,35]; this can propagate the damage to neighboring mitochondria and culminate in activation of calcium-dependent proteases (calpains) and lipases (cPLA2), inducing necrotic cell death [30,36]. The molecular nature of the PTP remains controversial, but current evidence implicates a matrix protein, Cyclophilin-D (Cyp-D), and two inner membrane proteins, adenine nucleotide translocase (ANT) and the phosphate carrier (PiC) [4,37–39].

An array of stress-responsive signaling pathways activated during early reoxygenation or in post-ischemic wound healing has been implicated in the regulation of these mitochondrial changes, and thus represents potential targets for therapeutic intervention.

2.2. The p38 Mitogen-Activated Protein Kinase Intracellular Signaling

A highly conserved component of myocyte stress-responsiveness in I/R involves signaling through a family of serine-threonine kinase effectors known as p38 mitogen-activated protein kinase (p38MAPK). Four separate p38MAPK isoforms, including p38α, p38β, p38γ, and p38δ, have been identified. Each p38 isoform phosphorylates a diverse array of intracellular proteins including stress-responsive transcription factors [40].

This signaling cascade ultimately converges in mitochondria to enhance oxidative stress and mitochondrial-dependent cardiomyocyte death [41–43]. Among the pro-apoptotic targets activated by p38Mapk in I/R, the tumor suppressor protein p53 and Bax play key roles in determining both acute cell injury and post-ischemic adverse remodeling [44–46]. Also, it has been demonstrated that p38 MAPK plays a causative role in the inhibition of the anti-apoptotic Bcl-2 protein [47]. Accordingly, inhibitors of p38 signaling have been shown to confer protection from IRI [48].

TH Inhibits p38MAPK under Stress Conditions

TH exhibits a prominent role in the regulation of p38MAPK. In the post-ischemic rat brain, thyroxine, T4, treatment was protective through its p38-targeted anti-apoptotic and anti-inflammatory mechanism [49]. In Langendorff-perfused rat heart models of I/R, long-term T4 pretreatment or acute T3 administration markedly improved post-ischemic recovery of left ventricular performance while reducing cardiomyocyte death markers and blunting the activation of p38MAPK [50,51]. As suggested by a subsequent study, this effect was mediated at least in part by the thyroid hormone receptor α1 (TRα1) [52]. Indeed, in a mouse model of AMI, pharmacological inhibition of TRα1 further depressed post-ischemic cardiac function and was accompanied by marked activation of p38MAPK [52].

2.3. Tumor Suppressor Protein p53

2.3.1. p53 and Cardiomyocyte Death: Direct Action

Tumor suppressor protein p53 accumulates in the myocardium after myocardial infarction, and plays an important role in the progression to heart failure. It is well established that p53 can trigger apoptosis through the mitochondrial pathway [53]. For example, it can trans-activate Bax, the pro-apoptotic member of the BCL-2 family that translocates from the cytosol to mitochondria, causing the release of apoptotic proteins [54,55]. Besides its classic role, a broader role in organ homeostasis is just beginning to be understood. It has recently been reported that in response to oxidative stress, p53 accumulates in the mitochondrial matrix and triggers mitochondrial PTPO and necrosis by physical interaction with the PTP regulator Cyclophilin D (Cyp-D) [56]. p53 also plays a critical role in other important processes that regulate mitochondrial integrity but are impaired in I/R, such as mitochondrial morphology and mitophagy [57,58].

2.3.2. p53 Regulation of Mitochondrial Morphology

Mitochondria change their morphology by undergoing either fusion or fission, resulting in either elongated, tubular, interconnected mitochondrial networks or fragmented, discontinuous mitochondria, respectively [59,60]. These two opposing processes are regulated by the mitochondrial fusion proteins: mitofusin (Mfn) 1, Mfn2, and optic atrophy protein 1(OPA1); and the mitochondrial fission proteins: dynamin-related protein 1 (Drp1) and human mitochondrial fission protein 1 (hFis1). The fine balance between mitochondrial fusion and fission within a cell may be upset by a variety of factors, including oxidative stress [61] and ischemia [34,62], which can predispose the cell to apoptosis and mitochondrial PTPO [63], critical mediators of IRI.

p53 affects the mitochondrial dynamic by two opposite mechanisms that disrupt the equilibrium between fission and fusion, promoting cell death. In one way, p53 may upregulate Drp1 with consequent activation of excessive mitochondrial fission [64]. Drp1, in turn, stabilizes p53 in the mitochondria to trigger necrosis [65]. On the other hand, p53 may promote indirect, Bax-mediated, excessive mitochondrial fusion leading to cell necrosis as well [66].

2.3.3. p53 Effect on Mitophagy

In response to stress, cells have developed mitophagy, a defense mechanism that involves selective sequestration and subsequent degradation of the dysfunctional mitochondrion [67]. In I/R, mitophagy functions as an early cardioprotective response, favoring the removal of damaged mitochondria before they can cause activation of cell death [58]. The E3 ubiquitin ligase Parkin was recently discovered to play an important role in targeting damaged mitochondria for removal via autophagy in cardiomyocytes [58]. The proposed mechanism involves Mfn2 activation and Parkin recruitment from the cytosol to depolarized mitochondria [68]. Interestingly, another report showed Parkin localization to depolarized mitochondria even in the absence of Mfn2, which could indicate the presence of alternative mechanisms for Parkin translocation [69].

In the mouse heart, p53 cytosolic accumulation induces mitochondrial dysfunction by binding to Parkin and disturbing its translocation to damaged mitochondria and their subsequent clearance by mitophagy [70]. On the contrary, p53 knock-down preserved mitophagic flux under ischemia without a change in cardiac tissue ATP content [71]. Analysis of autophagic mediators acting downstream of p53 revealed that the TP53-induced glycolysis and apoptosis regulator (TIGAR) mediated the inhibition of myocyte mitophagy responsible for impairment of mitochondrial integrity and subsequent apoptosis, and this process is closely involved in p53-dependent ventricular remodeling after myocardial infarction [71].

3. Promoters of Mitochondria-Mediated Cardioprotection in Ischemia/Reperfusion

3.1. The Reperfusion Injury Salvage Pathway

A central biochemical pathway involved in cytoprotection is the phosphoinositide 3-kinase (PI3K) pathway, also known as the reperfusion injury salvage kinase (RISK) pathway. This pathway consists of a tyrosine kinase receptor (RTK) whose activation results in the recruitment of PI3K. Next, PI3K activates Akt, which in turn phosphorylates downstream kinases [72]. Regarding the heart, the literature on Akt is extensive [73] and has largely established Akt as a key pro-survival kinase in normal cardiac homeostasis and in response to injury. Classically, Akt activation promotes survival via inhibition of pro-apoptotic Bcl-2 family proteins Bax and Bad, limiting mitochondrial outer membrane (OMM) permeabilization and thereby blocking release of cytochrome c and caspase-mediated apoptosis. The RISK pathway is also implicated in PTP regulation and preservation of mitochondrial membrane potential ($\Delta\Psi$m) [74]. The glycogen synthase kinase 3-β (GSK-3β) is a key downstream target of Akt and is inactive when phosphorylated. Thus, GSK-3β phosphorylation by Akt or other upstream mediators results in inhibition of GSK-3β-activated targets. For example, inactivation of GSK-3β by Akt reduces mitochondrial Bax recruitment [75] as well as PTPO [76,77]. Enhancement of p53 activity by GSK-3β and GSK-3β interaction with CypD may have a role in mPTP opening [78,79]. The use of GSK-3β inhibitors in the post-ischemic setting is hampered by the side effect of inhibiting the physiological function of GSK-3β [80]. To overcome this limitation, selective inhibition of GSK-3β mitochondria uptake has been reported as a promising and novel approach to cardioprotection from lethal reperfusion injury [81].

The recruitment of the RISK pathway also induces phosphorylation-dependent activation of the endothelial nitric oxide synthase (eNOS), which is expected to block PTPO through its release of nitric oxide (NO) [82]. In turn, NO triggers the opening of the mitochondrial ATP-dependent potassium channels (mitoKATP) [83], a cardioprotective process that has been causally related to post-conditioning [84]. Furthermore, an increase in NO availability may enhance mitochondrial protein S-nitrosylation (SNO) and promote cardioprotection [85,86]. Finally, the RISK pathway has also been shown to confer cardioprotection against IRI by modulating Mfn1-dependent mitochondrial morphology [86,87].

Role of Thyroid Hormone in the Activation of Reperfusion Injury Salvage Pathway

THs are critically involved in the activation of the RISK pathways in both physiological and stress conditions. Rapid T3-mediated activation of PI3K by cytosolic TRα1, and subsequent activation of the Akt-mTOR signaling pathway, has been proposed as one of the mechanisms by which TH regulates physiological cardiac growth [88]. T3 administration can prevent serum starvation-induced neonatal cardiomyocyte apoptosis via Akt [89]. *In vivo* T4 treatment has been shown to cause phosphorylation of Akt and downstream signaling targets such as GSK-3β and mTOR in rat heart ventricles [90]. The Akt-mediated cardioprotective action of TH was confirmed in an experimental model of rat myocardial ischemia, where early short-term treatment of T3 reduced myocytes apoptosis through activation of Akt [19]. In a recent study, TH was found to have a dose-dependent effect on Akt phosphorylation, which may be of physiological relevance [91]. Mild activation of Akt caused by the replacement dose of TH resulted in favorable effects, while further induction of Akt signaling by higher doses of TH was accompanied by increased mortality and activation of extracellular signal-regulated kinases (ERK), some of the most well-studied kinases in relation to pathological remodeling [92]. This study may be of important therapeutic relevance because it shows that TH replacement therapy may be sufficient to restore cardiac function, while excessive TH doses may be detrimental rather than beneficial.

3.2. Inhibition of p53 Signaling

Given the detrimental effects of p53 in the myocardial IRI, this molecule may be proposed as a central hub in stress-induced apoptosis and necrosis instigated in mitochondria and may act as a novel therapeutic target [93].

Role of Thyroid Hormone in the Inhibition of p53 Signaling

Thyroid hormone is a critical regulator of p53 activity. A p53-centered anti-apoptotic action of TH has been well characterized in tumor cells [94,95]. In a rat model of post-ischemic acute stroke, TH treatment reduced cerebral infarction while limiting cell death through modulation of the p53 targets Bax and BCl2 [49]. On the other hand, p53 is able to hamper TH signaling. Early studies showed that the physical interaction of thyroid hormone receptors (TRs) with p53 inhibited the binding of TRs to the TH-responsive elements (TREs) in a concentration-dependent manner and that this interaction negatively regulated the TRs' signaling pathways [96,97]. Although these data collectively suggest that the cross-talk between p53 and TH may play an important role in physiological and pathological conditions, its role in cardiac disease evolution is only beginning to be explored. A recent paper reported a critical role for TH in inhibiting the p53-dependent activation of mitochondrial-mediated cell death in a model of cardiac I/R [98]. In this study, the low-T3S following the ischemic insult was accompanied by an up-regulation of p53 and activation of its downstream events, such as Bax induction and mitochondrial impairment. Early T3 administration at near-physiological dose improved the recovery of post-ischemic cardiac performance. At the molecular level, T3 blunted p53 and Bax up-regulation in the area at risk (AAR), thus preserving mitochondrial function and decreasing apoptosis and necrosis extent in the AAR [98]. Similarly, in cardiomyocytes exposed to oxidative stress, T3 treatment reduced cell death, preserved mitochondrial biogenesis and membrane potential, and limited p53 upregulation [98,99].

3.3. Targeting Mitochondrial Oxidative Stress

In accordance with a role for mitochondrial dysfunction and ROS production in the pathogenesis of heart disease, it has been shown that targeted mitochondrial ROS scavenging reduces remodeling whereas non-targeted ROS treatment has no effect [32]. This is in agreement with the lack of benefit provided by non-targeted anti-oxidants in the clinical arena [100,101], and supports the general concept of compartmentalized signaling. This concept implies close vicinity of signaling molecules to provide local control over second messengers; in this regard, targeted ROS scavenging, which accumulates manifold at the microdomains of ROS formation in mitochondria, might be more efficient in the specific targeting of cellular ROS signaling. One relevant paper suggests that mitochondria-targeted Bendavia may be extremely effective in preventing reperfusion-induced damage to cardiac mitochondria [102]. Mitoquinone (mitoQ), a coenzyme Q analog, easily crosses phospholipid bilayers and is driven to concentrate within mitochondria by the large electrochemical membrane potential. The respiratory chain reduces mitoQ to its active ubiquinol antioxidant form to limit myocardial I/R injury [103]. The SS-31 (Szeto-Schiller) peptide is also of interest since it is cell-permeable and specifically targeted to inner mitochondrial membranes based on its residue sequence, with an anti-oxidant dimethyltyrosine moiety. SS-31 has been shown to be taken up by the heart in an *ex vivo* reperfusion system and was protective against I/R injury [104]. The peptides SS-02 and SS-31 were also protective against cardiac I/R injury when added during reperfusion [105].

Role of Thyroid Hormone in the Inhibition of Mitochondrial Oxidative Stress

It has recently been shown that TH has a mitochondria-targeted antioxidant protective effect under *in vitro* stress conditions and after myocardial infarction *in vivo* [98,99,106]. In cultured cardiomyocytes, T3 treatment decreased oxidative stress-induced cell death while maintaining mitochondrial function [99]. These effects were prevented by inhibitors of mitoKATP channel opening, suggesting that activation of the mitoKATP channel in rescued mitochondria is an important protective mechanism elicited by T3 against oxidative stress-mediated cell death [99]. In a post-ischemic HF model, TH administration during the post-infarction period leads to normalization of the myocardial performance index, reduction of ROS level, and stimulation of cytosolic and mitochondrial anti-oxidant defenses [106]. In an experimental AMI model, T3 supplementation reduced mitochondrial superoxide production and limited inner mitochondrial membrane depolarization, thus improving mitochondrial function and cell viability [99].

3.4. Inhibition of Mitochondrial Permeability Transition Pore Opening

Since the initial reports on the existence of mitochondrial cyclophilin in the late 1980s, a vast majority of studies have recognized the crucial role of Cyp-D in PTP regulation. In animal models, inhibition of Cyp-D by either pharmacologic targeting [107,108], genetic ablation [109,110], or RNA interference [111], provides strong protection from both reperfusion injury and post ischemic HF.

Although chronic pharmacological inhibition of CypD has been shown to cause metabolic reprogramming and worsening of pressure-induced HF [112], its acute inhibition to attenuate lethal IR injury holds great promise for reducing myocardial infarct size in humans [8,113]. Besides Cyp-D, several physiological regulators of mPTP function may be exploited to confer cardioprotection from I/R injury.

One important class of endogenous transducers of cell stress signals are the signal transducer and activator of transcription (STAT) proteins. Several STAT isoforms are expressed in the heart; among them, STAT3 is involved in the reduction of post-ischemic myocardial injury [114]. The infarct size reduction by ischemic post-conditioning is also attenuated in STAT3-KO mice [115]. STAT3 has been localized in mitochondria, where it contributes to cardioprotection by stimulating respiration and inhibiting the Ca^{2+}-induced mitochondrial PTPO [116].

Nitric oxide (NO) is another important signaling molecule that has been shown to reduce myocardial injury in a number of ischemia/reperfusion models. For example, brief periods of NO breathing reduced myocardial injury from ischemia/reperfusion in mice and pigs [117–119]. A critical process during NO-induced cardioprotection is to prevent mitochondrial PTPO potentially via targeting of the ANT component of the pore-forming complex [120].

Hypoxia inducible factor 1 α (HIF-1α) is an oxygen-sensitive transcription factor that enables aerobic organisms to adapt to hypoxia. This is achieved through the transcriptional activation of up to 200 genes, many of which are critical to cell survival [121]. Under normoxic conditions, the hydroxylation of HIF-1α by prolyl hydroxylase domain-containing (PHD) enzymes targets it for proteosomal degradation. However, under hypoxic conditions, PHD activity is inhibited, thereby allowing HIF-1α to accumulate and translocate to the nucleus, where it binds to the hypoxia-responsive element sequences of target gene promoters. Experimental studies suggest that stabilization of HIF-1α may protect the heart against the detrimental effects of acute I/R injury [121].

Role of TH in the Inhibition of Permeability Transition Pore Opening

The mechanisms underlying the myocyte-directed protective effect of HIF are not completely clear. A recent paper showed that HIF-1α stabilization, by either a pharmacological or genetic approach, protected the heart against acute IRI by inhibiting mitochondrial PTPO and decreasing mitochondrial oxidative stress [122]. Accordingly, T3 replacement has been shown to induce HIF-1α stabilization in a post-ischemic HF model, which was related to better preserved mitochondrial activity and cardiac performance [99].

3.5. Mitochondrial Biogenesis

Mitochondrial biogenesis has emerged as an important point in the multi-site control of mitochondrial function and a putative target for therapeutic intervention against cardiac IRI [123,124]. Mitochondrial biogenesis includes regulation of mitochondrial protein expression, their assembly within the mitochondrial network, and replication of mitochondrial DNA (mtDNA). Of the 1500 proteins representing the mitochondrial proteome, mtDNA provides 13 subunits of the oxidative phosphorylation system together with ribosomal and transfer RNAs; whereas more than 98% of the mitochondrial protein requirement is encoded by the nuclear genome [125]. Hence, a spatial and temporal coordination of nuclear and mitochondrial genomes is necessary to ensure that all mitochondrial components are available for correct assembly. The master regulator of the process is the nuclear-encoded peroxisome proliferator-activated receptor-γ coactivator-1α (PGC1-α). PGC-1α lacks DNA-binding activity but interacts and coactivates numerous transcription factors driving mitochondrial biogenesis, energy metabolism, fatty acid oxidation, and antioxidant activity [126]. In particular, PGC-1α activates nuclear transcription factors (NTFs) leading to upregulation of nuclear-encoded proteins. Nuclear-encoded proteins are imported into mitochondria through the outer-membrane (TOM) or inner-membrane (TIM) translocase transport machinery. Finally, nuclear- and mitochondrial-encoded subunits of the respiratory chain are assembled [127]. A downregulation of the entire pathway of mitochondrial biogenesis was reported both in AMI and in HF evolution [128,129]. Reduced PGC-1α activity and gene expression have been observed in several experimental models of pathologic cardiac hypertrophy, and HF [130,131] and has been involved in the pathogenesis of human heart disease [132]. It has been shown that in the heart, pathological stressors such as ischemia are associated with a downregulation of mitochondrial biogenesis via PGC-1α activity [133], and that impairment of the PGC-1α-mediated mitochondrial biogenesis increased heart vulnerability to IRI [134]. Accordingly, upregulation of the PGC-1α pathway confers protection against simulated I/R in cardiomyoblast cells [135]. Moreover, the induction of PGC-1α protein upregulates a broad spectrum of ROS detoxification systems, such as superoxide dismutase 2 (SOD2) and glutathione peroxidase-1 [136]. Hence, a putative mechanism whereby the mitochondrial biogenesis program may additionally augment tolerance to cardiac ischemia is via ROS detoxification.

During mitochondrial biogenesis, the coordinated transcription and replication of the mitochondrial genome is carried out via the nuclear-encoded mitochondrial transcription factor A (mtTFA), a downstream effector of PGC1-α signaling. It has long been recognized that post-ischemic adverse remodeling is frequently associated with qualitative and quantitative defects in mtDNA [137–139], and that a decline in mitochondrial function and mtDNA copy number play a major role in the development of post-ischemic heart disease [31,140]. In accordance, targeted disruption of mtTFA specifically within cardiac tissue resulted in a significant decrease in electron transport capacity, spontaneous cardiomyopathy, and cardiac disease [141,142]. Conversely, increasing the expression of mtTFA within cardiac tissue offered protection from adverse remodeling induced by myocardial infarction [143].

Given the causative role of mitochondrial dis-homeostasis in adverse cardiac remodeling, understanding the stimuli, signals, and transducers that govern mitochondrial biogenesis pathways may have critical significance in the treatment of ischemic cardiovascular disorders. In the last few years, the NAD^+-dependent protein deacetylase sirtuin 1 (SIRT1) has emerged as an important regulator of mitochondrial biogenesis [144,145]. Besides its epigenetic role in silencing of transcription by heterochromatin formation through histones modification, SIRT1 influences the activity of PGC-1α through a functional protein–protein interaction [146]. SIRT1 activation of PGC-1α enhances mitochondrial biogenesis, optimizes mitochondrial surface/volume ratio to reduce ROS production, and mounts an antioxidant defense [146,147]. Several lines of evidence show that SIRT1 has pivotal roles in cardiovascular function. Transgenic mice that overexpress SIRT1 in the heart are resistant to oxidative stress-related cardiac hypertrophy and ischemia/reperfusion injury [148,149]. In addition, the putative SIRT1 activator, resveratrol, a recognized mediator of mitochondrial biogenesis, can ameliorate heart ischemia or reperfusion injury, improve vascular functions, and ameliorate Ang II-induced cardiac remodeling [150,151].

Thyroid Hormone Is Key Regulator of Mitochondrial Biogenesis

Thyroid hormone plays a crucial role in regulation of mitochondrial biogenesis in both physiological and pathological conditions [24]. PGC-1α is rapidly and strongly induced by TH. PGC-1α expression and protein levels are increased 6 h after administration of T3, and this action is mediated by a TH responsive element (TRE) in the promoter [152–154]. In a rat model of post-ischemic HF, a low-T3S correlated with PGC-1α and mtTFA downregulation, which corresponded to decreased mitochondrial function in the border zone; T3 replacement rescued myocardial contractility and hemodynamic parameters, while maintaining the expression of PGC-1α and mtTFA and mitochondrial function [99]. Since the PGC-1α pathway is downregulated by p53 activation under oxidative stress conditions, the inhibitory role of T3 on p53 expression may be part of an additional and indirect mechanism by which TH controls PGC1-α levels in the post-cardiac ischemia setting [155].

The reduced PGC1-α level in the post-ischemic low-T3S is consistent with the activation of a fetal metabolic pathway observed in cardiomyopathy that is characterized by a preference for glucose over fat as a substrate for oxidative phosphorylation. Although such changes lower the oxygen consumed per ATP produced, the yield of ATP per substrate also decreases. Such inefficient metabolism lowers ATP and phosphocreatine levels and decreases metabolic reserve and flexibility, leading to pump dysfunction [156,157]. Therefore, T3 supplementation in low T3 post-ischemic cardiomyopathy may favor the normal mitochondrial homeostasis and metabolic flexibility of the heart, preventing adverse cardiac remodeling and HF evolution.

Thyroid-stimulated mitochondrial biogenesis appears to be mediated via specific TRs located in both the nuclear and mitochondrial compartments [21,22]. Wrutniak-Cabello *et al.* [158] reported the discovery in mitochondria of two *N*-terminally truncated forms of the T3 nuclear receptor, TRα1, with molecular weights of 43 and 28 kDa, respectively. While the function of p28 remains unknown, p43 is a T3-dependent transcription factor of the mitochondrial genome, acting through dimeric complexes involving at least two other truncated forms of nuclear receptors, mitochondria retinoid X receptor (mtRXR) and mitochondrial peroxisome proliferator-activated receptor (mtPPAR); p43 activation by T3 stimulates mitochondrial protein synthesis, respiratory chain activity, and mitochondriogenesis [23]. Similarly, Saelim *et al.* [159] reported that T3 bound TH truncated receptor isoforms (TRs) target mitochondria where they modulate inositol 1,4,5 trisphosphate (IP3)-mediated Ca^{2+} signaling [160] to inhibit apoptotic potency.

3.6. MicroRNAs

MicroRNAs (miRNAs) are a subset of regulatory molecules involved in several cellular processes of cardiac remodeling and heart failure (HF) [161–164], and have become an intriguing target for therapeutic interventions [165]. In response to diverse cardiac stresses such as myocardial I/R, miRNAs are reported to be up- or downregulated [166–169]. Some of them have recently attracted attention as regulators of mitochondrial function and mitochondrial cell death signaling in both myocardial I/R and *in vitro* models of oxidative stress [170–174].

Role of Thyroid Hormone in the Regulation of Cardioprotective miRNA

The miR-30 family members are abundantly expressed in the mature heart, but they are significantly downregulated in experimental I/R and *in vitro* after oxidative stress [174–176]. Li *et al.* [173] report that miR-30 family members are able to regulate apoptosis by targeting the mitochondrial fission machinery. In exploring the underlying molecular mechanism, they identified that miR-30 family members inhibited mitochondrial fission by suppressing the expression of p53 and its downstream target, dynamin-related protein 1 (Drp1) [174]. Therefore, maintenance of miR-30 levels in I/R may be regarded as cardioprotective. In a rat model of I/R, early short-term T3 supplementation at near-physiological dose maintained the post-ischemic level of miR-30a, leading to a depression of p53 and inhibition of p53 detrimental effects on mitochondria [98]. In turn, p53 is responsible for the post-ischemic inhibition of miR-499, another highly expressed cardiac miRNA with a key role in the regulation of mitochondrial dynamic [64]. MiR-499 levels are reduced in experimental ischemia as well as in anoxic cardiomyocytes, and this reduction is causally linked to apoptosis and the severity of myocardial infarction and cardiac dysfunction induced by I/R [64]. MiR-499 inhibits cardiomyocyte apoptosis through its suppression of calcineurin-mediated dephosphorylation of Drp1, thereby decreasing Drp1 accumulation in mitochondria and Drp1-mediated activation of the mitochondrial fission program [64].

4. Closing Remarks and Conclusions

In the last three decades, several biochemical pathways conveying I/R deleterious effects to the mitochondria have been characterized. In parallel, several endogenous protective molecules that enhance mitochondrial survival have been identified and, consequently, prevent progression to HF. As depicted in Figure 1, TH acts on both noxious and beneficial pathways to induce cardioprotection from IRI. Therefore, treatment of post-ischemic low-T3S appears to be a promising modality for reducing mitochondrial-driven IRI and preventing progression to HF. However, from a translational point of view, there are still some unsolved issues regarding the dose and timing of TH administration after AMI. To complicate the picture, a low-T3S in the very first hours after AMI is considered protective since it lowers the energetic demand and predisposes the heart to regenerative repair [177]. On the other hand, previous studies have demonstrated that post-MI LV remodeling, a major determinant of morbidity and mortality in overt HF [178,179], is an early process. As a consequence, it is expected that an efficacious intervention aimed at preventing the initial stages of remodeling would better contrast the progression towards HF [176]. In accordance, Henderson *et al.* [18] showed that L-T3 replacement, initiated one week after MI, improved ventricular performance without reversing cardiac remodeling. On the other hand, early T3 replacement limited post-ischemic cardiomyocyte loss and blunted adverse cardiac remodeling [19,98,99]. With TH administration, it is also critical to choose the right dose in order to limit cardiac remodeling and avoid the potentially adverse systemic effects (*i.e.*, thyrotoxicosis). In a previous study, an immediate long-term, but not controlled, supplementation of TH at a high dose in post-MI improved LV function and prevented cardiac remodeling, but also induced a thyrotoxic state [20], which in the long run may lead to heart dysfunction. These results were confirmed in a successive study demonstrating the dose-dependent bimodal effects of TH administration [91].

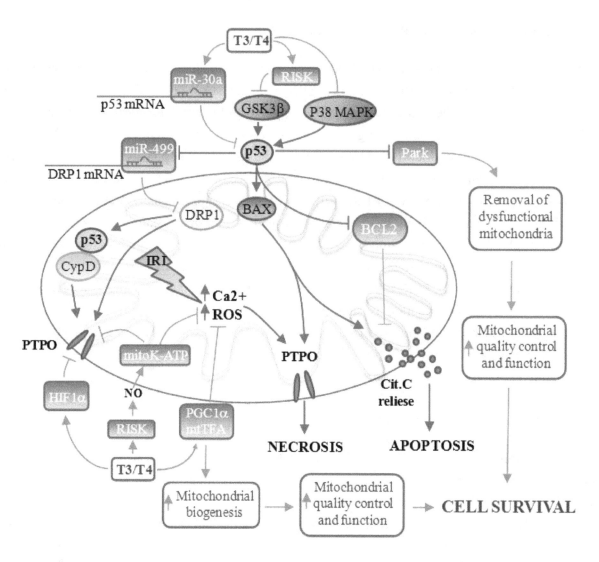

Figure 1. Schematic overview of the role of TH in the modulation of the mitochondrial pro-survival (blue connectors) or pro-death (red connectors) signaling networks that control cardiomyocyte fate in the I/R heart. CypD = Cyclophilin D; DRP1 = dynamin-related protein 1; GSK3β = glycogen synthase kinase 3-β; HIF1α = Hypoxia inducible factor 1 α, IRI = ischemia/reperfusion injuries; mitoK-ATP = mitochondrial ATP-dependent potassium channel; mtTFA = mitochondrial transcription factor A; Park = parkin; PTPO = permeability transition pore opening; PGC1-α = peroxisome proliferator-activated receptor-γ coactivator-1α; RISK = reperfusion injury salvage kinase.

In conclusion, if we exclude the hyperacute post-MI period, the available evidence suggests that TH should be administered at a physiological or near-physiological dose in the early phase of the post-ischemic wound healing following reactivation of the endogenous regenerative process in order to obtain the maximal protective effect.

Acknowledgments

This work was funded by the Tuscany Region Research Grant (DGR 1157/2011) "Study of the molecular, biochemical and metabolic mechanisms involved in the cardioprotective effect of T3".

Abbreviations

AMI = acute myocardial infarction; CypD = Cyclophilin D; DRP1 = dynamin-related protein; GSK3β = glycogen synthase kinase 3-β; HIF1α = Hypoxia inducible factor 1 α; IRI = ischemia/reperfusion injuries; Low T3 syndrome = Low-T3S; mitoK-ATP = mitochondrial ATP-dependent potassium channel; mtTFA = mitochondrial transcription factor A; Park = parkin; PGC1-α = peroxisome proliferator-activated receptor-γ coactivator-1α; PTPO = permeability transition pore opening; P38MAPK = P38 mitogen activated protein kinase; RISK = reperfusion injury salvage kinase.

References

1. Yellon, D.M.; Hausenloy, D.J. Myocardial reperfusion injury. *N. Engl. J. Med.* **2007**, *357*, 1121–1135.

2. Guzy, R.D.; Hoyos, B.; Robin, E.; Chen, H.; Liu, L.; Kyle, D.; Mansfield, K.D.; Simon, M.C.; Hammerling, U.; Schumacker, P.T. Mitochondrial complex III is required for hypoxia-induced ROS production and cellular oxygen sensing. *Cell Metab.* **2005**, *1*, 401–408.

3. Whelan, R.S.; Kaplinskiy, V.; Kitsis, R.N. Cell death in the pathogenesis of heart disease mechanisms and significance. *Annu. Rev. Physiol.* **2010**, *72*, 19–44.

4. Baines, C.P. The mitochondrial permeability transition pore and ischemia-reperfusion injury. *Basic Res. Cardiol.* **2009**, *104*, 181–188.

5. Marín-García, J.; Goldenthal, M.J. Mitochondrial centrality in heart failure. *Heart Fail. Rev.* **2008**, *13*, 137–150.

6. Galluzzi, L.; Kepp, O.; Kroemer, G. Mitochondria: Master regulators of danger signaling. *Nat. Rev. Mol. Cell Biol.* **2012**, *13*, 780–788.

7. Murry, C.E.; Jennings, R.B.; Reimer, K.A. Preconditioning with ischemia: A delay of lethal cell injury in ischemic myocardium. *Circulation* **1986**, *74*, 1124–1136.

8. Ovize, M.; Thibault, H.; Przyklenk, K. Myocardial conditioning: Opportunities for clinical translation. *Circ. Res.* **2013**, *113*, 439–450.

9. Gerdes, A.M.; Iervasi, G. Thyroid replacement therapy and heart failure. *Circulation* **2010**, *122*, 385–393.

10. Pingitore, A.; Chen, Y.; Gerdes, A.M.; Iervasi, G. Acute myocardial infarction and thyroid function: New pathophysiological and therapeutic perspectives. *Ann. Med.* **2012**, *44*, 745–757.

11. Mourouzis, I.; Forini, F.; Pantos, C.; Iervasi, G. Thyroid hormone and cardiac disease: From basic concepts to clinical application. *J. Thyroid Res.* **2011**, *2011*, doi:10.4061/2011/958626.

12. Nicolini, G.; Pitto, L.; Kusmic, C.; Balzan, S.; Sabatino, L.; Iervasi, G.; Forini, F. New insights into mechanisms of cardioprotection mediated by thyroid hormones. *J. Thyroid Res.* **2013**, *2013*, doi:10.1155/2013/264387.

13. Hamilton, M.A.; Stevenson, L.W.; Luu, M.; Walden, J.A. Altered thyroid hormone metabolism in advanced heart failure. *J. Am. Coll. Cardiol.* **1990**, *16*, 91–95.

14. Wiersinga, W.M.; Lie, K.I.; Touber, J.L. Thyroid hormones in acute myocardial infarction. *Clin. Endocrinol. (Oxf.)* **1981**, *14*, 367–374.

15. Friberg, L.; Drvota, V.; Bjelak, A.H.; Eggertsen, G.; Ahnve, S. Association between increased levels of reverse triiodothyronine and mortality after acute myocardial infarction. *Am. J. Med.* **2001**, *111*, 699–703.

16. Iervasi, G.; Pingitore, A.; Landi, P.; Raciti, M.; Ripoli, A.; Scarlattini, M.; L'Abbate, A.; Donato, L. Low-T3 syndrome: A strong prognostic predictor of death in patients with heart disease. *Circulation* **2003**, *107*, 708–713.

17. Pingitore, A.; Galli, E.; Barison, A.; Iervasi, A.; Scarlattini, M.; Nucci, D.; L'abbate, A.; Mariotti, R.; Iervasi, G. Acute effects of triiodothyronine (T3) replacement therapy in patients with chronic heart failure and low-T3 syndrome: A randomized, placebo-controlled study. *J. Clin. Endocrinol. Metab.* **2008**, *93*, 1351–1358.

18. Henderson, K.K.; Danzi, S.; Paul, J.T.; Leya, G.; Klein, I.; Samarel, A.M. Physiological replacement of t3 improves left ventricular function in an animal model of myocardial infarction-induced congestive heart failure. *Circ. Heart Fail.* **2009**, *2*, 243–252.

19. Chen, Y.F.; Kobayashi, S.; Chen, J.; Redetzke, R.A.; Said, S.; Liang, Q.; Gerdes, A.M. Short term triiodo-Lthyronine treatment inhibits cardiac myocyte apoptosis in border area after myocardial infarction in rats. *J. Mol. Cell. Cardiol.* **2008**, *44*, 180–187.

20. Pantos, C.; Mourouzis, I.; Markakis, K.; Tsagoulis, N.; Panagiotou, M.; Cokkinos, D.V. Long term thyroid hormone administration reshapes left ventricular chamber and improves cardiac function after myocardial infarction in rats. *Basic Res. Cardiol.* **2008**, *103*, 308–318.

21. Wrutniak-Cabello, C.; Casas, F.; Cabello, G. Thyroid hormone action in mitochondria. *J. Mol. Endocrinol.* **2001**, *26*, 67–77.

22. Goldenthal, M.J.; Ananthakrishnan, R.; Marín-García, J. Nuclear-mitochondrial cross-talk in cardiomyocyte T3 signaling: A time-course analysis. *J. Mol. Cell. Cardiol.* **2005**, *39*, 319–326.

23. Marín-García, J. Thyroid hormone and myocardial mitochondrial biogenesis. *Vascul. Pharmacol.* **2010**, *52*, 120–130.

24. Shintani-Ishida, K.; Inui, M.; Yoshida, K. Ischemia-reperfusion induces myocardial infarction through mitochondrial Ca^{2+} overload. *J. Mol. Cell. Cardiol.* **2012**, *53*, 233–239.

25. Herzig, S.; Maundrell, K.; Martinou, J.C. Life without the mitochondrial calcium uniporter. *Nat. Cell Biol.* **2013**, *15*, 1398–1400.

26. Tompkinsa, A.J.; Burwellb, L.; Digernessc, S.B.; Zaragozac, C.; Holmanc, W.L.; Brookesa, P.S. Mitochondrial dysfunction in cardiac ischemia-reperfusion injury: ROS from complex I, without inhibition. *BBA Mol. Basis Dis.* **2006**, *1762*, 223–231.

27. Dorn, G.W., II. Apoptotic and non-apoptotic programmed cardiomyocyte death in ventricular remodeling. *Cardiovasc. Res.* **2009**, *81*, 465–473.

28. Dröse, S.1.; Brandt, U. Molecular mechanisms of superoxide production by the mitochondrial respiratory chain. *Adv. Exp. Med. Biol.* **2012**, *748*, 145–169.

29. Becker, L.B. New concepts in reactive oxygen species and cardiovascular reperfusion physiology. *Cardiovasc. Res.* **2004**, *61*, 461–470.

30. Assaly, R.; d'Anglemont de Tassigny, A.; Paradis, S.; Jacquin, S.; Berdeaux, A.; Morin, D. Oxidative stress, mitochondrial permeability transition pore opening and cell death during hypoxia-reoxygenation in adult Cardiomyocytes. *Eur. J. Pharmacol.* **2012**, *675*, 6–14.

31. Ide, T.; Tsutsui, H.; Hayashidani, S.; Kang, D.; Suematsu, N.; Nakamura, K.; Utsumi, H.; Hamasaki, N.; Takeshita, A. Mitochondrial DNA damage and dysfunction associated with oxidative stress in failing hearts after myocardial infarction. *Circ. Res.* **2001**, *88*, 529–535.

32. Dai, D.F.; Chen, T.; Szeto, H.; Nieves-Cintrón, M.; Kutyavin, V.; Santana, L.F.; Rabinovitch, P.S. Mitochondrial targeted antioxidant Peptide ameliorates hypertensive cardiomyopathy. *J. Am. Coll. Cardiol.* **2011**, *58*, 73–82.

33. Baines, C.P. The cardiac mitochondrion: Nexus of stress. *Annu. Rev. Physiol.* **2010**, *72*, 61–80.

34. Brady, N.R.; Hamacher-Brady, A.; Gottlieb, R.A. Proapoptotic BCL-2 family members and mitochondrial dysfunction during ischemia/reperfusion injury, a study employing cardiac HL-1 cells and GFP biosensors. *Biochim. Biophys. Acta* **2006**, *1757*, 667–678.

35. Zorov, D.B.; Filburn, C.R.; Klotz, L.O.; Zweier, J.L.; Sollott, S.J. Reactive oxygen species (ROS)-induced ROS release: A new phenomenon accompanying induction of the mitochondrial permeability transition in cardiac myocytes. *J. Exp. Med.* **2000**, *192*, 1001–1014.

36. Garcia-Dorado, D.; Ruiz-Meana, M.; Inserte, J.; Rodriguez-Sinovas, A.; Piper, H.M. Calcium-mediated cell death during myocardial reperfusion. *Cardiovasc. Res.* **2012**, *94*, 168–180.

37. McStay, G.P.; Clarke, S.J.; Halestrap, A.P. Role of critical thiol groups on the matrix surface of the adenine nucleotide translocase in the mechanism of the mitochondrial permeability transition pore. *Biochem. J.* **2002**, *367*, 541–548.

38. Leung, A.W.C.; Varanyuwatana, P.; Halestrap, A.P. The mitochondrial phosphate carrier interacts with cyclophilin D and may play a key role in the permeability transition *J. Biol. Chem.* **2008**, *283*, 26312–26323.

39. Kwong, J.; Davis, C.P.; Baines, M.A.; Sargent, J.; Karch, X.; Wang, X.; Huang, T., Molkentin, J.D. Genetic deletion of the mitochondrial phosphate carrier desensitizes the mitochondrial permeability transition pore and causes cardiomyopathy. *Cell Death Differ.* **2014**, *21*, 1209–1217.

40. Paul, A.; Wilson, S.; Belham, C.M.; Robinson, C.J.; Scott, P.H.; Gould, G.W.; Plevin, R. Stress-activated protein kinases: Activation, regulation and function. *Cell Signal.* **1997**, *9*, 403–410.

41. Ma, X.L.; Kumar, S.; Gao, F.; Louden, C.S.; Lopez, B.L.; Christopher, T.A.; Wang, C.; Lee, J.C.; Feuerstein, G.Z.; Yue, T.L. Inhibition of p38 mitogen-activated protein kinase decreases cardiomyocyte apoptosis and improves cardiac function after myocardial ischemia and reperfusion. *Circulation* **1999**, *99*, 1685–1689.

42. Dhingra, S.; Sharma, A.K.; Singla, D.K.; Singal, P.K. p38 and ERK1/2 MAPKs mediate the interplay of TNF-α and IL-10 in regulating oxidative stress and cardiac myocyte apoptosis. *Am. J. Physiol. Heart Circ. Physiol.* **2007**, *293*, H3524–H3531.

43. Ashraf, M.I.; Ebner, M.; Wallner, C.; Haller, M.; Khalid, S.; Schwelberger, H.; Koziel, K.; Enthammer, M.; Hermann, M.; Sickinger, S.; *et al.* A p38MAPK/MK2 signaling pathway leading to redox stress, cell death and ischemia/reperfusion injury. *Cell Commun. Signal.* **2014**, *12*, doi:10.1186/1478-811X-12-6.

44. Ren, J.; Zhang, S.; Kovacs, A.; Wang, Y.; Muslin, A.J. Role of p38α MAPK in cardiac apoptosis and remodeling after myocardial infarction. *J. Mol. Cell. Cardiol.* **2005**, *38*, 617–623.

45. Capano, M.; Crompton, M. Bax translocates to mitochondria of heart cells during simulated ischaemia: Involvement of AMP-activated and p38 mitogen-activated protein kinases. *Biochem. J.* **2006**, *395*, 57–64.

46. Martin, E.D.; de Nicola, G.F.; Marber, M.S. New therapeutic targets in cardiology: p38 α mitogen-activated protein kinase for ischemic heart disease. *Circulation* **2012**, *126*, 357–368.

47. Kaiser, R.A.; Bueno, O.F.; Lips, D.J.; Doevendans, P.A.; Jones, F.; Kimball, T.F.; Molkentin, J.D. Targeted inhibition of p38 mitogen-activated protein kinase antagonizes cardiac injury and cell death following ischemia-reperfusion *in vivo*. *J. Biol. Chem.* **2004**, *279*, 15524–15530.

48. Jeong, C.W.; Yoo, K.Y.; Lee, S.H.; Jeong, H.J.; Lee, C.S.; Kim, S. Curcumin protects against regional myocardial ischemia/reperfusion injury through activation of RISK/GSK-3β and inhibition of p38 MAPK and JNK. *J. Cardiovasc. Pharmacol. Ther.* **2012**, *17*, 387–394.

49. Genovese, T.; Impellizzeri, D.; Ahmad, A.; Cornelius, C.; Campolo, M.; Cuzzocrea, S.; Esposito, E. Post ischaemic thyroid hormone treatment in a rat model of acute stroke. *Brain Res.* **2013**, *1513*, 92–102.

50. Pantos, C.; Malliopoulou, V.; Mourouzis, I.; Karamanoli, E.; Tzeis, S.M.; Carageorgiou, H.; Varonos, D.; Cokkinos, D.V. Long-term thyroxine administration increases HSP70 mRNA expression and attenuates p38 MAP kinase activity in response to ischaemia. *J. Endocrinol.* **2001**, *70*, 207–215.

51. Pantos, C.; Mourouzis, I.; Saranteas, T.; Clavé, G.; Ligeret, H.; Noack-Fraissignes, P.; Renard, P.Y.; Massonneau, M.; Perimenis, P.; Spanou, D.; *et al.* Thyroid hormone improves postischaemic recovery of function while limiting apoptosis: A new therapeutic approach to support hemodynamics in the setting of ischaemia-reperfusion? *Basic Res. Cardiol.* **2009**, *104*, 69–77.

52. Mourouzis, I.; Kostakou, E.; Galanopoulos, G.; Mantzouratou, P.; Pantos, C. Inhibition of thyroid hormone receptor α1 impairs post ischemic cardiac performance after myocardial infarction in mice. *Mol. Cell. Biochem.* **2013**, *379*, 97–105.

53. Vousden, K.H. p53, death star. *Cell* **2000**, *103*, 691–694.

54. Miyashita, T.; Reed, J. Tumor suppressor p53 is a direct transcriptional activator of the human bax gene. *Cell* **1995**, *80*, 293–299.

55. Long, X.; Boluyt, M.O.; Hipolito, M.; Lundberg, M.S.; Zheng, J.S.; O'Neill, L.; Cirielli, C.; Lakatta, E.G.; Crow, M.T. p53 and the hypoxia-induced apoptosis of cultured neonatal rat cardiac myocytes. *J. Clin. Investig.* **1997**, *99*, 2635–2643.

56. Vaseva, A.V.; Marchenko, N.D.; Ji, K.; Tsirka, S.E.; Holzmann, S.; Moll, U.M. p53 opens the mitochondrial permeability transition pore to trigger necrosis. *Cell* **2012**, *149*, 1536–1548.

57. Ong, S.B.; Hausenloy, D.J. Mitochondrial morphology and cardiovascular disease. *Cardiovasc. Res.* **2010**, *88*, 16–29.

58. Dieter, A.; Kubli, Å.B. Gustafsson mitochondria and mitophagy: The yin and yang of cell death control. *Circ. Res.* **2012**, *111*, 1208–1221.

59. Dimmer, K.S.; Scorrano, L. (De)constructing mitochondria: What for? *Physiology* **2006**, *21*, 233–241.

60. Hausenloy, D.J.; Scorrano, L. Targeting cell death. *Clin. Pharmacol. Ther.* **2007**, *82*, 370–373.

61. Shen, T.; Zheng, M.; Cao, C.; Chen, C.; Tang, J.; Zhang, W.; Cheng, H.; Chen, K.H.; Xiao, R.P. Mitofusin-2 is a major determinant of oxidative stress-mediated heart muscle cell apoptosis. *J. Biol. Chem.* **2007**, *282*, 23354–23361.

62. Ong, S.B.; Subrayan, S.; Lim, S.Y.; Yellon, D.M.; Davidson, S.M.; Hausenloy, D.J. Inhibiting mitochondrial fission protects the heart against ischemia/reperfusion injury. *Circulation* **2010**, *121*, 2012–2202.

63. Kong, D.; Xu, L.; Yu, Y.; Zhu, W.; Andrews, D.W.; Yoon, Y.; Kuo, T.H. Regulation of Ca^{2+}-induced permeability transition by Bcl-2 is antagonized by Drpl and hFis1. *Mol. Cell Biochem.* **2005**, *272*, 187–199.

64. Wang, J.; Jiao, J.; Li, Q.; Long, B.; Wang, K.; Liu, J.; Li, Y.; Li, P. miR-499 regulates mitochondrial dynamics by targeting calcineurin and dynamin-related protein-1. *Nat. Med.* **2011**, *17*, 71–78.

65. Guo, X.; Sesaki, H.H.; Qi, X. Drp1 stabilizes p53 on the mitochondria to trigger necrosis under oxidative stress conditions *in vitro* and *in vivo*. *Biochem. J.* **2014**, *461*, 137–146.

66. Whelan, R.S.; Konstantinidis, K.; Wei, A.C.; Chen, Y.; Reyna, D.E.; Jha, S.; Yang, Y.; Calvert, J.W.; Lindsten, T.; Thompson, C.B.; *et al.* Bax regulates primary necrosis through mitochondrial dynamics. *Proc. Natl. Acad. Sci. USA* **2012**, *109*, 6566–6571.

67. Wohlgemuth, S.E.; Calvani, R.; Marzetti, E. The interplay between autophagy and mitochondrial dysfunction in oxidative stress-induced cardiac aging and pathology. *J. Mol. Cell. Cardiol.* **2014**, *71*, 62–70.

68. Chen, Y.; Dorn, G.W., II. PINK1-phosphorylated mitofusin 2 is a Parkin receptor for culling damaged mitochondria. *Science* **2013**, *340*, 471–475.

69. Narendra, D.; Tanaka, A.; Suen, D.F.; Youle, R.J. Parkin is recruited selectively to impaired mitochondria and promotes their autophagy. *J. Cell Biol.* **2008**, *183*, 795–803.

70. Hoshino, A.; Mita, Y.; Okawa, Y.; Ariyoshi, M.; Iwai-Kanai, E.; Ueyama, T.; Ikeda, K.; Ogata, T.; Matoba, S. Cytosolic p53 inhibits Parkin-mediated mitophagy and promotes mitochondrial dysfunction in the mouse heart. *Nat. Commun.* **2013**, *4*, doi:10.1038/ncomms3308.

71. Hoshino, A.; Matoba, S.; Iwai-Kanai, E.; Nakamura, H.; Kimata, M.; Nakaoka, M.; Katamura, M.; Okawa, Y.; Ariyoshi, M.; Mita, Y.; *et al.* p53-TIGAR axis attenuates mitophagy to exacerbate cardiac damage after ischemia. *J. Mol. Cell. Cardiol.* **2012**, *52*, 1175–1184.

72. Cohen, P.; Frame, S. The renaissance of GSK3B. *Nat. Rev. Mol. Cell Biol.* **2001**, *2*, 769–776.

73. Sussman, M.A.; Völkers, M.; Fischer, K.; Bailey, B.; Cottage, C.T.; Din, S.; Gude, N.; Avitabile, D.; Alvarez, R.; Sundararaman, B.; *et al.* Myocardial AKT: The omnipresent nexus. *Physiol. Rev.* **2011**, *91*, 1023–1070.

74. Hausenloy, D.J.; Yellon, D.M. New directions for protecting the heart against ischaemia–reperfusion injury: Targeting the Reperfusion Injury Salvage Kinase (RISK)-pathway. *Cardiovasc. Res.* **2004**, *61*, 448–460.

75. Linseman, D.A.; Butts, B.D.; Precht, T.A.; Phelps, R.A.; Le, S.S.; Laessig, T.A.; Bouchard, R.J.; Florez-McClure, M.L.; Heidenreich, K.A. Glycogen synthase kinase-3β phosphorylates Bax and promotes its mitochondrial localization during neuronal apoptosis. *J. Neurosci.* **2004**, *24*, 9993–10002.

76. Juhaszova, M.; Zorov, D.B.; Kim, S.H.; Pepe, S.; Fu, Q.; Fishbein, K.W.; Ziman, B.D.; Wang, S.; Ytrehus, K.; Antos, C.L.; *et al.* Glycogen synthase kinase-3β mediates convergence of protection signaling to inhibit the mitochondrial permeability transition pore. *J. Clin. Investig.* **2004**, *113*, 1535–1549.

77. Gomez, L.; Paillard, M.; Thibault, H.; Derumeaux, G.; Ovize, M. Inhibition of GSK3β by postconditioning is required to prevent opening of the mitochondrial permeability transition pore during reperfusion. *Circulation* **2008**, *117*, 2761–2768.

78. Watcharasit, P.; Bijur, G.N.; Song, L.; Zhu, J.; Chen, X.; Jope, R.S. Glycogen synthase kinase-3b(GSK3b) binds to and promotes the actions of p53. *J. Biol. Chem.* **2003**, *278*, 48872–48879.

79. Rasola, A.; Sciacovelli, M.; Chiara, F.; Pantic, B.; Brusilow, W.S.; Bernardi, P. Activation of mitochondrial ERK protects cancer cells from death through inhibition of the permeability transition. *Proc. Natl. Acad. Sci. USA* **2010**, *107*, 726–731.

80. Phukan, S.; Babu, V.S.; Kannoji, A.; Hariharan, R.; Balaji, V.N. GSK3β: Role in therapeutic landscape and development of modulators. *Br. J. Pharmacol.* **2010**, *160*, 1–19.

81. Tanno, M.; Kuno, A.; Ishikawa, S.; Miki, T.; Kouzu, H.; Yano, T.; Murase, H.; Tobisawa, T.; Ogasawara, M.; Horio, Y.; *et al.* Translocation of Glycogen Synthase Kinase-3β (GSK-3β), a trigger of permeability transition, is kinase activity dependent and mediated by interaction with voltage-dependent anion channel 2 (VDAC2). *J. Biol. Chem.* **2014**, *289*, 29285–29296.

82. Gross, G.J.; Hsu, A.; Pfeiffer, A.W.; Nithipatikom, K. Roles of endothelial nitric oxide synthase (eNOS) and mitochondrial permeability transition pore (MPTP) in epoxyeicosatrienoic acid (EET)-induced cardioprotection against infarction in intact rat hearts. *J. Mol. Cell. Cardiol.* **2013**, *59*, 20–29.

83. Sasaki, N.; Sato, T.; Ohler, A.; O'Rourke, B.; Marbán, E. Activation of mitochondrial ATP-dependent potassium channels by nitric oxide. *Circulation* **2000**, *101*, 439–445.

84. Penna, C.; Rastaldo, R.; Mancardi, D.; Raimondo, S.; Cappello, S.; Gattullo, D.; Losano, G.; Pagliario, P. Post-conditioning induced cardioprotection requires signaling through a redox-sensitive mechanism, mitochondrial ATP-sensitive K$^+$ channel and protein kinase C activation. *Basic Res. Cardiol.* **2006**, *101*, 180–189.

85. Gucek, M.; Murphy, E. What can we learn about cardioprotection from the cardiac mitochondrial proteome? *Cardiovasc. Res.* **2010**, *88*, 211–218.

86. Burwell, L.S.; Brookes, P.S. Mitochondria as a target for the cardioprotective effects of nitric oxide in ischemia-reperfusion injury. *Antioxid. Redox Signal.* **2008**, *10*, 579–599.

87. Ong, S.B.; Hall, A.R.; Dongworth, R.K.; Kalkhoran, S.; Pyakurel, A.; Scorrano, L.; Hausenloy, D.J. Akt protects the heart against ischaemia/reperfusion injury by modulating mitochondrial morphology. *Thromb. Haemost.* **2015**, *113*, 513–516.

88. Kenessey, A.; Ojamaa, K. Thyroid hormone stimulates protein synthesis in the cardiomyocyte by activating the Akt-mTOR and p70S6Kpathways. *J. Biol. Chem.* **2006**, *28*, 20666–20672.

89. Kuzman, J.A.; Gerdes, A.M.; Kobayashi, S.; Liang, Q. Thyroid hormone activates Akt and prevents serum starvation-induced cell death in neonatal rat cardiomyocytes. *J. Mol. Cell. Cardiol.* **2005**, *39*, 841–844.

90. Kuzman, J.A.; Vogelsang, K.A.; Thomas, T.A.; Gerdes, A.M. L-Thyroxine activates Akt signaling in the heart. *J. Mol. Cell. Cardiol.* **2005**, *39*, 251–258.

91. Mourouzis, I.; Mantzouratou, P.; Galanopoulos, G.; Kostakou, E.; Roukounakis, N.; Kokkinos, A.D.; Cokkinos, D.V.; Pantos, C. Dose-dependent effects of thyroid hormone on post-ischemic cardiac performance: Potential involvement of Akt and ERK signalings. *Mol. Cell. Biochem.* **2012**, *363*, 235–243.

92. Kehat, I.; Davis, J.; Tiburcy, M.; Accornero, F.; Saba-El-Leil, M.K.; Maillet, M.; York, A.J.; Lorenz, J.N.; Zimmermann, W.H.; Meloche, S.; *et al.* Extracellular signal-regulated kinases 1 and 2 regulate the balance between eccentric and concentric cardiac growth. *Circ. Res.* **2010**, *108*, 176–183.

93. Naito, A.T.; Okada, S.; Minamino, T.; Iwanaga, K.; Liu, M.L.; Sumida, T.; Nomura, S.; Sahara, N.; Mizoroki, T.; Takashima, A.; *et al.* Promotion of chip-mediated p53 degradation protects the heart from ischemic injury. *Circ. Res.* **2010**, *106*, 1692–1702.

94. Lin, H.Y.; Davis, P.J.; Tang, H.Y.; Mousa, S.A.; Luidens, M.K.; Hercbergs, A.H.; Davis, F.B. The pro-apoptotic action of stilbene-induced COX-2 in cancer cells: Convergence with the anti-apoptotic effect of thyroid hormone. *Cell Cycle* **2009**, *8*, 1877–1882

95. Lin, H.Y.; Tang, H.Y.; Keating, T.; Wu, Y.H.; Shih, A.; Hammond, D.; Sun, M.; Hercbergs, A.; Davis, F.B.; Davis, P.J. Resveratrol is pro-apoptotic and thyroid hormone is anti-apoptotic in glioma cells: Both actions are integrin and ERK mediated. *Carcinogenesis* **2008**, *29*, 62–69.

96. Yap, N.; Yu, C.L.; Cheng, S.Y. Modulation of thetranscriptional activity ofthyroid hormone receptor by the tumor suppressor p53. *Proc. Natl. Acad. Sci. USA* **1996**, *93*, 4273–4277.

97. Bhat, M.K.; Yu, C.l.; Yap, N.; Zhan, Q.; Hayashi, Y.; Seth, P. Tumor suppressor p53 is a negative regulator in thyroid hormone receptor signaling pathways. *J. Biol. Chem.* **1997**, *272*, 28989–28993.

98. Forini, F.; Kusmic, C.; Nicolini, G.; Mariani, L.; Zucchi, R.; Matteucci, M.; Iervasi, G.; Pitto, L. Triiodothyronine prevents cardiac ischemia/reperfusion mitochondrial impairment and cell loss by regulating miR30a/p53 axis. *Endocrinology* **2014**, *155*, 4581–4590.

99. Forini, F.; Lionetti, V.; Ardehali, H.; Pucci, A.; Cecchetti, F.; Ghanefar, M.; Nicolini, G.; Ichikawa, Y.; Nannipieri, M.; Recchia, F.A.; *et al.* Early long-term L-T3 replacement rescues mitochondria and prevents ischemic cardiac remodelling in rats. *J. Cell. Mol. Med.* **2011**, *15*, 514–524.

100. Yusuf, S.; Dagenais, G.; Pogue, J.; Bosch, J.; Sleight, P. Vitamin E supplementation and cardiovascular events in high-risk patients. The heart outcomes prevention evaluation study investigators. *N. Engl. J. Med.* **2000**, *342*, 154–160.

101. Hare, J.M.; Mangal, B.; Brown, J.; Fisher, C., Jr.; Freudenberger, R.; Colucci, W.S.; Mann, D.L.; Liu, P.; Givertz, M.M.; Schwarz, R.P.; OPT-CHF Investigators. Impact of oxypurinol in patients with symptomatic heart failure: Results of the OPT-CHF study. *J. Am. Coll. Cardiol.* **2008**, *5*, 2301–2309.

102. Brown, D.A.; Hale, S.L.; Baines, C.P.; del Rio, C.L.; Hamlin, R.L.; Yueyama, Y.; Kijtawornrat, A.; Yeh, S.T.; Frasier, C.R.; Stewart, L.M.; *et al.* Reduction of early reperfusion injury with the mitochondria-targeting peptide bendavia. *J. Cardiovasc. Pharmacol. Ther.* **2014**, *19*, 121–132.

103. Adlam, V.J.; Harrison, J.C.; Porteous, C.M.; James, A.M.; Smith, R.A.; Murphy, M.P.; Sammut, I.A. Targeting an antioxidant to mitochondria decreases cardiac ischemia-reperfusion injury. *FASEB J.* **2005**, *19*, 1088–1095.

104. Szeto, H.H. Mitochondria-targeted cytoprotective peptides for ischemia-reperfusion injury. *Antiox. Redox Signal.* **2008**, *10*, 601–619.

105. Zhao, K.; Zhao, G.M.; Wu, D.; Soong, Y.; Birk, A.V.; Schiller, P.W.; Szeto, H.H. Cell-permeable peptide antioxidants targeted to inner mitochondrial membrane inhibit mitochondrial swelling, oxidative cell death, and reperfusion injury. *J. Biol. Chem.* **2004**, *279*, 34682–34690.

106. De Castro, A.L.; Tavares, A.V.; Campos, C.; Fernandes, R.O.; Siqueira, R.; Conzatti, A.; Bicca, A.M.; Fernandes, T.R.; Sartório, C.L.; Schenkel, P.C.; *et al.* Cardioprotective effects of thyroid hormones ina rat model of myocardial infarction are associated with oxidative stress reduction. *Mol. Cell. Endocrinol.* **2014**, *391*, 22–29.

107. Di Lisa, F.; Menabò, R.; Canton, M.; Barile, M.; Bernardi, P. Opening of the mitochondrial permeability transition pore causes depletion of mitochondrial and cytosolic NAD^+ and is a causative event in the death of myocytes in postischemic reperfusion of the heart. *J. Biol. Chem.* **2001**, *276*, 2571–2575.

108. Clarke, S.J.; McStay, G.P.; Halestrap, A.P. Sanglifehrin A acts as a potent inhibitor of the mitochondrial permeability transition and reperfusion injury of the heart by binding to cyclophilin-D at a different site from cyclosporin A. *J. Biol. Chem.* **2002**, *277*, 34793–34799.

109. Nakayama, H.; Chen, X.; Baines, C.P.; Klevitsky, R.; Zhang, X.; Zhang, H.; Jaleel, N.; Chua, B.H.; Hewett, T.E.; Robbins, J.; *et al.* Ca^{2+}- and mitochondrial-dependent cardiomyocyte necrosis as a primary mediator of heart failure. *J. Clin. Investig.* **2007**, *117*, 2431–2444.

110. Nakagawa, T.; Shimizu, S.; Watanabe, T.; Yamaguchi, O.; Otsu, K.; Yamagata, H.; Inohara, H.; Kubo, T.; Tsujimoto, Y. Cyclophilin D-dependent mitochondrial permeability transition regulates some necrotic but not apoptotic cell death. *Nature* **2005**, *434*, 652–658.

111. Kato, M.; Akao, M.; Matsumoto-Ida, M.; Makiyama, T.; Iguchi, M.; Takeda, T.; Shimizu, S.; Kita, T. The targeting of cyclophilin D by RNAi as a novel cardioprotective therapy: Evidence from two-photon imaging. *Cardiovasc. Res.* **2009**, *83*, 335–344.

112. Elrod, J.W.; Wong, R.; Mishra, S.; Vagnozzi, R.J.; Sakthievel, B.; Goonasekera, S.A.; Karch, J.; Gabel, S.; Farber, J.; Force, T.; *et al.* Cyclophilin D controls mitochondrial pore-dependent Ca^{2+} exchange, metabolic flexibility, and propensity for heart failure in mice. *J. Clin. Investig.* **2010**, *120*, 3680–3687.

113. Piot, C.; Croisille, P.; Staat, P.; Thibault, H.; Rioufol, G.; Mewton, N.; Elbelghiti, R.; Cung, T.T.; Bonnefoy, E.; Angoulvant, D.; *et al.* Effect of cyclosporine on reperfusion injury in acute myocardial infarction. *N. Engl. J. Med.* **2008**, *359*, 473–448.

114. Fuglesteg, B.N.; Suleman, N.; Tiron, C.; Kanhema, T.; Lacerda, L.; Andreasen, T.V.; Sack, M.N.; Janassen, A.K.; Mjos, O.D.; Opie, L.H.; *et al.* Signal transducer and activator of transcription 3 is involved in the cardioprotective signaling pathway activated by insulin therapy at reperfusion. *Bas. Res. Cardiol.* **2008**, *103*, 444–453.

115. Lacerda, L.; Somers, S.; Opie, L.H.; Lecour, S. Ischemic postconditioning protect against reperfusion injury via SAFE pathway. *Cardiovasc. Res.* **2009**, *84*, 201–208.

116. Boengler, K.; Hilfiker-Kleiner, D.; Heusch, G.; Schulz, R. Inhibition of permeability transition pore opening by mitochondrial STAT3 and its role in myocardial ischemia/reperfusion. *Basic Res. Cardiol.* **2010**, *105*, 771–785.

117. Hataishi, R.; Rodrigues, A.C.; Neilan, T.G.; Morgan, J.G.; Buys, E.; Shiva, S.; Tambouret, R.; Jassal, D.S.; Raher, M.J.; Furutani, E.; *et al*. Inhaled nitric oxide decreases infarction size and improves left ventricular function in a murine model of myocardial ischemia-reperfusion injury. *Am. J. Physiol. Heart Circ. Physiol.* **2006**, *291*, H379–H384.

118. Nagasaka, Y.; Fernandez, B.O.; Garcia-Saura, M.F.; Petersen, B.; Ichinose, F.; Bloch, K.D.; Feelisch, M.; Zapol, W.M. Brief periods of nitric oxide inhalation protect against myocardial ischemia-reperfusion injury. *Anesthesiology* **2008**, *109*, 675–682.

119. Liu, X.; Huang, Y.; Pokreisz, P.; Vermeersch, P.; Marsboom, G.; Swinnen, M.; Verbeken, E.; Santos, J.; Pellens, M.; Gillijns, H.; *et al*. Nitric oxide inhalation improves microvascular flow and decreases infarction size after myocardial ischemia and reperfusion. *J. Am. Coll. Cardiol.* **2007**, *50*, 808–817.

120. Wang, G.; Liem, D.A.; Vondriska, T.M.; Honda, H.M.; Korge, P.; Pantaleon, D.M.; Qiao, X.; Wang, Y.; Weiss, J.N.; Ping, P. Nitric oxide donors protect murine myocardium against infarction via modulation of mitochondrial permeability transition. *Am. J. Physiol. Heart Circ. Physiol.* **2005**, *288*, H1290–H1295.

121. Ong, S.G.; Hausenloy, D.J. Hypoxia-inducible factor as a therapeutic target for cardioprotection. *Pharmacol. Ther.* **2012**, *136*, 69–81.

122. Ong, S.G.; Lee, W.H.; Theodorou, L.; Kodo, K.; Lim, S.Y.; Shukla, D.H.; Briston, T.; Kiriakidis, S.; Ashcroft, M.; Davidson, S.M.; *et al*. HIF-1 reduces ischaemia-reperfusion injury in the heart by targeting the mitochondrial permeability transition pore. *Cardiovasc. Res.* **2014**, *104*, 24–36.

123. Benard, G.; Bellance, N.; Jose, C.; Melser, S.; Nouette-Gaulain, K.; Rossignol, R. Multi-site control and regulation of mitochondrial energy production. *Biochim. Biophys. Acta* **2010**, *1797*, 698–709.

124. McLeod, C.J.; Pagel, I.; Sack, M.N. The mitochondrial biogenesis regulatory program adaptation to ischemia-A putative target for therapeutic intervention. *Trends Cardiovasc. Med.* **2005**, *15*, 118–123.

125. Hock, M.B.; Kralli, A. Transcriptional control of mitochondrial biogenesis and function. *Annu. Rev. Physiol.* **2009**, *71*, 177–203.

126. Ventura-Clapier, R.; Garnier, A.; Veksler, V. Transcriptional control of mitochondrial biogenesis: The central role of PGC-1α. *Cardiovasc. Res.* **2008**, *79*, 208–217.

127. Ventura-Clapier, R.; Garnier, A.; Veksler, V.; Joubert, F. Bioenergetics of the failing heart. *Biochim. Biophys. Acta* **2011**, *1813*, 1360–1372.

128. Garnier, A.; Fortin, D.; Deloménie, C.; Momken, I.; Veksler, V.; Ventura-Clapier, R. Depressed mitochondrial transcription factors and oxidative capacity in rat failing cardiac and skeletal muscles. *J. Physiol.* **2003**, *551*, 491–501.

129. Watson, P.A.; Reusch, J.E.; McCune, S.A.; Leinwand, L.A.; Luckey, S.W.; Konhilas, J.P. Restoration of CREB function is linked to completion and stabilization of adaptive cardiac hypertrophy in response to exercise. *Am. J. Physiol.* **2007**, *293*, H246–H259.

130. Lehman J.J.; Kelly, D.P. Transcriptional activation of energy metabolic switches in the developing and hypertrophied heart. *Clin. Exp. Pharmacol. Physiol.* **2002**, *29*, 339–345.

131. Arany, Z.; Novikov, M.; Chin, S.; Ma, Y.; Rosenzweig, A.; Spiegelman, B.M. Transverse aortic constriction leads to accelerated heart failure in mice lacking PPARγ coactivator 1α. *Proc. Natl. Acad. Sci. USA* **2006**, *103*, 10086–10091.

132. Sihag, S.; Li, A.Y.; Cresci, S.; Sucharov, C.C.; Lehman, J.J. PGC-1α and ERRα target gene down-regulation is a signature of the failing human heart *J. Mol. Cell. Cardiol.* **2009**, *46*, 201–212.

133. Ahuja, P.; Zhao, P.; Angelis, E.; Ruan, H.; Korge, P.; Olson, A.; Wang, Y.; Jin, E.S.; Jeffrey, F.M.; Portman, M.; *et al.* Myc controls transcriptional regulation of cardiac metabolism and mitochondrial biogenesis in response to pathological stress in mice. *J. Clin. Investig.* **2010**, *120*, 1494–1505.

134. Yan, W.; Zhang, H.; Liu, P.; Wang, H.; Liu, J.; Gao, C.; Liu, Y.; Lian, K.; Yang, L.; Sun, L.; *et al.* Impaired mitochondrial biogenesis due to dysfunctional adiponectin-AMPK-PGC-1α signaling contributing to increased vulnerability in diabetic heart. *Basic Res. Cardiol.* **2013**, *108*, doi:10.1007/s00395-013-0329-1.

135. Sun, L.; Zhao, M.; Yu, X.J.; Wang, H.; He, X.; Liu, J.K.; Zang, W.J. Cardioprotection by acetylcholine: A novel mechanism via mitochondrial biogenesis and function involving the PGC-1α pathway. *J. Cell. Physiol.* **2013**, *228*, 1238–1248.

136. St-Pierre, J.; Lin, J.; Krauss, S.; Tarr, P.T.; Yang, R.; Newgard, C.B.; Spiegelman, B.M. Bioenergetic analysis of peroxisome proliferator-activated receptor gamma coactivators 1α and 1β (PGC-1α and PGC-1β) in muscle cells. *J. Biol. Chem.* **2003**, *278*, 26597–26603.

137. Kajander, O.A.; Karhunen, P.J.; Jacobs, H.T. The relationship between somatic mtDNA rearrangements, human heart disease and aging. *Hum. Mol. Genet.* **2002**, *11*, 317–324.

138. Naya, F.J.; Black, B.L.; Wu, H.; Bassel-Duby, R.; Richardson, J.A.; Hill, J.A.; Olson, E.N. Mitochondrial deficiency and cardiac sudden death in mice lacking the MEF2A transcription factor. *Nat. Med.* **2002**, *8*, 1303–1309.

139. Lebrecht, D.; Setzer, B.; Ketelsen, U.P.; Haberstroh, J.; Walker, U.A. Timedependent and tissue-specific accumulation of mtDNA and respiratory chain defects in chronic doxorubicin cardiomyopathy. *Circulation* **2003**, *108*, 2423–2429.

140. Ide, T.; Tsutsui, H.; Kinugawa, S.; Utsumi, H.; Kang, D.; Hattori, N.; Uchida, K.; Arimura, K.; Egashira, K.; Takeshita, A. Mitochondrial electron transport complex I is a potential source of oxygen free radicals in the failing myocardium. *Circ. Res.* **1999**, *85*, 357–363.

141. Li, H.; Wang, J.; Wilhelmsson, H.; Hansson, A.; Thoren, P.; Duffy, J.; Rustin, P.; Larsson, N.G. Genetic modification of survival in tissue-specific knockout mice with mitochondrial cardiomyopathy. *Proc. Natl. Acad. Sci. USA* **2000**, *97*, 3467–3472.

142. Wang, J.; Wilhelmsson, H.; Graff, C.; Li, H.; Oldfors, A.; Rustin, P.; Bruning, J.C.; Kahn, C.R.; Clayton, D.A.; Barsh, G.S.; *et al.* Dilated cardiomyopathy and atrioventricular conduction blocks induced by heart-specific inactivation of mitochondrial DNA gene expression. *Nat. Genet.* **1999**, *21*, 133–137.

143. Ikeuchi, M.; Matsusaka, H.; Kang, D.; Matsushima, S.; Ide, T.; Kubota, T.; Fujiwara, T.; Hamasaki, N.; Takeshita, A.; Sunagawa, K.; *et al.* Overexpression of mitochondrial transcription factor a ameliorates mitochondrial deficiencies and cardiac failure after myocardial infarction. *Circulation* **2005**, *112*, 683–669.

144. Guarente, L. Sirtuins in aging and disease. *Cold Spring Harb. Symp. Quant. Biol.* **2007**, *72*, 483–488.

145. Nakagawa, T.; Guarente, L. Sirtuins at a glance. *J. Cell Sci.* **2011**, *124*, 833–838.

146. Aquilano, K.; Vigilanza, P.; Baldelli, S.; Pagliei, B.; Rotilio, G.; Ciriolo, M.R. Peroxisome proliferator-activated receptor γ co-activator 1α (PGC-1α) and sirtuin 1 (SIRT1) reside in mitochondria. Possible direct function ion mitochondrila biogenesis. *J. Biol. Chem.* **2010**, *285*, 21590–21599.

147. Nemoto, S.; Fergusson, M.M.; Finkel, T. SIRT1 functionally interacts with the metabolic regulator and transcriptional coactivator PGC-1α. *J. Biol. Chem.* **2005**, *280*, 16456–16460.

148. Alcendor, R.R.; Gao, S.; Zhai, P.; Zablocki, D.; Holle, E.; Yu, X.; Tian, B.; Wagner, T.; Vatner, S.F.; Sadoshima, J. Sirt1 regulates aging and resistance to oxidative stress in the heart. *Circ. Res.* **2007**, *100*, 1512–1521.

149. Hsu, C.P.; Zhai, P.; Yamamoto, T.; Maejima, Y.; Matsushima, S.; Hariharan, N.; Shao, D.; Takagi, H.; Oka, S.; Sadoshima, J. Silent information regulator 1 protects the heart from ischemia/reperfusion. *Circulation* **2010**, *122*, 2170–2182.

150. Orallo, F.; Alvarez, E.; Camina, M.; Leiro, J.M.; Gomez, E.; Fernandez, P. The possible implication of trans-Resveratrol in the cardioprotective effects of long-term moderate wine consumption. *Mol. Pharmacol.* **2002**, *61*, 294–302.

151. Biala, A.; Tauriainen, E.; Siltanen, A.; Shi, J.; Merasto, S.; Louhelainen, M.; Martonen, E.; Finckenberg, P.; Muller, D.N.; Mervaala, E. Resveratrol induces mitochondrial biogenesis and ameliorates Ang II-induced cardiac remodeling in transgenic rats harboring human renin and angiotensinogen genes. *Blood Press.* **2010**, *19*, 196–205.

152. Weitzel, J.M.; Iwen, K.A. Coordination of mitochondrial biogenesis by thyroid hormone. *Mol. Cell. Endocrinol.* **2011**, *342*, 1–7.

153. Venditti, P.; Bari, A.; di Stefano, L.; Cardone, A.; della Ragione, F.; D'Esposito, M.; di Meo, S. Involvement of PGC-1, NRF-1, and NRF-2 in metabolic response by rat liver to hormonal and environmental signals. *Mol. Cell. Endocrinol.* **2009**, *305*, 22–29.

154. Wulf, A.; Harneit, A.; Kröger, M.; Kebenko, M.; Wetzel, M.G.; Weitzel, J.M. T3-mediated expression of PGC-1α via a far upstream located thyroid hormone response element. *Mol. Cell. Endocrinol.* **2008**, *287*, 90–95.

155. Villeneuve, C.L.; Guilbeau-Frugier, C.; Sicard, P.; Lairez, O.; Ordener, C.; Duparc, T.; de Paulis, D.; Couderc, B.; Spreux-Varoquaux, O.; Tortosa, F.; *et al.* p53-PGC-1α pathway mediates oxidative mitochondrial damage and cardiomyocyte necrosis induced by monoamine oxidase-A up-regulation: Role in chronic left ventricular dysfunction in mice. *Antioxid. Redox Signal.* **2013**, *18*, 5–18.

156. Ingwall, J.S. Energy metabolism in heart failure and remodelling. *Cardiovasc. Res.* **2009**, *81*, 412–419.

157. Ardehali, H.; Sabbah, H.N.; Burke, M.A.; Sarma, S.; Liu, P.P.; Cleland, J.G.; Maggioni, A.; Fonarow, G.C.; Abel, E.D.; Campia, U.; *et al.* Targeting myocardial substrate metabolism in heart failure: Potential for new therapies. *Eur. J. Heart Fail.* **2012**, *14*, 120–129.

158. Wrutniak-Cabello, C.; Carazo, A.; Casas, F.; Cabello, G. Triiodothyronine mitochondrial receptors: Import and molecular mechanisms. *J. Soc. Biol.* **2008**, *202*, 83–92.

159. Saelim, N.; Holstein, D.; Chocron, E.S.; Camacho, P.; Lechleiter, J.D. Inhibition of apoptotic potency by ligand stimulated thyroid hormone receptors located in mitochondria. *Apoptosis* **2007**, *12*, 1781–1794.

160. Saelim, N.; John, L.M.; Wu, J.; Park, J.S.; Bai, Y.; Camacho, P.; Lechleiter, J.D. Nontranscriptional modulation of intracellular Ca^{2+} signaling by ligand stimulated thyroid hormone receptor. *J. Cell Biol.* **2004**, *167*, 915–924.

161. Van Rooij, E.; Sutherland, L.B.; Qi, X.; Richardson, J.A.; Hill, J.; Olson, E.N. Control of stress-dependent cardiac growth and gene expression by a microRNA. *Science* **2007**, *316*, 575–579, doi:10.1126/science.1139089.

162. Barringhaus, K.G.; Zamore, P.D. MicroRNAs: Regulating a change of heart. *Circulation* **2009**, *119*, 2217–2224.

163. Divakaran, V.; Mann, D.L. The emerging role of microRNAs in cardiac remodeling and heart failure. *Circ. Res.* **2008**, *103*, 1072–1083.

164. Thum, T.; Galuppo, P.; Wolf, C.; Fiedler, J.; Kneitz, S.; van Laake, L.W.; Doevendans, P.A.; Mummery, C.L.; Borlak, J.; Haverich, A.; *et al.* MicroRNAs in the human heart: A clue to fetal gene reprogramming in heart failure. *Circulation* **2007**, *116*, 258–267.

165. Van Rooij, E.; Marshall, W.; Olson, E. Toward microRNA-based therapeutics for heart disease the sense in antisense. *Circ. Res.* **2008**, *103*, 919–928.

166. Van Rooij, E.; Sutherland, L.B.; Liu, N.; Williams, A.H.; McAnally, J.; Gerard, R.D.; Richardson, J.A.; Olson, E.N. A signature pattern of stress-responsive micrornas that can evoke cardiac hypertrophy and heart failure. *Proc. Natl. Acad. Sci. USA* **2006**, *103*, 18255–18260.

167. Van Rooij, E.; Sutherland, L.B.; Thatcher, J.E.; diMaio, J.M.; Naseem, R.H.; Marshall, W.S.; Hill, J.A.; Olson, E.N. Dysregulation of microRNAs after myocardial infarction reveals a role of miR-29 in cardiac fibrosis. *Proc. Natl. Acad. Sci. USA* **2008**, *105*, 13027–13032.

168. Roy, S.; Khanna, S.; Hussain, S.R.; Biswas, S.; Azad, A.; Rink, C.; Gnyawali, S.; Shilo, S.; Nuovo, G.J.; Sen, C.K. MicroRNA expression in response to murine myocardial infarction: miR-21 regulates fibroblast metalloprotease-2 via phosphatase and tensin homologue. *Cardiovasc. Res.* **2009**, *82*, 21–29.

169. Ren, X.P.; Wu, J.; Wang, X.; Sartor, M.A.; Qian, J.; Jones, K.; Nicolaou, P.; Pritchard, T.J.; Fan, G.C. MicroRNA-320 is involved in the regulation of cardiac ischemia/reperfusion injury by targeting heat-shock protein 20. *Circulation* **2009**, *119*, 2357–2366.

170. Sripada, L.; Tomar, D.; Singh, R. Mitochondria: One of the destinations of miRNAs. *Mitochondrion* **2012**, *12*, 593–599.

171. Ye, Y.; Perez-Polo, J.R.; Qian, J.; Birnbaum, Y. The role of microRNA in modulating myocardial ischemia-reperfusion injury. *Physiol. Genomics* **2011**, *43*, 534–542.

172. Aurora, A.B.; Mahmoud, A.I.; Luo, X.; Johnson, B.A.; van Rooij, E.; Matsuzaki, S.; Humphries, K.M.; Hill, J.A.; Bassel-Duby, R.; Sadek, H.A.; *et al.* MicroRNA-214 protects the mouse heart from ischemic injury by controlling Ca^{2+} overload and cell death. *J. Clin. Investig.* **2012**, *122*, 1222–1232.

173. Wang, X.; Zhang, X.; Ren, X.P.; Chen, J.; Liu, H.; Yang, J.; Medvedovic, M.; Hu, Z.; Fan, G.C. MicroRNA494 targeting both proapoptotic and antiapoptotic proteins protects against ischemia/reperfusion-induced cardiac injury. *Circulation* **2010**, *122*, 1308–1318.

174. Li, J.; Donath, S.; Li, Y.; Qin, D.; Prabhakar, B.; Li, P. miR-30 regulates mitochondrial fission through targeting p53 and the dynamin-related protein-1 pathway. *PLoS Genet.* **2010**, *6*, e1000795.

175. Duisters, R.F.; Tijsen, A.J.; Schroen, B.; Leenders, J.J.; Lentink, V.; van der Made, I.; Herias, V.; van Leeuwen, R.E.; Schellings, M.W.; Barenbrug, P.; *et al.* miR-133 and miR-30 regulate connective tissue growth factor: Implications for a role of microRNAs in myocardial matrix remodeling. *Circ. Res.* **2009**, *104*, 170–178.

176. Gambacciani, C.; Kusmic, C.; Chiavacci, E.; Meghini, F.; Rizzo, M.; Mariani, L.; Pitto, L. miR-29a and miR-30c negatively regulate DNMT3a in cardiac ischemic tissues: Implications for cardiac remodelling. *microRNA Diagn. Ther.* **2013**, *2013*, 34–44.

177. Pantos, C.; Mourouzis, I.; Cokkinos, D.V. Thyroid hormone and cardiac repair/regeneration: From Prometheus myth to reality? *Can. J. Physiol. Pharmacol.* **2012**, *90*, 977–987.

178. Pfeffer, M.A.; Braunwald, E. Ventricular remodeling after myocardial infarction. Experimental observations and clinical implications. *Circulation* **1990**, *81*, 1161–1172.

179. Sigurdsson, A.; Eriksson, S.V.; Hall, C.; Kahan, T.; Swedberg, K. Early neurohormonal effects of trandolapril in patients with left ventricular dysfunction and a recent acute myocardial infarction: A double-blind, randomized, placebo-controlled multicentre study. *Eur. J. Heart Fail.* **2001**, *3*, 69–78.

10

Mevalonate Pathway Blockade, Mitochondrial Dysfunction and Autophagy

Paola Maura Tricarico [1,*], Sergio Crovella [1,2] and Fulvio Celsi [2]

[1] Department of Medicine, Surgery and Health Sciences, University of Trieste, Piazzale Europa 1, 34128 Trieste, Italy; E-Mail: sergio.crovella@burlo.trieste.it

[2] Institute for Maternal and Child Health "Burlo Garofolo", via dell'Istria 65/1, 34137 Trieste, Italy; E-Mail: fulvio.celsi@gmail.com

* Author to whom correspondence should be addressed; E-Mail: paola.tricarico@burlo.trieste.it

Academic Editors: Lars Olson, Jaime M. Ross and Giuseppe Coppotelli

Abstract: The mevalonate pathway, crucial for cholesterol synthesis, plays a key role in multiple cellular processes. Deregulation of this pathway is also correlated with diminished protein prenylation, an important post-translational modification necessary to localize certain proteins, such as small GTPases, to membranes. Mevalonate pathway blockade has been linked to mitochondrial dysfunction: especially involving lower mitochondrial membrane potential and increased release of pro-apoptotic factors in cytosol. Furthermore a severe reduction of protein prenylation has also been associated with defective autophagy, possibly causing inflammasome activation and subsequent cell death. So, it is tempting to hypothesize a mechanism in which defective autophagy fails to remove damaged mitochondria, resulting in increased cell death. This mechanism could play a significant role in Mevalonate Kinase Deficiency, an autoinflammatory disease characterized by a defect in Mevalonate Kinase, a key enzyme of the mevalonate pathway. Patients carrying mutations in the *MVK* gene, encoding this enzyme, show increased inflammation and lower protein prenylation levels. This review aims at analysing the correlation between mevalonate pathway defects, mitochondrial dysfunction and defective autophagy, as well as inflammation, using Mevalonate Kinase Deficiency as a model to clarify the current pathogenetic hypothesis as the basis of the disease.

Keywords: autophagy; mevalonate pathway; mitochondrial dysfunction; inflammation; Mevalonate Kinase Deficiency; statins

1. Mevalonate Pathway

The mevalonate pathway, fundamental for cholesterol synthesis, is one of the most important metabolic networks in the cell; it provides essential cell constituents, such as cholesterol, and some of its branches produce key metabolites, such as geranylgeranyl pyrophosphate and farnesyl pyrophosphate, necessary for normal cell metabolism.

The first step of the mevalonate pathway is the synthesis of 3-hydroxy-3-methylglutaryl-CoA (HMG-CoA) from three molecules of acetyl-CoA, firstly by a condensation reaction forming acetoacetyl-CoA through acetoacetyl-CoA thiolase (EC 2.3.1.9) and subsequently through a second condensation between acetoacetyl-CoA and a third acetyl-CoA molecule catalysed by HMG-CoA synthase (EC 2.3.3.10) (Figure 1a, 1). In the second step, HMG-CoA is reduced to mevalonate acid by NADPH, a reaction catalysed by the HMG-CoA reductase (HMGR) enzyme (EC 1.1.1.88 and EC 1.1.1.34). HMGR is the rate-limiting enzyme for the mevalonate pathway and is one of the most finely regulated enzymes [1]. Regulation begins at the transcriptional level; if cholesterol or other sterol isoprenoids are in shortage, sterol regulatory element binding proteins (SREBP) are activated and they bind to sterol regulatory elements (SREs) present on the HMGR promoter, increasing its transcription [2,3]. Cholesterol also regulates the degradation of HMGR, promoting its association with gp78, an ubiquitin-E3 ligase that directs the enzyme towards proteasome 26s. HMGR is also regulated at the post-translational level, by phosphorylation mediated through AMP-activated protein kinase (AMPK). This enzyme is sensitive to the AMP:ATP ratio, and is activated by increased AMP concentration, thus in casea of metabolic stress, it deactivates HMGR, reducing cellular metabolism [4] (Figure 1a, 2).

The third key enzyme of the mevalonate pathway is the one responsible for converting mevalonic acid into mevalonate-5-phosphate, a key pathway intermediate. Mevalonate kinase (EC 2.7.1.36) (MVK) catalyses this conversion, using ATP as a phosphate donor and energy source. Furthermore, this enzyme is finely regulated, firstly at transcriptional level in a similar manner of HMGR: SREs are present at the MVK promoter and increases its transcription upon cholesterol shortage [5]. In addition, MVK presents feedback inhibition from some of the mevalonate pathway substrates, specifically geranylgeranyl pyrophosphate and farnesyl pyrophosphate, demonstrating that non-sterol isoprenoid could have a key role in regulation of this enzyme [6] (Figure 1a, 3).

In the fourth step of the mevalonate pathway, Mevalonate-5-phosphate is then converted into mevalonate-5-pyrophosphate by phosphomevalonate kinase (EC 2.7.4.2), using again ATP as phosphate and energy donor. Differently from MVK, this enzyme does not present feedback inhibition from its products [6]. However, various compounds were recently found to be inhibitors for this enzyme, suggesting novel mechanisms to inhibit the mevalonate pathway [7] and more interestingly, phosphomevalonate kinase appears also to be regulated by cholesterol shortage, as for mevalonate kinase and HMGR [8]. Indeed, cholesterol shortage induces increases in all the three first enzymes of the mevalonate pathway, thus guaranteeing a continued supply of this key membrane component (Figure 1a, 4).

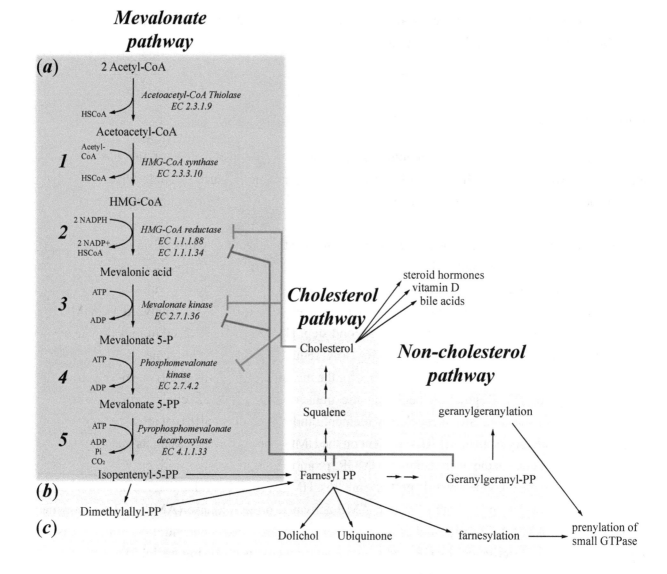

Figure 1. Schematic representation of the mevalonate pathway divided into: (**a**) The mevalonate pathway that produces mevalonate 5-PP and then isppententenyl 5-PP; (**b**) The cholesterol pathway that produces cholesterol, which in turn induces the formation of steroid hormones, vitamin D and bile acids; and (**c**) The non-cholesterol pathway important for the production of farnesyl-PP and geranylgeranyl-PP that induces respectively farnesylation and geranylgeranylation of small GTPase.

The fifth enzyme of the mevalonate pathway is pyrophosphomevalonate decarboxylase or diphosphomevalonate decarboxylase (EC 4.1.1.33). It converts mevalonate-5-pyrophosphate into isopentenyl-5-pyrophosphate (IPP), the final product of mevalonate pathway and the starting substrate for successive biosyntheticals reactions, especially cholesterol and isoprenoid production. This enzyme performs two key reactions: firstly, it phosphorylates mevalonate-5-pyrophosphate generating an intermediate product that, secondly, it is dephosphorylated and decarboxylated, obtaining thus IPP as a final product (Figure 1a, 5).

The mevalonate pathway, as described above, generates a key intermediate for cholesterol production, a fundamental constituent of cell membranes. Moreover, cholesterol is also converted to steroid hormones, regulating different cellular pathways, vitamin D and bile acid production (Figure 1b). IPP is the first step also in other, non-cholesterol, reactions; it is important for the production of farnesyl-pyrophosphate (FPP). FPP is converted in dolichols, used to assemble carbohydrate chains in glycoproteins, or in ubiquinones (or coenzyme Q10), electron transporters in mitochondria; or it is used to farnesylate or geranylate proteins, thus targeting them to cell membranes (Figure 1c). In summary, the mevalonate pathway is responsible for numerous cellular processes and the key enzymes described above undergo different regulation to maintain a constant supply of IPP.

2. Exogenous Mevalonate Pathway Blockade

The principal compounds that induce exogenous mevalonate pathway blockade are the statins, which are a class of compounds that act as competitive inhibitors of 3-hydroxy-3-methylglutaryl coenzyme-A (HMG-CoA) reductase, a key enzyme of the mevalonate pathway, which converts HMG-CoA into mevalonic acid. Statins, in general, are able to bind to a portion of HMG-CoA binding site, thus blocking the access of this substrate to the active site of the enzyme; effectively reducing the rate of mevalonate productions [9,10].

In 1976 Endo and coauthors discovered the first statin, isolated from *Penicillium citrinium* [11]. Subsequently, over the last two decades, several statins have been identified and classified in several ways. The most commonly used classification divides them into statins produced by fungi (such as Lovastatin, Simvastatin) and statins synthetically made (such as Atorvastatin, Fluvastatin).

All statins share a conserved HMG-like moiety covalently linked to a more or less extended hydrophobic group.

By blocking HMG-CoA reductase, statins induce a decrease in cholesterol level and simultaneously other by-products of the mevalonate pathway such as farnesyl pyrophosphate (FPP), geranylgeranyl pyrophosphate (GGPP), dolichols and coenzyme Q10 [12,13]. As reviewed in Winter-Vann and Casey (2005), inhibition of HMG-CoA reductase has a pleiotropic effect, due to the different affinities of key enzymes in the mevalonate pathway. FPP, the main metabolite in this pathway, could be converted to cholesterol through squalene synthase and this enzyme has a Km for the substrate of about 2 μM. GGPP synthase, instead, could convert FPP to GGPP, with a Km of 1 μM; GGPP is attached to different proteins (the majority of which pertain to the Rab family) to ensure their correct localization. On the other hand, protein farnesyl trasferase (FTase) uses FPP to attach a farnesyl group to specific proteins, such as the family of small GTPase proteins (Ras and Rho GTPases), with a Km of 5 nM. Therefore, inhibition of HMG-CoA reductase lowers FPP levels and the first consequence is a reduction in cholesterol levels; following that, GGPP levels are reduced, causing mislocalization and loss of activity of specific proteins. Instead, due to the high affinity of FTase towards FPP, farnesylation levels of key cellular enzymes remain stable [14].

Indeed, a widely adopted view considers the pleiotropic effects of statins independent of lowering cholesterol levels, but rather connected to a lack of these prenylated proteins [12]. In the last few years there has been an increase in interest of these pleiotropic effects, because of their possible main responsibility for statin anti-cancer and immunomodulatory effects [15–18].

For all these reasons, the role of statins are debatable, and there are many studies describing statins as drugs for treatment of a variety of disease such as hypercholesterolemia, cancer, cardiovascular diseases, inflammatory diseases [19–24].

Furthermore, statins are used as a pharmacological compound to biochemically reproduce some features of Mevalonate Kinase Deficiency (MKD)—a pathology characterized by a defect in a key enzyme of mevalonate pathway [13,25,26]. In some studies, mevalonate pathway blockade, obtained in neuronal and monocytic cell lines by statin (Lovastatin) administration, induces an increase of apoptosis correlated to mitochondrial damage [27–29].

Also, Van der Burgh and co-workers have recently demonstrated that mevalonate pathway blockade, obtained in monocytic cell line by statin (Simvastatin) administration, produces mitochondrial damage and autophagy impairment, related to a decrease in protein prenylation levels [25,30].

2.1. Mitochondrial Dysfunction and Statin

Mevalonate pathway blockade, obtained by treatment with statins, has been linked to mitochondrial dysfunction, specifically by lowering mitochondrial membrane potential and increasing release of pro-apoptotic factors.

Usually, mitochondrial dysfunction is associated with intrinsic apoptosis, also known as the mitochondrial apoptotic pathway. This pathway is characterized by activation of caspase-9 and -3, and inhibition or activation of anti- or pro-apoptotic Bcl-2 family members. Furthermore, mitochondrial membrane potential decreases, causing release of pro-apoptotic factors, oxidative stress and then cell death [31].

In a biochemical MKD model, obtained by Lovastatin treatment in neuroblastoma cell lines, we observed mitochondrial dysfunction correlated to increased intrinsic apoptosis, also confirmed by activation of caspase-3 and -9 [27,28]; furthermore, in monocyte cell lines, we observed a similar increase in oxidative stress [29].

Mitochondrial dysfunction, caused by statins, could be related to oxidative stress, shortage of prenylated proteins or both. In fact, it was observed that the block of mevalonate pathway, obtained by statin (Simvastin) treatment in endothelial cancer cell lines, resulted in G1 cell cycle arrest, apoptosis, DNA damage and cellular stress [32].

Another study showed that simvastatin, in lung cancer cells, inhibited the proliferation and significantly increased oxidative stress, in particular augmenting reactive oxygen species (ROS) production and the activity of total superoxide dismutase (SOD) and in particular the mitochondrial form, superoxide dismutase 2 (SOD2) [33].

Strong oxidative stress, which induces mitochondrial dysfunction, could be due to the action of statins on the mevalonate pathway, decreasing coenzyme Q10 and dolichol levels, considered as anti-oxidants defense systems.

Coenzyme Q10 is a product of the mevalonate pathway and is an important electron transporter of the mitochondrial respiratory chain. A decrease in coenzyme Q10 levels, caused by mevalonate pathway blockade, could result in an abnormal mitochondrial respiratory function causing mitochondrial and oxidative damage [34].

Dolichol, a polyprenol compound, is an important free-radical scavenger in cell membranes [35]. Ciosek and co-workers observed a significant decrease in dolichol levels after Lovastatin administration in *in vivo* models [36]; a lack of this compound might cause oxidative stress and mitochondrial damage [13,37].

Nevertheless, mitochondrial dysfunction caused by statins could also be related to a decrease in prenylated protein levels; indeed, statins treatment could lead to a reduction in cholesterol level, and also in farnesyl pyrophosphate (FPP) and in geranylgeranyl pyrophosphate (GGPP). Xia and co-workers have demonstrated that apoptosis induced by Lovastatin treatment, in human AML cells is connected to a decrease in GGPP and, to a lesser extent, related to a FPP decrease [38].

Agarwal and co-workers also observed the close correlation between decrease in prenylated proteins levels, apoptosis and mitochondrial damage in Lovastatin-treated colon cancer cells. The treatment caused a decrease in expression of anti-apoptotic protein Bcl-2 and an increase of pro-apoptotic protein such as Bax; the subsequent addition of GGPP prevented Lovastatin apoptosis, confirming a key role of prenylated proteins levels [39].

Recently, Van der Burgh and co-workers have demonstrated that, in simvastatin-treated cells, mitochondria clearance is reduced, with lower oxygen consumption and glycolysis rate. These conditions suggested that accumulation of damaged mitochondria could be the trigger for NACHT, LRR and PYD domains-containing protein 3 (NALP3) inflammasome activation. The authors also speculate that prenylated proteins could be the main mediators of statin adverse effects [25,30].

Further confirmations that statins treatment could impair mitochondrial activity come from two recent studies done using a completely different model, *C. elegans*. In the first paper, the authors show that animals resistant to statin treatment have an increased mitochondrial unfolded protein response (UPRmt) which, they speculate, could lower protein turnover and thus lessening the need for protein prenylation [40]. In the second paper, the authors demonstrate that statin abrogates the *C. elegans* ability to sense mitochondrial damage and that this ability could be partially rescued through GGPP subministration [41]. Taken together, these results demonstrate once more the key role of protein prenylation in mitochondrial homeostasis.

A mitochondrial-specific effect of statin, probably mediated through lowering prenylated proteins, suggests that this class of compound could be considered as anti-cancer drugs. However, further studies are necessary to completely clarify the variety of effects of these drugs and at present, only hypotheses have been raised to explain actions of statins on cellular survival.

2.2. Autophagy and Statins

Mevalonate pathway blockade has been linked to defective autophagy, possibly causing inflammasome activation and subsequent cell death. Autophagy (macroautophagy) is the main catabolic mechanism involved in the turnover of cytoplasmic components and selective removal of damaged or redundant organelles (such as mitochondria, peroxisomes and endoplasmic reticulum), through the lysosome machinery. Initial steps include the formation of phagophore or pre-autophagosome, an isolated membrane able to elongate and forming the autophagosome, a double-membrane compartment that sequesters the cytoplasmic materials. Subsequently, the fusion of autophagosome with lysosome forms the autolysosome, where the captured material is degraded [42] (Figure 2).

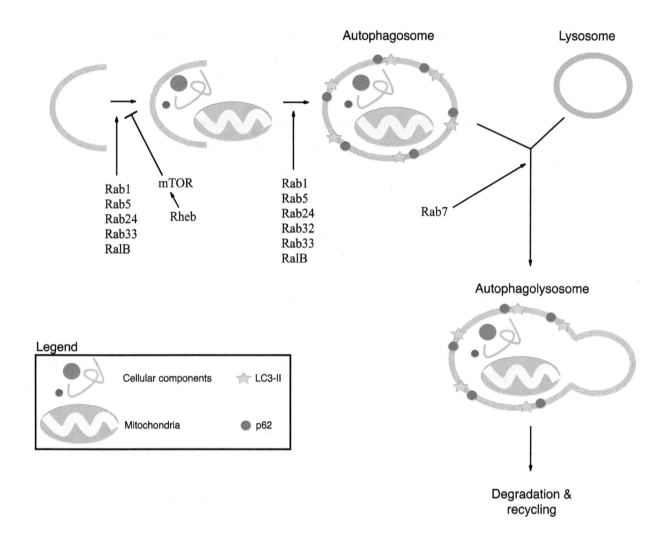

Figure 2. Schematic representation of macroautophagy mechanism and its main actors. Macroautophagy delivers cellular components and damaged or redundant organelles (such as mitochondria), to the lysosome through the intermediary of a double membrane-bound vesicle, referred to as an autophagosome. Autophagy is initiated by the formation of the isolation membrane that induces the formation of autophagosome. Subsequently, the autophagosome fuses with the lysosome to form an autolysosome. Finally all the material is degraded in the autophagolysosome and recycled. The p62 protein interacts with damaged proteins in the cells, and the complexes are then selectively tied to the autophagosome through LC3-II. Rabs, Rheb and RalB are autophagy-related protein important for the regulation of macroautophagy mechanism.

Autophagy involves numerous molecular mediators called autophagy-related (ATG) proteins; among these, prenylation of proteins appears to be one of the key regulation mechanisms [43]. Specifically, different small GTPase are indicated as ATG proteins: Rabs, Rheb, RalB. Rabs are crucial proteins for developing subdomains on membranes to facilitate maturation; recent studies have shown that some Rabs are essential for autophagy. The best known Rabs at the present time are: Rab1, able to regulate the autophagosome formation; Rab5, an early endosome protein, responsible for autophagosome membrane elongation and autophagosome formation, regulating Beclin1-Vps34-Atg6 class III PI3-kinase complex;

Rab7, a late endosome protein, responsible for autophagosome maturation, promoting the microtubule plus-end-directed transport and facilitating fusion of autophagosome with lysosome; Rab24, normally present in reticular distribution around the nucleus, is important for autophagosome maturation; Rab32, generally present in mitochondria, regulates the membrane trafficking, and is required for autophagosome formation; Rab33 modulates autophagosome formation [44,45] (Figure 2).

Ras homology enriched in brain (Rheb) directly binds and selectively activates the multiprotein complex 1 of mammalian target of rapamycin (mTORC1) [46] which is composed of mTOR, a negative regulator of autophagy, and mLST8 [47,48]. mTOR activity inhibits mammalian autophagy and indeed a recent study demonstrated that autophagy impairment is correlated to mTORC1 hyperactivation in β-cell [49] (Figure 2).

RalB localizes in nascent autophagosome and is activated due to nutrient deprivation and, thanks to the binding to its effector Exo84, induces the assembly of active Beclin1-VPS34 and ULK1. The resulting complex induces the isolation of pre-autophagosomal membrane and maturation of autophagosomes [50,51] (Figure 2).

All these proteins require prenylation for their activation, either farnesylated or geranylgeranylated; indeed statins, blocking the mevalonate pathway and causing a decrease in prenylated proteins levels, could play a regulatory role in autophagy. Nevertheless, the statin effects in autophagy remain poorly understood.

Recently, Van der Burgh and co-workers have observed defective autophagy in statin-treated monocytes, correlated to damaged mitochondria and NALP3 inflammasome activation [25]. The same authors have subsequently demonstrated that statin treatment increases levels of unprenylated RhoA, which in turn activates protein kinase B (PKB) possibly playing a role in statin-induced autophagy blockade [30].

On the contrary, other studies show that treatment with statins induces an increase in autophagy levels, and for this reason, statins could be considered as anti-cancer drugs. Indeed, a study showed that statins, such as Cerivastatin, Pitavastatin and Fluvastatin, are the most potent autophagy inducing agents in human cancer cells; the authors, however, did not analyze levels of p62, thus the possibility that autophagy is increased but subsequentrly blocked was not examined [52].

Another study demonstrated that statin induces autophagy through depleting cellular levels of geranylgeranyl diphosphonate (GGPP), independently of the decreased activity in two major small G proteins, Rheb and Ras [53]. However, the authors did not examine all autophagic pathways, thus the observations are not conclusive and further investigations are needed.

Lastly, Wei and co-workers observed that simvastatin inhibits the Rac1-mTOR pathway and thereby increases autophagy, in coronary arterial myocytes [54].

All these results show that the role of statin in autophagy is related to GGPP and prenylated proteins levels, thus being important actors in this mechanism. Indeed, cellular differences in GGPP and prenylated proteins levels could explain the contradictory findings in the studies described above. However, further studies are necessary to clarify the mechanism of action and the molecular targets involved in statin-modulated autophagy.

3. Endogenous Mevalonate Pathway Blockade

The mevalonate pathway could also be blocked by enzymatic defects due to mutations in genes involved in this pathway. In particular, a rare disease involving mutations on *MVK* gene (12q24.11) has been described: Mevalonate Kinase Deficiency (MKD). Currently, 82 mutations of the *MVK* gene have been reported in the Human Gene Mutation Database [55].

MKD possesses two distinct phenotypes: a milder one, also called Hyper IgD Syndrome (HIDS; OMIM#260920), in which the patients suffer recurrent fevers, have skin rashes, hepatosplenomegalia and generally a sustained inflammatory response; and a severe, rarer, one, called Mevalonic Aciduria (MA; OMIM #610377), characterized by the involvement of the Central Nervous System, with cerebellar ataxia, psychomotor retardation and also, as in HIDS, recurrent fever attacks [56].

Residual MVK enzymatic activity marks the boundary between HIDS and MA, with MA patients having less than 1% activity, while HIDS between 1% and 7% of activity [57]. Initially, disease pathogenesis was thought to derive from low cholesterol levels, being MVK a central enzyme in the mevalonate pathway. However, patients, either with HIDS or MA, showed normal cholesterol levels, probably due to dietary intake. Subsequently, accumulation of Mevalonic acid was indicated as responsible for the MKD phenotype. Still, a small clinical trial, involving two MA patients, using statin (Lovastatin) to reduce Mevalonic acid, resulted in worsening of the symptoms [58]; on the contrary, Simvastatin appeared to be beneficial for treating HIDS patients [56]. Thus, the hypothesis pointing to Mevalonic acid levels as causative for MKD does not explain completely the disease's manifestations. Celec and Behuliak in 2008 hypothesized that MVK dysfunctions could diminish non-steroid isoprenoids, causing oxidative stress and ultimately leading to chronic hyperinflammation [13].

The shortage of isoprenoids, correlated to a severe reduction in protein prenylation, in particular of geranylgeranyl pyrophosphate (GGPP), has been linked with the activation of caspase-1 and thereby with the production of IL-1β [59,60].

In particular, the IL-1 family is strongly supposed to play a fundamental role in MKD inflammatory processes, indeed, several biological therapies have successfully targeted these molecules [61–63].

In a previous work it has been shown that, in monocytes from MKD patients, a key component of the inflammation machinery is NACHT, LRR and PYD domains-containing protein 3 (NALP3) [64]; NALP3 interacts with another protein, pyrin domain (PYD) of apoptosis-associated speck-like protein containing a CARD domain (ASC), constituting the inflammasome platform. The CARD domain recruits pro-caspase-1, which self-cleaves into active caspase-1 and then converts pro-IL-1β to active IL-1β, activating one of the main pathways of inflammation [65,66].

However it remains an open question how isoprenoid shortage, as in MKD and in presence of the biochemical block, activates NALP3 and the inflammasome pathway.

Recently Van der Burgh and co-workers have demonstrated that, in MKD patients' cells and in statin-treated monocytes, autophagy is impaired and specifically mitochondria clearance is slowed, suggesting that accumulation of damaged mitochondria could be the trigger to NALP3 inflammasome activation [25]. The same group has recently reported that statin treatment increases levels of unprenylated Ras homolog gene family member A (RhoA), which in turn activates PKB, representing then the hypothetical starting point for autophagy. The authors also demonstrated that levels of unprenylated RhoA correlate with IL-1b release, thus partially confirming this hypothetical link [25,30].

4. Autophagy, Inflammation and Damaged Mitochondria

An emerging concept in recent years tightly associates autophagy with inflammation regulation mechanisms. Autophagy can regulate different aspects of the immune response: it is involved in the degradation of bacteria/virus engulfed by the cell, it regulates Pattern Recognition Receptors (PRRs) and can act as their effector, it can process Antigens for MHC presentation and finally autophagy can regulate inflammasome activation and secretion of different cytokines [67]. The first three mechanisms have been extensively described by Deretic (2013) [68], and will be briefly discussed here.

Autophagy can be envisaged as a mechanism to clear the cytosol from invading intracellular pathogens, either bacteria or viruses, which are engulfed in autophagic membranes and targeted to lysosomes to be degraded. This process is facilitated by sequestosome 1/p62-like receptors (SLRs) that recognize pathogens and facilitate their encasement in autophagosomes, possessing an LC3 interacting region.

Furthermore, autophagy could be an effector for PRRs, degrading targets marked by toll-like receptors (TLRs) or it can help in delivering ligands to TLRs, as for TLR7 [68].

Antigen processing for MHC II presentation represents another important mechanism regulated by autophagy. Indeed, autophagy is crucial for viral immunosurvelliance and is also inhibited by HIV-1 by upregulating mTOR in dendritic cells [69,70]. Moreover, autophagy is required for positive selection of naïve T cells in thymus, whereas knocking-out key autophagy proteins results in autoimmune syndromes [71].

How autophagy regulates inflammasome activation is currently a subject of numerous studies and a general consensus has not been yet reached. However, two hypotheses are at the moment explored: a first one suggesting that autophagy regulates processing of IL-1b and other pro-inflammatory molecules; the second proposing that autophagy removes damaged mitochondria, thus dampening NALP3 activation. It is possible that those two processes are not mutually exclusive and act in parallel to maintain the inflammatory status in "inactive" condition.

Direct regulation of IL-1b processing by inflammasomes has been demonstrated in macrophages and *in vivo* where treatment with rapamycin (autophagy inducer) decreases its secreted and circulating levels [72]. Further confirmation came from the work of Shi and co-authors (2012), in which they demonstrate how inflammasome activation induces autophagy and autophagosomes formation containing inflammasomes components such as ASC or absent in melanoma 2 (AIM2), in a self-limiting process. IL-1b does not possess a "canonical" secretory signature and it is translated in the cytosol, via polyribosomes linked to the cytoskeleton [73–75]. Later it was demonstrated that secretion of IL-1b is dependent on its localization in lysosome-associated vesicles and agents that regulates autophagy can modulate its release [72,76]. These works clearly show the regulation of IL-1b processing by autophagy.

Other studies put autophagy upstream of inflammasome activation. Reactive oxygen species (ROS) can activate NALP3 inflammasome and damaged mitochondria are the main source for ROS. Mitophagy, a specialized form of autophagy, constantly removes damaged mitochondria, thus lowering ROS levels. If cells are challenged with 3-methyladenine, a blocker of mitophagy, NALP3 activation is increased and redistributed near mitochondria-ER contact points, working as a sensor for mitochondrial damage [77].

Moreover, mitochondrial DNA (mtDNA) can work as NALP3 activation inducer, thus sensing mitochondrial damage and 3-MA could increase NALP3 activation caused by mtDNA [78,79].

These data show a possible pipeline: decreased mitophagy leading to increased ROS and mtDNA in cytosol, leading to increased NALP3 activation.

The two mechanisms described above are not necessarily self-exclusive. It is then possible that autophagy machinery collaborates in dampening inflammation and a disturbance in mitochondria homeostasis could lead to exacerbating inflammation.

In MKD is it then possible that a disturbance in autophagy mechanisms causes damage in mitochondria, impairing their recycling and thus increasing ROS levels; this, in turn, increases activation of inflammation. This chain of events still remains to be verified; however exploring this mechanism could represent a novel strategy to fight this debilitating disease.

5. Conclusive Remarks

MKD is an orphan drug disease, so many efforts are being made in search of potential targets for novel treatments tailored to prevent, or at least to diminish, apoptosis in MKD patients. Several studies reported *in vitro* administration of natural and synthetic isoprenoids to restore the mevalonate pathway in cell cultures (both models and patients' derived monocytes) treated with statins to biochemically mimic the genetic defect.

As described above, a possible link exists between defective protein prenylation and mitochondrial dysfunction, supposedly made by autophagy (Figure 3).

Furthermore, it remains to be determined how autophagy is impaired in MKD. Protein prenylation seems to be one of the regulation mechanisms involved in autophagy. Compounds able to restore protein prenylation could be considered as potential therapy to tackle MKD; unfortunatly such compounds are at the present time, not actively researched. Other strategies, such as modulation of farnesyl protein transferase could be exploited to fight MKD.

For all these reasons, our review aimed at recalling the attention of the scientific community on another possible mechanism at the basis of MKD pathogenesis, and intends to point out that autophagy should be considered when trying to design novel therapeutic strategies to fight cell death in MKD patients.

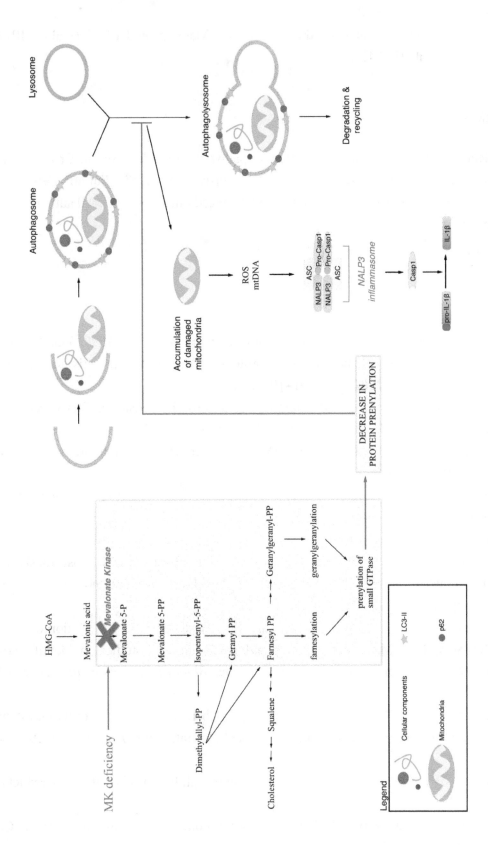

Figure 3. Schematic representation of a possibile link between defective protein prenylation, mitochondrial dysfunction and autophagy. Mevalonate Kinase Deficiency is characterized by a block of the mevalonate pathway induces by mutation in a gene that encodes for Mevalonate Kinase. Blockade of the mevalonate pathway induces decrease in protein prenylation that could alter the macroautophagy mechanism and in particular mitochondrial degradation and recycling. Accumulation of damaged mitochondria induces ROS production and mtDNA release. All these events are important for the activation of NALP3 inflammasome that cleaves and activates IL-1b.

Acknowledgments

This study was supported by a grant from the Institute for Maternal and Child Health—IRCCS "Burlo Garofolo"—Trieste, Italy (RC 42/2011).

Author Contributions

Paola Maura Tricarico wrote "Exogenous Mevalonate pathway blockade"; Sergio Crovella wrote "Endogenous mevalonate pathway blockade" and "Conclusive remarks"; Fulvio Celsi wrote "Mevalonate pathway" and "Autophagy, inflammation and damaged mitochondria". All authors revised and assembled the paper.

References

1. Goldstein, J.L.; Brown, M.S. Regulation of the mevalonate pathway. *Nature* **1990**, *343*, 425–430.
2. Horton, J.D. Sterol regulatory element-binding proteins: Transcriptional activators of lipid synthesis. *Biochem. Soc. Trans.* **2002**, *30*, 1091–1095.
3. Weber, L.W.; Boll, M.; Stampfl, A. Maintaining cholesterol homeostasis: Sterol regulatory element-binding proteins. *World J. Gastroenterol.* **2004**, *10*, 3081–3087.
4. Burg, J.S.; Espenshade, P.J. Regulation of HMG-CoA reductase in mammals and yeast. *Progress Lipid Res.* **2011**, *50*, 403–410.
5. Murphy, C.; Murray, A.M.; Meaney, S.; Gåfvels, M. Regulation by SREBP-2 defines a potential link between isoprenoid and adenosylcobalamin metabolism. *Biochem. Biophys. Res. Commun.* **2007**, *355*, 359–364.
6. Hinson, D.D.; Chambliss, K.L.; Toth, M.J.; Tanaka, R.D.; Gibson, K.M. Post-translational regulation of mevalonate kinase by intermediates of the cholesterol and nonsterol isoprene biosynthetic pathways. *J. Lipid Res.* **1997**, *38*, 2216–2223.
7. Boonsri, P.; Neumann, T.S.; Olson, A.L.; Cai, S.; Herdendorf, T.J.; Miziorko, H.M.; Hannongbua, S.; Sem, D.S. Molecular docking and NMR binding studies to identify novel inhibitors of human phosphomevalonate kinase. *Biochem. Biophys. Res. Commun.* **2013**, *430*, 313–319.
8. Olivier, L.M.; Chambliss, K.L.; Gibson, K.M.; Krisans, S.K. Characterization of phosphomevalonate kinase: Chromosomal localization, regulation, and subcellular targeting. *J. Lipid Res.* **1999**, *40*, 672–679.
9. Istvan, E.S.; Deisenhofer, J. Structural mechanism for statin inhibition of HMG-CoA reductase. *Science* **2001**, *292*, 1160–1164.
10. Corsini, A.; Maggi, F.M.; Catapano, A.L. Pharmacology of competitive inhibitors of HMG-CoA reductase. *Pharmacol. Res.* **1995**, *31*, 9–27.
11. Endo, A.; Kuroda, M.; Tsujita, Y. ML-236A, ML-236B, and ML-236C, new inhibitors of cholesterogenesis produced by Penicillium citrinium. *J. Antibiot. (Tokyo)* **1976**, *29*, 1346–1348.

12. Alegret, M.; Silvestre, J.S. Pleiotropic effects of statins and related pharmacological experimental approaches. *Methods Find Exp. Clin. Pharmacol.* **2006**, *28*, 627–656.

13. Celec, P.; Behuliak, M. The lack of non-steroid isoprenoids causes oxidative stress in patients with mevalonic aciduria. *Med. Hypotheses* **2008**, *70*, 938–940.

14. Winter-Vann, A.M.; Casey, P.J. Post-prenylation-processing enzymes as new targets in oncogenesis. *Nat. Rev. Cancer* **2005**, *5*, 405–412.

15. Wong, W.W.; Dimitroulakos, J.; Minden, M.D.; Penn, L.Z. HMG-CoA reductase inhibitors and the malignant cell: The statin family of drugs as triggers of tumor-specific apoptosis. *Leukemia* **2002**, *16*, 508–519.

16. Sassano, A.; Platanias, L.C. Statins in tumor suppression. *Cancer Lett.* **2008**, *260*, 11–9.

17. Osmak, M. Statins and cancer: Current and future prospects. *Cancer Lett.* **2012**, *324*, 1–12.

18. Blum, A.; Shamburek, R. The pleiotropic effects of statins on endothelial function, vascular inflammation, immunomodulation and thrombogenesis. *Atherosclerosis* **2009**, *203*, 325–330.

19. Olsson, A.G.; Istad, H.; Luurila, O.; Ose, L.; Stender, S.; Tuomilehto, J.; Wiklund, O.; Southworth, H.; Pears, J.; Wilpshaar, J.W.; *et al.* Effects of rosuvastatin and atorvastatin compared over 52 weeks of treatment in patients with hypercholesterolemia. *Am. Heart J.* **2002**, *144*, 1044–1051.

20. Cardwell, C.R.; Mc Menamin, Ú.; Hughes, C.M.; Murray, L.J. Statin use and survival from lung cancer: A population-based cohort study. *Cancer Epidemiol. Biomarkers Prev.* **2015**, *24*, 833–841.

21. Shepherd, J.; Blauw, G.J.; Murphy, M.B.; Bollen, E.L.; Buckley, B.M.; Cobbe, S.M.; Ford, I.; Gaw, A.; Hyland, M.; Jukema, J.W.; *et al.* PROSPER study group. Pravastatin in elderly individuals at risk of vascular disease (PROSPER): A randomised controlled trial. *Lancet* **2002**, *23*, 360, 1623–1630.

22. Dursun, S.; Çuhadar, S.; Köseoğlu, M.; Atay, A.; Aktaş, S.G. The anti-inflammatory and antioxidant effects of pravastatin and nebivolol in rat aorta. *Anadolu Kardiyol. Derg.* **2014**, *14*, 229–233.

23. Leung, B.P.; Sattar, N.; Crilly, A.; Prach, M.; McCarey, D.W.; Payne, H.; Madhok, R.; Campbell, C.; Gracie, J.A.; Liew, F.Y.; *et al.* A novel anti-inflammatory role for simvastatin in inflammatory arthritis. *J. Immunol.* **2003**, *170*, 1524–1530.

24. Barsante, M.M.; Roffê, E.; Yokoro, C.M.; Tafuri, W.L.; Souza, D.G.; Pinho, V.; Castro, M.S.; Teixeira, M.M. Anti-inflammatory and analgesic effects of atorvastatin in a rat model of adjuvant-induced arthritis. *Eur. J. Pharmacol.* **2005**, *516*, 282–289.

25. Van der Burgh, R.; Nijhuis, L.; Pervolaraki, K.; Compeer, E.; Jongeneel, L.H.; van Gijn, M.; Coffer, P.J.; Murphy, M.P.; Mastroberardino, P.G.; Frenkel, J.; *et al.* Defects in mitochondrial clearance predispose human monocytes to interleukin-1β hypersecretion. *J. Biol. Chem.* **2014**, *289*, 5000–5012.

26. Kuijk, L.M.; Beekman, J.M.; Koster, J.; Waterham, H.R.; Frenkel, J.; Coffer, P.J. HMG-CoA reductase inhibition induces IL-1β release through Rac1/PI3K/PKB-dependent caspase-1 activation. *Blood* **2008**, *112*, 3563–3573.

27. Marcuzzi, A.; Tricarico, P.M.; Piscianz, E.; Kleiner, G.; Brumatti, L.V.; Crovella, S. Lovastatin induces apoptosis through the mitochondrial pathway in an undifferentiated SH-SY5Y neuroblastoma cell line. *Cell Death Dis.* **2013**, *4*, e585, doi:10.1038/cddis.2013.112.

28. Marcuzzi, A.; Zanin, V.; Piscianz, E.; Tricarico, P.M.; Vuch, J.; Girardelli, M.; Monasta, L.; Bianco, A.M.; Crovella, S. Lovastatin-induced apoptosis is modulated by geranylgeraniol in a neuroblastoma cell line. *Int. J. Dev. Neurosci.* **2012**, *30*, 451–456.

29. Tricarico, P.M.; Kleiner, G.; Valencic, E.; Campisciano, G.; Girardelli, M.; Crovella, S.; Knowles, A.; Marcuzzi, A. Block of the mevalonate pathway triggers oxidative and inflammatory molecular mechanisms modulated by exogenous isoprenoid compounds. *Int. J. Mol. Sci.* **2014**, *15*, 6843–6856.

30. Van der Burgh, R.; Pervolaraki, K.; Turkenburg, M.; Waterham, H.R.; Frenkel, J.; Boes, M. Unprenylated RhoA contributes to IL-1β hypersecretion in mevalonate kinase deficiency model through stimulation of Rac1 activity. *J. Biol. Chem.* **2014**, *289*, 27757–27765.

31. Tricarico, P.M.; Marcuzzi, A.; Piscianz, E.; Monasta, L.; Crovella, S.; Kleiner, G. Mevalonate kinase deficiency and neuroinflammation: Balance between apoptosis and pyroptosis. *Int. J. Mol. Sci.* **2013**, *14*, 23274–23288.

32. Schointuch, M.N.; Gilliam, T.P.; Stine, J.E.; Han, X. Zhou, C.; Gehrig, P.A.; Kim, K.; Bae-Jump, V.L. Simvastatin, an HMG-CoA reductase inhibitor, exhibits anti-metastatic and anti-tumorigenic effects in endometrial cancer. *Gynecol. Oncol.* **2014**, *134*, 346–355.

33. Li, Y.; Fu, J.; Yuan, X.; Hu, C. Simvastatin inhibits the proliferation of A549 lung cancer cells through oxidative stress and up-regulation of SOD2. *Pharmazie* **2014**, *69*, 610–614.

34. Tavintharan, S.; Ong, C.N.; Jeyaseelan, K.; Sivakumar, M.; Lim, S.C.; Sum, C.F. Reduced mitochondrial coenzyme Q10 levels in HepG2 cells treated with high-dose simvastatin: A possible role in statin-induced hepatotoxicity? *Toxicol. Appl. Pharmacol.* **2007**, *223*, 173–179.

35. Bergamini, E.; Bizzarri, R.; Cavallini, G.; Cerbai, B.; Chiellini, E.; Donati, A.; Gori, Z.; Manfrini, A.; Parentini, I.; Signori, F.; *et al.* Ageing and oxidative stress: A role for dolichol in the antioxidant machinery of cell membranes? *J. Alzheimers Dis.* **2004**, *6*, 129–135.

36. Ciosek, C.P.; Magnin, D.R.; Harrity, T.W.; Logan, J.V.; Dickson, J.K.; Gordon, E.M.; Hamilton, K.A.; Jolibois, K.G.; Kunselman, L.K.; Lawrence, R.M.; *et al.* Lipophilic 1,1-bisphosphonates are potent squalene synthase inhibitors and orally active cholesterol lowering agents *in vivo*. *J. Biol. Chem.* **1993**, *268*, 24832–24837.

37. Sirvent, P.; Mercier, J.; Lacampagne, A. New insights into mechanisms of statin-associated myotoxicity. *Curr. Opin. Pharmacol.* **2008**, *8*, 333–338.

38. Xia, Z.; Tan, M.M.; Wong, W.W.; Dimitroulakos, J.; Minden, M.D.; Penn, L.Z. Blocking protein geranylgeranylation is essential for lovastatin-induced apoptosis of human acute myeloid leukemia cells. *Leukemia (Baltimore)* **2001**, *15*, 1398–1407.

39. Agarwal, B.; Bhendwal, S.; Halmos, B.; Moss, S.F.; Ramey, W.G.; Holt, P.R. Lovastatin augments apoptosis induced by chemotherapeutic agents in colon cancer cells. *Clin. Cancer Res.* **1999**, *5*, 2223–2229.

40. Rauthan, M.; Ranji, P.; Aguilera Pradenas, N.; Pitot, C.; Pilon, M. The mitochondrial unfolded protein response activator ATFS-1 protects cells from inhibition of the mevalonate pathway. *Proc. Natl. Acad. Sci. USA* **2013**, *110*, 5981–5986

41. Liu, Y.; Samuel, B.S.; Breen, P.C.; Ruvkun, G. Caenorhabditis elegans pathways that surveil and defend mitochondria. *Nature* **2014**, *508*, 406–410.

42. Levine, B.; Kroemer, G. Autophagy in the pathogenesis of disease. *Cell* **2008**, *132*, 27–42.

43. Longatti, A.; Tooze, S.A. Vesicular trafficking and autophagosome formation. *Cell Death Differ.* **2009**, *16*, 956–965.

44. Zhu, Y.; Casey, P.J.; Kumar, A.P.; Pervaiz, S. Deciphering the signaling networks underlying simvastatin-induced apoptosis in human cancer cells: Evidence for non-canonical activation of RhoA and Rac1 GTPases. *Cell Death Dis.* **2013**, *4*, e568, doi:10.1038/cddis.2013.103.

45. Hutagalung, A.H.; Novick, P.J. Role of Rab GTPases in membrane traffic and cell physiology. *Physiol. Rev.* **2011**, *91*, 119–149.

46. Sciarretta, S.; Zhai, P.; Shao, D.; Maejima, Y.; Robbins, J.; Volpe, M.; Condorelli, G.; Sadoshima, J. Rheb is a critical regulator of autophagy during myocardial ischemia: Pathophysiological implications in obesity and metabolic syndrome. *Circulation* **2012**, *125*, 1134–1146.

47. Ravikumar, B.; Futter, M.; Jahreiss, L.; Korolchuk, V.I.; Lichtenberg, M.; Luo, S.; Massey, D.C.; Menzies, F.M.; Narayanan, U.; Renna, M.; *et al.* Mammalian macroautophagy at a glance. *J. Cell Sci.* **2009**, *122*, 1707–1711.

48. Hall, M.N. mTOR-what does it do? *Transplant. Proc.* **2008**, *40*, S5–S8.

49. Bartolomé, A.; Kimura-Koyanagi, M.; Asahara, S.; Guillén, C.; Inoue, H.; Teruyama, K.; Shimizu, S.; Kanno, A.; García-Aguilar, A.; Koike, M.; Uchiyama, Y.; *et al.* Pancreatic β-cell failure mediated by mTORC1 hyperactivity and autophagic impairment. *Diabetes* **2014**, *63*, 2996–3008.

50. Bodemann, B.O.; Orvedahl, A.; Cheng, T.; Ram, R.R.; Ou, Y.H.; Formstecher, E.; Maiti, M.; Hazelett, C.C.; Wauson, E.M.; Balakireva, M.; Camonis, J.H.; *et al.* RalB and the exocyst mediate the cellular starvation response by direct activation of autophagosome assembly. *Cell* **2011**, *144*, 253–267.

51. Bento, C.F.; Puri, C.; Moreau, K.; Rubinsztein, D.C. The role of membrane-trafficking small GTPases in the regulation of autophagy. *J. Cell Sci.* **2013**, *126*, 1059–1069.

52. Jiang, P.; Mukthavaram, R.; Chao, Y.; Nomura, N.; Bharati, I.S.; Fogal, V.; Pastorino, S.; Teng, D.; Cong, X.; Pingle, S.C.; Kapoor, S.; *et al. In vitro* and *in vivo* anticancer effects of mevalonate pathway modulation on human cancer cells. *Br. J. Cancer* **2014**, *111*, 1562–1571.

53. Araki, M.; Maeda, M.; Motojima, K. Hydrophobic statins induce autophagy and cell death in human rhabdomyosarcoma cells by depleting geranylgeranyl diphosphate. *Eur. J. Pharmacol.* **2012**, *674*, 95–103.

54. Wei, Y.M.; Li, X.; Xu, M.; Abais, J.M.; Chen, Y.; Riebling, C.R.; Boini, K.M.; Li, P.L.; Zhang, Y. Enhancement of autophagy by simvastatin through inhibition of Rac1-mTOR signaling pathway in coronary arterial myocytes. *Cell Physiol. Biochem.* **2013**, *31*, 925–937.

55. Stenson, P.D.; Mort, M.; Ball, E.V.; Shaw, K.; Phillips, A.; Cooper, D.N. The Human Gene Mutation Database: Building a comprehensive mutation repository for clinical and molecular genetics, diagnostic testing and personalized genomic medicine. *Hum. Genet.* **2014**, *133*, 1–9.

56. Simon, A.; Kremer, H.P.; Wevers, R.A.; Scheffer, H.; de Jong, J.G.; van der Meer, J.W.; Drenth, J.P. Mevalonate kinase deficiency: Evidence for a phenotypic continuum. *Neurology* **2004**, *62*, 994–997.

57. Hoffmann, G.F.; Charpentier, C.; Mayatepek, E.; Mancini, J.; Leichsenring, M.; Gibson, K.M.; Divry, P.; Hrebicek, M.; Lehnert, W.; Sartor, K.; *et al.* Clinical and biochemical phenotype in 11 patients with mevalonic aciduria. *Pediatrics* **1993**, *91*, 915–921.

58. Haas, D.; Hoffmann, G.F. Mevalonate kinase deficiencies: From mevalonic aciduria to hyperimmunoglobulinemia D syndrome. *Orphanet. J. Rare Dis.* **2006**, *1*, 13.

59. Mandey, S.H.; Kuijk, L.M.; Frenkel, J.; Waterham, H.R. A role for geranylgeranylation in interleukin-1β secretion. *Arthritis Rheum.* **2006**, *54*, 3690–3695.

60. Kuijk, L.M.; Mandey, S.H.; Schellens, I.; Waterham, H.R.; Rijkers, G.T.; Coffer, P.J.; Frenkel, J. Statin synergizes with LPS to induce IL-1β release by THP-1 cells through activation of caspase-1. *Mol. Immunol.* **2008**, *45*, 2158–2165.

61. Cailliez, M.; Garaix, F.; Rousset-Rouvière, C.; Bruno, D.; Kone-Paut, I.; Sarles, J.; Chabrol, B.; Tsimaratos, M. Anakinra is safe and effective in controlling hyperimmunoglobulinaemia D syndrome-associated febrile crisis. *J. Inherit. Metab. Dis.* **2006**, *29*, 763.

62. Bodar, E.J.; Kuijk, L.M.; Drenth, J.P.; van der Meer, J.W.; Simon, A.; Frenkel, J. On-demand anakinra treatment is effective in mevalonate kinase deficiency. *Ann. Rheum. Dis.* **2011**, *70*, 2155–2158.

63. Galeotti, C.; Meinzer, U.; Quartier, P.; Rossi-Semerano, L.; Bader-Meunier, B.; Pillet, P.; Koné-Paut, I. Efficacy of interleukin-1-targeting drugs in mevalonate kinase deficiency. *Rheumatology (Oxford)* **2012**, *51*, 1855–1859.

64. Pontillo, A.; Paoluzzi, E.; Crovella, S. The inhibition of mevalonate pathway induces upregulation of NALP3 expression: New insight in the pathogenesis of mevalonate kinase deficiency. *Eur. J. Hum. Genet.* **2010**, *18*, 844–847.

65. Lamkanfi, M.; Dixit, V.M. The inflammasomes. *PLoS Pathog.* **2009**, *5*, e1000510.

66. Martinon, F.; Mayor, A.; Tschopp, J. The inflammasomes: Guardians of the body. *Annu. Rev. Immunol.* **2009**, *27*, 229–265.

67. Deretic, V.; Saitoh, T.; Akira, S. Autophagy in infection, inflammation and immunity. *Nat. Rev. Immunol.* **2013**, *13*, 722–737.

68. Lee, H.K.; Lund, J.M.; Ramanathan, B.; Mizushima, N.; Iwasaki, A. Autophagy-Dependent Viral Recognition by Plasmacytoid Dendritic Cells. *Science* **2007**, *315*, 1398–1401.

69. Paludan, C.; Schmid, D.; Landthaler, M.; Vockerodt, M.; Kube, D.; Tuschl, T.; Münz, C. Endogenous MHC class II processing of a viral nuclear antigen after autophagy. *Science* **2005**, *307*, 593–596.

70. Blanchet, F.P.; Moris, A.; Nikolic, D.S.; Lehmann, M.; Cardinaud, S.; Stalder, R.; Garcia, E.; Dinkins, C.; Leuba, F.; Wu, L.; *et al.* Human immunodeficiency virus-1 inhibition of immunoamphisomes in dendritic cells impairs early innate and adaptive immune responses. *Immunity* **2010**, *32*, 654–669.

71. Nedjic, J.; Aichinger, M.; Emmerich, J.; Mizushima, N.; Klein, L. Autophagy in thymic epithelium shapes the T-cell repertoire and is essential for tolerance. *Nature* **2008**, *455*, 396–400.

72. Harris, J.; Hartman, M.; Roche, C.; Zeng, S.G.; O'Shea, A.; Sharp, F.A.; Lambe, E.M.; Creagh, E.M.; Golenbock, D.T.; Tschopp, J.; *et al.* Autophagy Controls IL-1 Secretion by Targeting Pro-IL-1 for Degradation. *J. Biol. Chem.* **2011**, *286*, 9587–9597.

73. Auron, P.E.; Webb, A.C.; Rosenwasser, L.J.; Mucci, S.F.; Rich, A.; Wolff, S.M.; Dinarello, C.A. Nucleotide sequence of human monocyte interleukin 1 precursor cDNA. *Proc. Natl. Acad. Sci. USA* **1984**, *81*, 7907–7911.

74. Matsushima, K.; Taguchi, M.; Kovacs, E.J.; Young, H.A.; Oppenheim, J.J. Intracellular localization of human monocyte associated interleukin 1 (IL 1) activity and release of biologically active IL 1 from monocytes by trypsin and plasmin. *J. Immunol.* **1986**, *136*, 2883–2891.

75. Shi, C.S.; Shenderov, K.; Huang, N.N.; Kabat, J.; Abu-Asab, M.; Fitzgerald, K.A.; Sher, A.; Kehrl, J.H. Activation of autophagy by inflammatory signals limits IL-1β production by targeting ubiquitinated inflammasomes for destruction. *Nat. Immunol.* **2012**, *13*, 255–263.

76. Andrei, C.; Dazzi, C.; Lotti, L.; Torrisi, M.R.; Chimini, G.; Rubartelli, A. The secretory route of the leaderless protein interleukin 1β involves exocytosis of endolysosome-related vesicles. *Mol. Biol. Cell* **1999**, *10*, 1463–1475.

77. Zhou, R.; Yazdi, A.S.; Menu, P.; Tschopp, J. A role for mitochondria in NLRP3 inflammasome activation. *Nature* **2011**, *469*, 221–225.

78. Shimada, K.; Crother, T.R.; Karlin, J.; Dagvadorj, J.; Chiba, N.; Chen, S.; Ramanujan, V.K.; Wolf, A.J.; Vergnes, L.; *et al.* Oxidized Mitochondrial DNA Activates the NLRP3 Inflammasome during Apoptosis. *Immunity* **2012**, *36*, 401–414.

79. Ding, Z.; Liu, S.; Wang, X.; Khaidakov, M.; Dai, Y.; Mehta, J.L. Oxidant stress in mitochondrial DNA damage, autophagy and inflammation in atherosclerosis. *Sci. Rep.* **2013**, *3*, 1077.

11

Mitochondrial Optic Atrophy (OPA) 1 Processing is Altered in Response to Neonatal Hypoxic-Ischemic Brain Injury

Ana A. Baburamani [1,†], Chloe Hurling [1,†], Helen Stolp [1], Kristina Sobotka [2], Pierre Gressens [1,3,4], Henrik Hagberg [1,2] and Claire Thornton [1,*]

[1] Centre for the Developing Brain, Division of Imaging Sciences and Biomedical Engineering, King's College London, St. Thomas' Hospital, SE1 7EH London, UK;
E-Mails: ana.baburamani@kcl.ac.uk (A.A.B.); chloe.hurling@kcl.ac.uk (C.H.); helen.stolp@kcl.ac.uk (H.S.); pierre.gressens@inserm.fr (P.G.); henrik.hagberg@kcl.ac.uk (H.H.)

[2] Perinatal Center, Institute for Clinical Sciences and Physiology & Neuroscience, Sahlgrenska Academy, University of Gothenburg, 41685 Gothenburg, Sweden;
E-Mail: kristina.sobotka@gu.se

[3] Inserm, U 1141, 75019 Paris, France

[4] University Paris Diderot, Sorbonne Paris Cité, UMRS 1141, 75019 Paris, France

[†] These authors contributed equally to this work.

[*] Author to whom correspondence should be addressed; E-Mail: claire.thornton@kcl.ac.uk

Academic Editors: Jaime M. Ross and Giuseppe Coppotelli

Abstract: Perturbation of mitochondrial function and subsequent induction of cell death pathways are key hallmarks in neonatal hypoxic-ischemic (HI) injury, both in animal models and in term infants. Mitoprotective therapies therefore offer a new avenue for intervention for the babies who suffer life-long disabilities as a result of birth asphyxia. Here we show that after oxygen-glucose deprivation in primary neurons or in a mouse model of HI, mitochondrial protein homeostasis is altered, manifesting as a change in mitochondrial morphology and functional impairment. Furthermore we find that the mitochondrial fusion and cristae regulatory protein, OPA1, is aberrantly cleaved to shorter forms. OPA1 cleavage is normally regulated by a balanced action of the proteases Yme1L and Oma1. However, in primary neurons or after HI *in vivo*, protein expression of Yme1L is also reduced, whereas no change is observed in Oma1 expression. Our data strongly suggest that alterations in mitochondria-shaping proteins are an early event in the pathogenesis of neonatal HI injury.

Keywords: mitochondria; OPA1; Oma1; Yme1L; oxygen-glucose deprivation (OGD); hypoxia-ischaemia; neonatal brain injury

1. Introduction

Moderate to severe hypoxic-ischemic encephalopathy (HIE), caused by a lack of oxygen or blood flow to the brain around the time of birth, affects 1.5 in every 1000 live births in the UK and far more in the developing world [1–3]. The consequences for babies and parents affected by HIE are devastating; 15%–20% of infants will die in the postnatal period and a further 25% will develop severe and long-lasting neurological impairments [4].

In infants and in animal models of hypoxic-ischemic injury (HI) there is an initial depletion of ATP, phosphocreatine and glucose within the brain followed by a transient recovery to almost physiological levels [5]. However, a second, rapid energy failure facilitates the majority of cell death [6–8]. We and others have shown that HI triggers multiple signaling events such as NMDA/AMPA receptor activation, release of reactive oxygen species and increase in intracellular calcium [9–12]. In addition, cell death after neonatal brain injury is characterized morphologically by a mixed necrotic–necroptotic–apoptotic phenotype depending on time post injury and brain region [10,13,14]. However, data from our lab and others strongly suggest that the common thread linking these diverse mechanisms is mitochondrial dysfunction [15,16].

It is well established that in animal models of neonatal HI, mitochondrial respiration and calcium homeostasis are impaired [17–19]. More recently, it was determined that mitochondrial outer membrane permeabilization (MOMP) mediated mitochondrial dysfunction in rodent neonatal HI models [20]. In response to HI, the Bcl-2 family member Bax is activated and translocates to the mitochondria where it complexes and forms a pore with Bak allowing passage of cytochrome c and apoptosis inducing factor (AIF) into the cytosol. Once released AIF and cytochrome c initiate a cascade resulting in activation of caspases, degradation of DNA and ultimately cell death [21]. As such, genetic and pharmacological inhibition of Bax is protective from HI in immature brain [20,22,23]. In addition to Bax-mediated MOMP, mitochondrial ultrastructure is also altered in response to neonatal HI insult [10] and a wide range of mitochondrial morphologies are observed [13]. We therefore hypothesize that such environmental stress may alter mitochondrial dynamics, particularly in the proteins which regulate fission and fusion. Optic Atrophy 1 (OPA1), a dynamin-related guanosine triphosphatase protein, plays a pivotal role in conducting inner-membrane mitochondrial fusion and therefore regulates both mitochondrial cristae junction formation and fusion of distinct mitochondria [24–26]. Here we present data analyzing the effect of *in vitro* oxygen-glucose deprivation (OGD) and *in vivo* HI on the processing of OPA1.

2. Results

2.1. OGD in C17.2 Cells Alters Mitochondrial Function and Morphology

OGD is a widely used *in vitro* technique to mimic aspects of cell death observed in *in vivo* HI injury. We performed OGD on mouse primary cortical neurons and examined mitochondrial morphology and membrane potential in live cells throughout the insult using JC-1 dye. Aggregates of JC-1 accumulate in mitochondria in which the membrane potential is maintained, exhibiting red fluorescence, whereas the appearance of diffuse green JC-1 monomers throughout the cell indicates dissipation of membrane potential. Neurons were preloaded with JC-1 before exposure to OGD. Mitochondria were clearly visible in the processes of control cells and generally of uniform size (Figure 1a,b, Con). However after 90 min OGD, we observed an increase in green monomeric JC-1 suggesting impaired membrane potential and altered morphology with both mitochondrial aggregates and rounded puncta (Figure 1a,b, OGD). Similar findings were observed in a recent study of rat cortical neurons exposed to OGD [27], where control mitochondria were found to be tubular and OGD-exposed mitochondria rounded or poorly labelled. In order to quantify these changes, we performed time-lapse imaging on isolated neurons and calculated the changes in mitochondrial length over time. We found a significant decrease in the average mitochondrial length after 30 min of OGD (Figure 1c). After 90 min OGD we returned the cultures to growth medium and analyzed them at subsequent time points for the effect of the insult on mitochondrial health. We found that 24 h post insult, citrate synthase activity was significantly reduced indicating impaired TCA cycle function (Figure 1d). This suggests that neurons which survive the initial insult may subsequently exhibit impaired mitochondrial function.

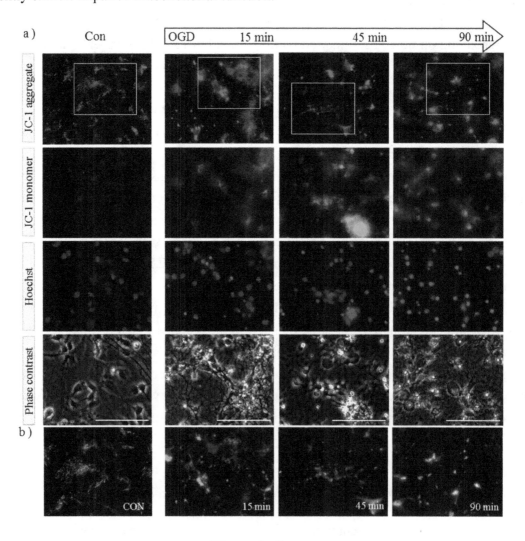

Figure 1. *Cont.*

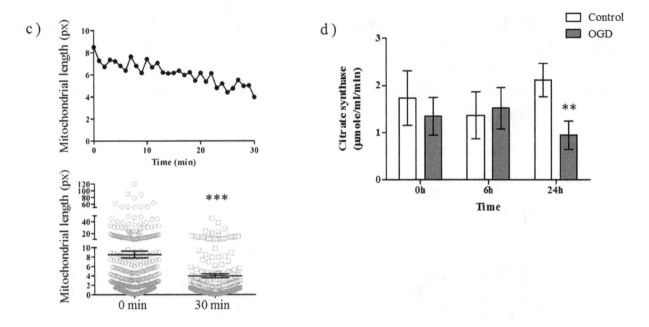

Figure 1. Oxygen-glucose deprivation (OGD) alters mitochondrial membrane potential, morphology and function in primary cortical neurons. (**a**) Primary mouse cortical neurons were loaded with JC-1 dye and Hoechst before exposure to OGD. Cells were imaged live before (Con) and at 15, 45 and 90 min during OGD. Both mitochondrial morphology (as observed in red, top row) and membrane potential (increased green signal, second row) are altered during exposure to OGD. Scale bar represents 100 μm; Figures are representative of three individual experiments: (**b**) Enlargement (3×) of regions defined by white boxes in (**a**). As the experiment progresses, mitochondria morphology appears to alter from tubular structures to round punctate or larger aggregations; (**c**) Primary neurons loaded with JC-1 were imaged every minute during OGD followed by analyses of mitochondrial length. Data shown are an average of 360 mitochondria per time point, and mitochondria from the first and last time points analyzed by student's *t*-test in the panel below, *** $p < 0.001$; (**d**) Primary neurons were subjected to 90 min of OGD followed by up to 24 h incubation in normal growth medium. Lysates were assayed for citrate synthase activity at time points shown following the insult. Data is shown ± SD, $n = 4$–6 independent litters, determined by two-way ANOVA followed by a Bonferroni *post-hoc* test, ** $p < 0.01$ for interaction and treatment.

2.2. OPA1 Processing Is Altered after OGD

As there was a distinct alteration in mitochondrial morphology in response to OGD, we examined the expression of key genes involved in mitochondrial fission and fusion. Primary neurons were either untreated or exposed to OGD and RNA extracted at 0, 6 and 24 h post insult. Expression of fission genes (*Drp-1, Fis-1*) and fusion genes (*Mitofusin 1, Mitofusin 2* and *OPA1*) after OGD were compared with expression in control untreated neurons. We found that there was a small but significant decrease in the expression of *OPA1* mRNA comparing treatment groups (Figure 2a, $a = 0.0296$, two-way ANOVA for treatment). To further analyze changes in OGD-mediated OPA1 expression, we generated whole cell lysates from control and OGD-treated neurons and determined OPA1 protein expression by western blot at 0, 6 and 24 h post insult. There was a small decrease in the expression of OPA1 apparent at the 6 h timepoint (Figure 2b). Interestingly, OGD appeared to induce the generation of a smaller band and alter the distribution of remaining OPA1 immunoreactivity. There was a proportional shift towards expression of smaller OPA1 moieties most pronounced at 6 h after OGD, compared with control OPA1 expression. (Figure 2b, arrowheads).

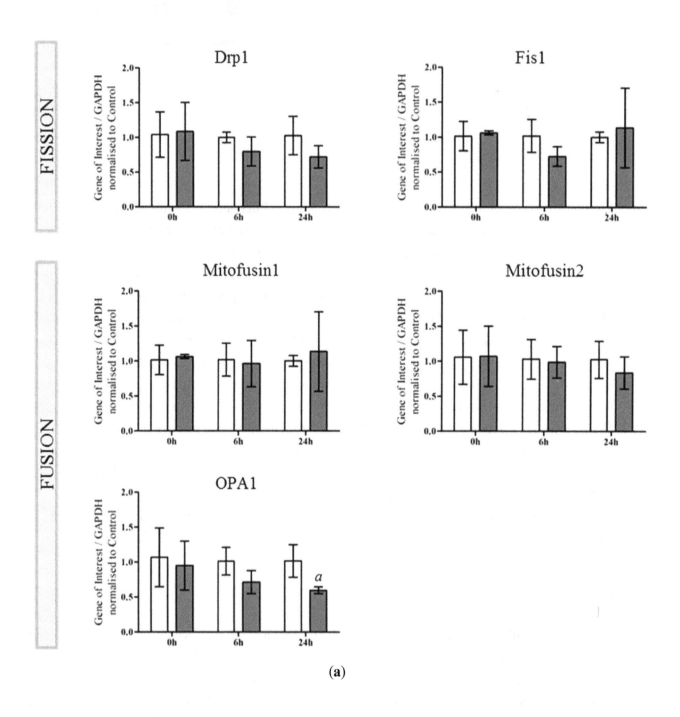

(a)

Figure 2. *Cont.*

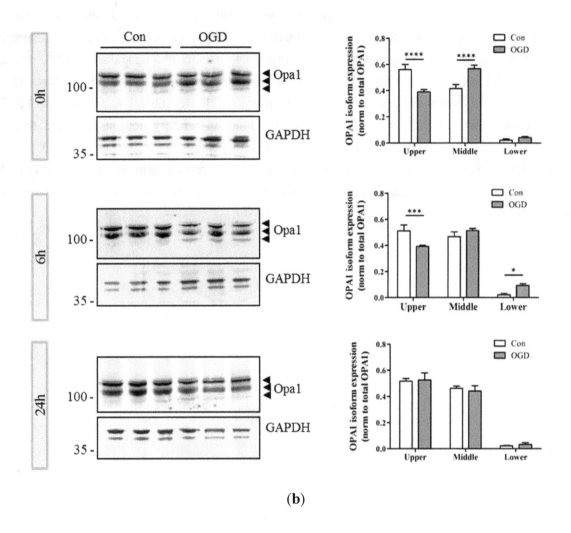

(b)

Figure 2. OPA1 processing is altered after OGD (**a**) mRNA generated from control (white bars) and OGD-treated (grey bars) primary neurons was analyzed by qRT-PCR for changes in expression of fission (*Drp1, Fis1*) and fusion genes (*Mitofusin 1* and *2, OPA1*). There was a small but significant decrease in OPA1 expression in response to OGD exposure ($a = 0.0296$). Mean data shown ± SD ($n = 4$–5 independent litters), significance determined by two way ANOVA; (**b**) Protein lysates were generated from primary neurons either immediately after 90 min OGD (0 h) or following 6 or 24 h recovery. Proteins were resolved by SDS-PAGE and OPA1 analyzed by western blot. Equal protein loading was determined by GAPDH expression. Size distribution of the OPA1 immunoreactivity is expressed as a proportion of total OPA1 (arrowheads). There was a significant increase in the expression of the OPA1 lower band at 0 and 6 h, significance determined by two-way ANOVA for treatment and band. If there was a significant interaction, a Bonferroni *post-hoc* was performed. Data are mean ± SD ($n = 3$ independent litters), * $p < 0.05$, *** $p < 0.001$, **** $p < 0.0001$.

2.3. OGD Reduces Yme1L Protein Expression in Primary Neurons

Alternative splicing of OPA1 generates eight isoforms which depending on variant, will contain S1 and S2 cleavage sites, or an S1 site alone [28]. Previous studies have demonstrated that cleavage at S2 by the intermembrane space AAA-protease Yme1L produces a balance of long and short OPA1 products, optimal for OPA1 function [24,29]. When mitochondrial membrane potential is lost, Oma1, a zinc-metalloprotease which resides on the inner membrane, cleaves OPA1 at the S1 site [30,31]. We therefore examined the expression of Yme1L and Oma1 in primary neurons exposed to OGD. Although gene expression of *Yme1L* was not altered significantly in response to OGD (Yme1L $p = 0.0506$; Figure 3a), there was a discernible decrease in Yme1L protein expression at the end of OGD (Figure 3b). Conversely, no changes were apparent for either the gene (Figure 3c) or protein expression (Figure 3d) of Oma1.

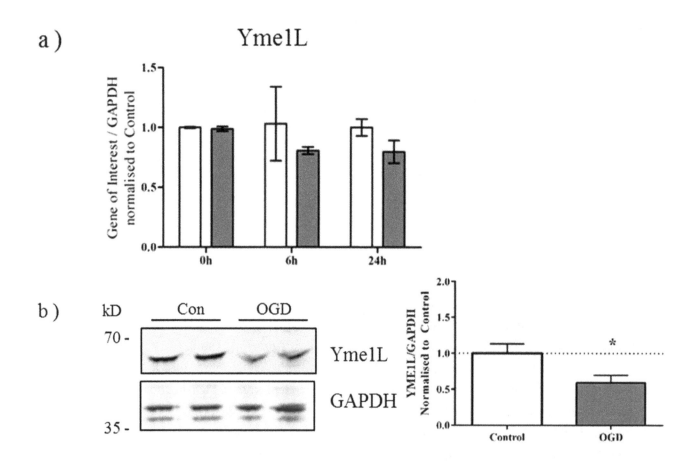

Figure 3. *Cont.*

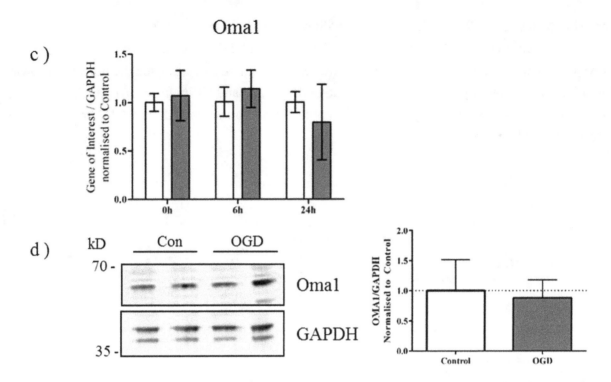

Figure 3. Yme1L protein expression is reduced after OGD (**a**) mRNA generated from control and OGD-treated primary neurons was analyzed by qRT-PCR for changes in expression of Yme1L. Data shown ± SD, *n* = 3–4 independent litters; (**b**) Protein lysates were generated from primary neurons immediately following OGD and analyzed by western blot for expression of Yme1L. Equal protein loading was determined by GAPDH expression which was used for the quantification (right hand panel). Figure is representative of three individual litters, * $p < 0.05$ determined by students *t*-test; (**c**) Oma1 gene expression or (**d**) Oma1 protein expression was determined as above with GAPDH for equal loading. Data was analyzed as above. Figure is representative of three individual litters.

2.4. Alterations in OPA1 Processing Are Apparent in Vivo after HI

Finally we determined if these effects occurred *in vivo* in an animal model of term HI. We used the well-characterized Vannucci HI model in mouse P9 pups, which recapitulates aspects of delayed cell death in human perinatal HI [32,33]. Following unilateral carotid artery ligation, pups are exposed to hypoxia for 75 min before returning to normoxia. This allows both hypoxic (contralateral hemisphere) and hypoxic-ischemic (ipsilateral hemisphere) brain tissue to be sampled from the same animal. Brain tissue was harvested at 0, 24 and 48 h post injury, mitochondrial fractions isolated and OPA1, Yme1L and Oma1 analyzed by western blot (Figure 4a). We found that the bias towards cleaved OPA1 was clearly visible in the hypoxic-ischemic samples from the earliest time point, with a significant decrease of upper band intensity correlating with a significant increase in middle band intensity (Figure 4a, 0 h). Furthermore an additional band of a lower molecular weight was clearly visible in the 24 (Figure 4b) and 48 h (Figure 4c) HI samples. We quantified the upper, middle and lower molecular weight OPA1 bands as a proportion of total OPA1 and observed a significant decrease in the upper band after HI but not hypoxia alone, which was accompanied by a significant increase in the expression of the lower form (Figure 4b). In addition to changes in OPA1, there was a distinct trend towards a decrease in Yme1L expression at 0 (Figure 4a) and 24 h (Figure 4b) which appeared to be resolved by 48 h. Throughout the time course of the experiment, Oma1 expression did not appear to vary (Figure 4a–c). In summary, our data suggest that OGD *in vitro* and HI injury *in vivo* result in cleavage of OPA1 to lower molecular weight forms. This observation correlates with an OGD- or HI-mediated decrease in Yme1L expression.

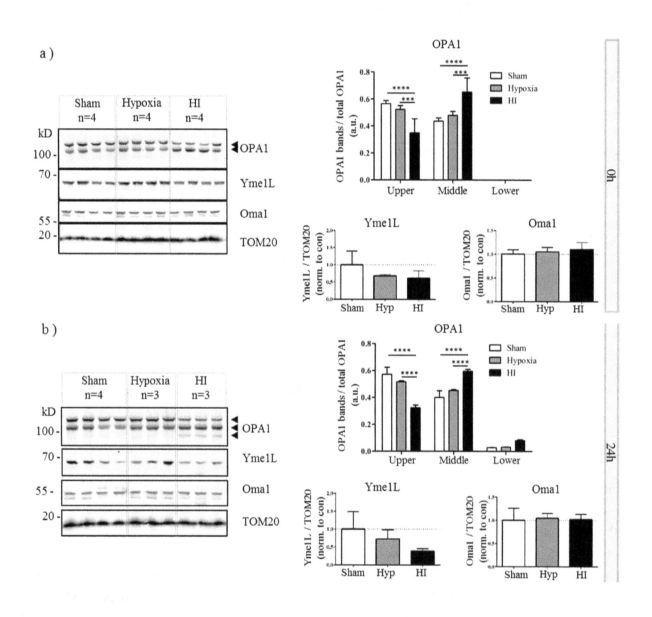

Figure 4. *Cont.*

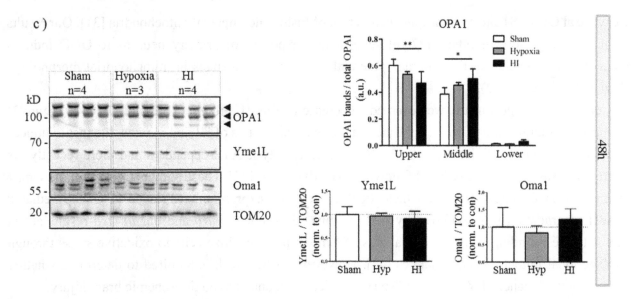

Figure 4. Aberrant processing of OPA1 *in vivo*. Mitochondrial fractions were generated from hypoxic-ischemic (HI), hypoxia alone or sham control mice. Proteins were resolved by SDS-PAGE and analyzed by western blot for OPA1, Yme1L and Oma1 at 0 (**a**), 24 (**b**) and 48 h (**c**) following HI. Tom20 was used as a loading control for mitochondria (bottom panel). Total OPA1 expression was determined by densitometry and OPA1 isoforms or cleavage products expressed as a proportion of that total. Arrowheads indicate alternate forms of OPA1. Mean data shown ± SD. OPA1 significance was determined by two-way ANOVA for band size and treatment followed by a Bonferroni *post-hoc* test * $p < 0.05$, ** $p < 0.01$, *** $p < 0.001$, **** $p < 0.0001$. YME1L and Oma1 data were analyzed with a one-way ANOVA.

3. Discussion

Dysregulation of energy metabolism is a common feature in a number of human diseases including diabetes, cardiovascular and neurodegenerative disorders [34–36]. It is therefore unsurprising the mitochondria are center stage in the development of neonatal brain injury, due to additional high energy demands of the immature brain as it develops [15], and protecting mitochondrial function represents a valid target for future therapeutic intervention. Here we present data suggesting that the homeostasis of inner mitochondrial membrane proteins is disrupted in response to OGD *in vitro* and HI *in vivo* and that alterations in protein function are due largely to post-translational modification.

Although we only identified small changes in OPA1 gene expression, our major finding is that OPA1 is rapidly cleaved to shorter forms in response to hypoxia-ischemia. Shortened forms of OPA1 are reported to occur as a result of environmental stress, resulting in fragmented mitochondria [37,38]. Furthermore, actively altering the balance of long (L-OPA1) and short (S-OPA1) forms may favor mitochondrial fission [39], agreeing with the appearance of small punctate mitochondria apparent during the OGD insult in primary neurons (Figure 1).

OPA1 cleavage occurs due to the actions of the ATP-dependent protease Yme1L and the ATP-independent protease Oma1 [30,31]. Yme1L cleaves OPA1 at the S2 site and subsequent products remain fusion-competent [24,29]. However, loss of mitochondrial membrane potential results in cleavage at OPA1 S1 site by Oma1 and generation of fusion-incompetent mitochondria [31]. Our results (Figure 1) and those of others [27,40] suggest that exposure of primary neurons to OGD induces a decrease in mitochondrial membrane potential coupled with changes in mitochondrial morphology (Figure 1, Con *vs*. OGD).

Concomitantly, post insult, we observed a decrease in Yme1L protein expression *in vitro* (Figure 3) and *in vivo* (Figure 4). It is well established that in animal models of HI and *in vitro*, the insult induces a rapid depletion of cellular ATP [8,33,41]. Yme1L activity is ATP-dependent and more recently, its expression was found to be reduced following oxidative stress [42]. These authors also identified Oma1 as an ATP-independent protease which regulated Yme1L expression; resistance to Oma1-mediated Yme1L degradation was conferred by ATP binding. Both our *in vitro* and our *in vivo* results are in line with these findings suggesting that loss of Yme1L may sensitize cells to oxidative stress through dysfunctional mitochondrial dynamics [43]. However, further work is required to determine whether disrupting the balance of Yme1L and Oma1 is critical in neonatal hypoxic-ischemic brain injury.

In the development of neonatal brain injury in response to HI insult, we and others have documented the induction of apoptosis resulting in cytochrome c release from permeabilized mitochondria [13,44–46]. However, the majority of cytochrome c is held within the cristae, relying on cristae reconfiguration to allow it access to move into the intermembrane space once apoptosis is induced. In addition to its role in fusion, OPA1 controls the integrity of the cristae [25] and inhibition of OPA1 leads to cristae disorganization [26]. Our data suggest the possibility that OPA1 processing may be an early but key step in the propagation of neuronal cell death induced by neonatal hypoxic-ischemic injury. Interestingly, during revision of our manuscript, Sanderson and colleagues identified release of cytochrome c and appearance of degraded OPA1 in the cytosol in response to OGD/reperfusion in primary neurons [47] providing further evidence for our hypothesis. Our future studies will therefore center on the roles of Yme1L and Oma1 in the regulation of OPA1 in order to highlight whether prevention of such cleavage is neuroprotective in neonatal hypoxic-ischemic injury.

4. Experimental Section

4.1. Research Ethics Statement

All animal use was in accordance with local rules (King's College London, Animal Welfare and Ethical Review Board, London, UK) and with the regulations and guidance issued under the Animals (Scientific Procedures) Act (1986) covered by Home Office personal and project licenses.

4.2. Primary Cortical Neuron Preparation

C57/Bl6 pregnant mice (Charles Rivers, Margate, UK) at embryonic day 13.5–15.5 were killed by schedule 1 methods. Embryonic cerebral cortices were dissected and tissue from the same litter pooled. Primary cortical neurons were prepared as described previously [48], plated at a density of 2×10^6 cells/6 cm plate and maintained in neurobasal medium (Life Technologies, Paisley, UK) containing B27® (Life Technologies), L-Glutamine (Sigma, Gillingham, UK) and Streptomycin/ AmphotericinB (Life Technologies,). Cultures were maintained at 37 °C, 5% CO_2.

4.3. Neonatal Hypoxia-Ischemia

C57/Bl6 mice (Charles River) at postnatal day 9 (P9) were subjected to unilateral hypoxia-ischemia, essentially according to the Rice–Vannucci model that results in a focal ischemic injury allowing for comparison between an HI (ipsilateral) and hypoxia alone (contralateral) hemisphere [32,33]. Briefly, mice were anesthetized with isoflurane (4.5% for induction and 2% for maintenance) in a mixture of nitrous oxide and oxygen (1:1), with the duration of anesthesia being <5 min per pup. The left common carotid artery was isolated and ligated. Pups recovered for 1–2 h in the parent cage. Litters were placed in a chamber with a humidified hypoxic gas mixture (10% oxygen in nitrogen, 36 °C) for 75 min. Sham control mice were not subjected to surgery or hypoxic chamber. After hypoxic exposure, pups were returned to their biological dams until the conclusion of the experiment. Both females and males pups were used and treatment groups contained pups from at least 3 independent litters.

4.4. Oxygen-Glucose Deprivation (OGD) of Primary Neurons

Primary neurons were cultured for a minimum of 6 days (DIV6) prior to treatment then loaded with JC-1 (5 µM; Life Technologies) and Hoechst (10 µg/mL; Sigma) for 30 min, 37 °C, 5% CO_2. Growth medium was replaced with de-gassed, glucose-free, Neurobasal-A medium (Life Technologies) and culture plates mounted on the EVOS/Chamlide microscope (Life Technologies) where they were maintained at 37 °C in a 95% N_2/5% CO_2 environment for the duration of the OGD. Following OGD, medium was replaced with standard Neurobasal medium (containing additions described above) and cultures returned to 5% CO_2 incubation. For control plates, medium was replaced with standard Neurobasal media at the start of the OGD plates and replaced again with media after 90 min. Cells were collected at 0, 6 or 24 h following treatment.

4.5. MTT Assay

Primary cortical neurons were assayed for mitochondrial reductase activity using the MTT (3-(4,5-Dimethylthiazol-2-yl-)-2,5-diphenyl-2H-tetrazolium bromide; Sigma) assay as described previously [49].

4.6. Citrate Synthase Assay

Primary neurons were lysed in CelLytic MT Cell Lysis Reagent (Sigma), protein concentration determined by BCA assay (Thermo Scientific, Loughborough, UK) and were assayed for enzymatic activity using Citrate Synthase Assay Kit (Sigma) according to manufacturer's instructions. Eight micrograms of total protein was used per reaction on a 96-well plate and independent samples were measured in duplicate. Absorbance was read at 412 nm on a SPECTROstar Nano plate reader using MARS analysis software (BMG Labtech, Aylesbury, UK). Baseline absorbance was measured every 30 s for 5 min, and following addition of oxaloacetic acid, total activity was measured every 10 min for 60 min.

4.7. qRT-PCR

RNA was harvested using the Direct-zol RNA MiniPrep kit (Zymo Research, through Cambridge Biosciences, Cambridge UK) as per manufacturer's instructions. Total RNA (100 ng) was analysed using Taqman gene expression assays and RNA-to-CT kit (Life Technologies) on a StepOneplus Cycler (Life Technologies). Data were normalized to the expression of GAPDH and to controls for each time point using the $2^{-\Delta\Delta Ct}$ method [50]. The following primer pairs were used: *GAPDH* (Mm99999915), *DRP1* (Dmn1; Mm01342903), *Fis1* (Mm00481580), *Mitofusin1* (Mm00612599), *Mitofusin2* (Mm00500120), *OPA1* (Mm01349707), *Oma1* (Mm01260328) and *Yme1L* (Mm00496843) from Life Technologies.

4.8. Subcellular Fractionation

For preparation of mitochondrial fractions, mice were sacrificed at 0, 24 and 48 h post HI and brains rapidly dissected into ice-cold subcellular fractionation buffer (250 mM sucrose, 20 mM HEPES pH 7.4, 10 mM KCL, 1.5 mM MgCl$_2$, 1 mM EDTA, 1 mM EGTA, 1 mM DTT, 1× protease inhibitor cocktail). Samples were homogenized in a 2 mL dounce homogenizer on ice, passed through a 27 G needle and incubated on ice for 20 min. The suspension was centrifuged (720× *g*, 5 min) to remove the nuclear fraction and any unbroken cells. The resulting supernatant was centrifuged (15,000× *g*, 15 min) to obtain a mitochondrial pellet and a cytosolic supernatant.

4.9. Western Blot

For protein analysis primary neurons were lysed in HEPES buffer A (50 mM HEPES (pH 7.5), 50 mM sodium fluoride, 5 mM sodium pyrophosphate, 1 mM EDTA, +1× protease inhibitors (Sigma)) containing 1% (*v/v*) Triton X-100 (Sigma). Protein from cell lysates (50 μg) and mitochondrial fractions from brain lysates (30 μg) were resolved on 4%–12% gel (*w/v*) NuPAGE BisTris gels in MOPs buffer (ThermoFisher Scientific, Hemel Hempstead, UK) and transferred to polyvinylidene fluoride membrane (PVDF, Millipore, Beeston, UK) in NuPAGE transfer buffer (Life Technologies). Membranes were blocked in 5% skim-milk in Tris-buffered saline with 0.1% Tween 20 (TBS-T) and incubated overnight with the following antibodies: anti-mouse OPA1 (1:1000, Cat# 612606, BD Biosciences, Oxford, UK), anti-rabbit YME1 (1:1000, Cat# 11510-1-AP, ProteinTech, Manchester, UK), anti-rabbit OMA1 (for primary neurons; 1:1000, Cat# NBP1-56970, Novusbio, UK and for mitochondrial fractions from brain lysates; 1:750, Cat# 17116-1-AP, ProteinTech), anti-mouse GAPDH (1:2000, Cat# G8795 Sigma) and for mitochondrial fractions Tom20 (1:750, Cat# sc-11415, Santa Cruz Biotechnology, Wembley, UK). Secondary antibodies: Li-cor IRDye Goat anti-rabbit 800 or Goat anti-mouse 680 secondary antibodies were used at 1:10,000 and incubated for 2 h at room temperature. Membranes were imaged on a Li-Cor Odyssey Infrared Imaging System (Li-Cor Imaging Biotechnology UK Ltd., Cambridge, UK) using the manufacturer's Image Studio software for band quantification.

4.10. Data Analysis

Data are expressed as mean ± SD. All primary neuronal culture experiments were performed on 3–6 independent litters as stated in the figure legends. Mitochondrial length was analyzed using Squassh (segmentation and quantification of subcellular shapes) software, part of the Mosaic toolkit in Image J [51]. All statistical analyses were performed using GraphPad Prism 6 Software (GraphPad Software, San Diego, CA, USA). All data were assessed for normality. Data was assessed either by a Student's t-test or for multiple conditions, with a two-way ANOVA. If significant, a Bonferroni *post-hoc* analysis was conducted. Analyses used are detailed in table and figure captions. * $p < 0.05$, ** $p < 0.01$, *** $p < 0.001$, **** $p < 0.0001$.

5. Conclusions

We have determined that in primary neurons, mitochondrial membrane potential, morphology and function are impaired in response to OGD. Furthermore, we present the first data suggesting that in a mouse model of neonatal HI, the expression of mitochondrial shaping proteins, such as OPA1 and Yme1L, are altered; *in vitro* and *in vivo*, OPA1 is cleaved to shorter forms and Yme1L expression is reduced. Further studies are required to determine the molecular pathways regulating these events.

Acknowledgments

We gratefully acknowledge the support of the Department of Perinatal Imaging and Health and financial support from Wellcome Trust (WT094823), the Medical Research Council, Action Medical Research, Swedish Medical Research Council (VR 2012-3500), Brain Foundation (HH), Ahlen Foundation (HH), ALF-GBG (426401), ERA-net (EU;VR 529-2014-7551) and the Leducq Foundation (DSRRP34404) to enable this study to be completed. CH was supported by the King's Bioscience Institute and the Guy's and St Thomas' Charity Prize PhD Programme in Biomedical and Translational Science. In addition, the authors acknowledge financial support from the Department of Health via the National Institute for Health Research (NIHR) comprehensive Biomedical Research Centre Award to Guy's & St Thomas' NHS Foundation Trust in partnership with King's College London and King's College Hospital NHS Foundation Trust.

Author Contributions

Claire Thornton conceived and designed the experiments; Ana A. Baburamani, Chloe Hurling and Claire Thornton performed the experiments; Ana A. Baburamani, Chloe Hurling, Helen Stolp, Kristina Sobotka, Pierre Gressens and Henrik Hagberg analyzed the data; Helen Stolp contributed reagents/materials/analysis tools; Ana A. Baburamani, Chloe Hurling, Helen Stolp, Kristina Sobotka, Pierre Gressens and Henrik Hagbergcontributed to the preparation of the manuscript.

References

1. Evans, K.; Rigby, A.S.; Hamilton, P.; Titchiner, N.; Hall, D.M. The relationships between neonatal encephalopathy and cerebral palsy: A cohort study. *J. Obstet. Gynaecol.* **2001**, *21*, 114–120.

2. Smith, J.; Wells, L.; Dodd, K. The continuing fall in incidence of hypoxic-ischaemic encephalopathy in term infants. *BJOG* **2000**, *107*, 461–466.

3. Lawn, J.E.; Bahl, R.; Bergstrom, S.; Bhutta, Z.A.; Darmstadt, G.L.; Ellis, M.; English, M.; Kurinczuk, J.J.; Lee, A.C.; Merialdi, M.; *et al.* Setting research priorities to reduce almost one million deaths from birth asphyxia by 2015. *PLoS Med.* **2011**, *8*, e1000389.

4. Vannucci, R.C.; Perlman, J.M. Interventions for perinatal hypoxic-ischemic encephalopathy. *Pediatrics* **1997**, *100*, 1004–1014.

5. Azzopardi, D.; Wyatt, J.S.; Cady, E.B.; Delpy, D.T.; Baudin, J.; Stewart, A.L.; Hope, P.L.; Hamilton, P.A.; Reynolds, E.O. Prognosis of newborn infants with hypoxic-ischemic brain injury assessed by phosphorus magnetic resonance spectroscopy. *Pediatr. Res.* **1989**, *25*, 445–451.

6. Blumberg, R.M.; Cady, E.B.; Wigglesworth, J.S.; McKenzie, J.E.; Edwards, A.D. Relation between delayed impairment of cerebral energy metabolism and infarction following transient focal hypoxia-ischaemia in the developing brain. *Exp. Brain Res.* **1997**, *113*, 130–137.

7. Gilland, E.; Bona, E.; Hagberg, H. Temporal changes of regional glucose use, blood flow, and microtubule-associated protein 2 immunostaining after hypoxia-ischemia in the immature rat brain. *J. Cereb. Blood Flow Metab.* **1998**, *18*, 222–228.

8. Lorek, A.; Takei, Y.; Cady, E.B.; Wyatt, J.S.; Penrice, J.; Edwards, A.D.; Peebles, D.; Wylezinska, M.; Owen-Reece, H.; Kirkbride, V.; *et al.* Delayed ("secondary") cerebral energy failure after acute hypoxia-ischemia in the newborn piglet: Continuous 48-hour studies by phosphorus magnetic resonance spectroscopy. *Pediatr. Res.* **1994**, *36*, 699–706.

9. Hagberg, H.; Thornberg, E.; Blennow, M.; Kjellmer, I.; Lagercrantz, H.; Thiringer, K.; Hamberger, A.; Sandberg, M. Excitatory amino acids in the cerebrospinal fluid of asphyxiated infants: Relationship to hypoxic-ischemic encephalopathy. *Acta Paediatr.* **1993**, *82*, 925–929.

10. Puka-Sundvall, M.; Gajkowska, B.; Cholewinski, M.; Blomgren, K.; Lazarewicz, J.W.; Hagberg, H. Subcellular distribution of calcium and ultrastructural changes after cerebral hypoxia-ischemia in immature rats. *Brain Res. Dev. Brain Res.* **2000**, *125*, 31–41.

11. Van den Tweel, E.R.; Nijboer, C.; Kavelaars, A.; Heijnen, C.J.; Groenendaal, F.; van Bel, F. Expression of nitric oxide synthase isoforms and nitrotyrosine formation after hypoxia-ischemia in the neonatal rat brain. *J. Neuroimmunol.* **2005**, *167*, 64–71.

12. Wallin, C.; Puka-Sundvall, M.; Hagberg, H.; Weber, S.G.; Sandberg, M. Alterations in glutathione and amino acid concentrations after hypoxia-ischemia in the immature rat brain. *Brain Res. Dev. Brain Res.* **2000**, *125*, 51–60.

13. Northington, F.J.; Zelaya, M.E.; O'Riordan, D.P.; Blomgren, K.; Flock, D.L.; Hagberg, H.; Ferriero, D.M.; Martin, L.J. Failure to complete apoptosis following neonatal hypoxia-ischemia manifests as "continuum" phenotype of cell death and occurs with multiple manifestations of mitochondrial dysfunction in rodent forebrain. *Neuroscience* **2007**, *149*, 822–833.

14. Portera-Cailliau, C.; Price, D.L.; Martin, L.J. Excitotoxic neuronal death in the immature brain is an apoptosis-necrosis morphological continuum. *J. Comp. Neurol.* **1997**, *378*, 70–87.

15. Hagberg, H.; Mallard, C.; Rousset, C.I.; Thornton, C. Mitochondria: Hub of injury responses in the developing brain. *Lancet Neurol.* **2014**, *13*, 217–232.

16. Thornton, C.; Rousset, C.I.; Kichev, A.; Miyakuni, Y.; Vontell, R.; Baburamani, A.A.; Fleiss, B.; Gressens, P.; Hagberg, H. Molecular mechanisms of neonatal brain injury. *Neurol. Res. Int.* **2012**, *2012*, doi:10.1155/2012/506320.

17. Gilland, E.; Puka-Sundvall, M.; Hillered, L.; Hagberg, H. Mitochondrial function and energy metabolism after hypoxia-ischemia in the immature rat brain: Involvement of NMDA-receptors. *J. Cereb. Blood Flow Metab.* **1998**, *18*, 297–304.

18. Puka-Sundvall, M.; Wallin, C.; Gilland, E.; Hallin, U.; Wang, X.; Sandberg, M.; Karlsson, J.; Blomgren, K.; Hagberg, H. Impairment of mitochondrial respiration after cerebral hypoxia-ischemia in immature rats: Relationship to activation of caspase-3 and neuronal injury. *Brain Res. Dev. Brain Res.* **2000**, *125*, 43–50.

19. Rosenberg, A.A.; Parks, J.K.; Murdaugh, E.; Parker, W.D., Jr. Mitochondrial function after asphyxia in newborn lambs. *Stroke* **1989**, *20*, 674–679.

20. Wang, X.; Carlsson, Y.; Basso, E.; Zhu, C.; Rousset, C.I.; Rasola, A.; Johansson, B.R.; Blomgren, K.; Mallard, C.; Bernardi, P.; *et al.* Developmental shift of cyclophilin D contribution to hypoxic-ischemic brain injury. *J. Neurosci.* **2009**, *29*, 2588–2596.

21. Zhu, C.; Wang, X.; Huang, Z.; Qiu, L.; Xu, F.; Vahsen, N.; Nilsson, M.; Eriksson, P.S.; Hagberg, H.; Culmsee, C.; *et al.* Apoptosis-inducing factor is a major contributor to neuronal loss induced by neonatal cerebral hypoxia-ischemia. *Cell Death Differ.* **2007**, *14*, 775–784.

22. Gibson, M.E.; Han, B.H.; Choi, J.; Knudson, C.M.; Korsmeyer, S.J.; Parsadanian, M.; Holtzman, D.M. BAX contributes to apoptotic-like death following neonatal hypoxia-ischemia: Evidence for distinct apoptosis pathways. *Mol. Med.* **2001**, *7*, 644–655.

23. Wang, X.; Han, W.; Du, X.; Zhu, C.; Carlsson, Y.; Mallard, C.; Jacotot, E.; Hagberg, H. Neuroprotective effect of Bax-inhibiting peptide on neonatal brain injury. *Stroke* **2010**, *41*, 2050–2055.

24. Song, Z.; Chen, H.; Fiket, M.; Alexander, C.; Chan, D.C. OPA1 processing controls mitochondrial fusion and is regulated by mRNA splicing, membrane potential, and Yme1L. *J. Cell Biol.* **2007**, *178*, 749–755.

25. Frezza, C.; Cipolat, S.; Martins de Brito, O.; Micaroni, M.; Beznoussenko, G.V.; Rudka, T.; Bartoli, D.; Polishuck, R.S.; Danial, N.N.; De Strooper, B.; *et al.* OPA1 controls apoptotic cristae remodeling independently from mitochondrial fusion. *Cell* **2006**, *126*, 177–189.

26. Olichon, A.; Baricault, L.; Gas, N.; Guillou, E.; Valette, A.; Belenguer, P.; Lenaers, G. Loss of OPA1 perturbates the mitochondrial inner membrane structure and integrity, leading to cytochrome c release and apoptosis. *J. Biol. Chem.* **2003**, *278*, 7743–7746.

27. Wappler, E.A.; Institoris, A.; Dutta, S.; Katakam, P.V.; Busija, D.W. Mitochondrial dynamics associated with oxygen-glucose deprivation in rat primary neuronal cultures. *PLoS ONE* **2013**, *8*, e63206.

28. Delettre, C.; Griffoin, J.M.; Kaplan, J.; Dollfus, H.; Lorenz, B.; Faivre, L.; Lenaers, G.; Belenguer, P.; Hamel, C.P. Mutation spectrum and splicing variants in the *OPA1* gene. *Hum. Genet.* **2001**, *109*, 584–591.

29. Griparic, L.; Kanazawa, T.; van der Bliek, A.M. Regulation of the mitochondrial dynamin-like protein Opa1 by proteolytic cleavage. *J. Cell Biol.* **2007**, *178*, 757–764.

30. Ehses, S.; Raschke, I.; Mancuso, G.; Bernacchia, A.; Geimer, S.; Tondera, D.; Martinou, J.C.; Westermann, B.; Rugarli, E.I.; Langer, T. Regulation of OPA1 processing and mitochondrial fusion by m-AAA protease isoenzymes and OMA1. *J. Cell Biol.* **2009**, *187*, 1023–1036.

31. Head, B.; Griparic, L.; Amiri, M.; Gandre-Babbe, S.; van der Bliek, A.M. Inducible proteolytic inactivation of OPA1 mediated by the OMA1 protease in mammalian cells. *J. Cell Biol.* **2009**, *187*, 959–966.

32. Rice, J.E., 3rd; Vannucci, R.C.; Brierley, J.B. The influence of immaturity on hypoxic-ischemic brain damage in the rat. *Ann. Neurol.* **1981**, *9*, 131–141.

33. Vannucci, R.C.; Vannucci, S.J. A model of perinatal hypoxic-ischemic brain damage. *Ann. N. Y. Acad. Sci.* **1997**, *835*, 234–249.

34. Biala, A.K.; Dhingra, R.; Kirshenbaum, L.A. Mitochondrial dynamics: Orchestrating the journey to advanced age. *J. Mol. Cell. Cardiol.* **2015**, *83*, 37–43.

35. Lin, M.T.; Beal, M.F. Mitochondrial dysfunction and oxidative stress in neurodegenerative diseases. *Nature* **2006**, *443*, 787–795.

36. Supale, S.; Li, N.; Brun, T.; Maechler, P. Mitochondrial dysfunction in pancreatic β cells. *Trends Endocrinol. Metab.* **2012**, *23*, 477–487.

37. Duvezin-Caubet, S.; Jagasia, R.; Wagener, J.; Hofmann, S.; Trifunovic, A.; Hansson, A.; Chomyn, A.; Bauer, M.F.; Attardi, G.; Larsson, N.G.; *et al.* Proteolytic processing of OPA1 links mitochondrial dysfunction to alterations in mitochondrial morphology. *J. Biol. Chem.* **2006**, *281*, 37972–37979.

38. Ishihara, N.; Fujita, Y.; Oka, T.; Mihara, K. Regulation of mitochondrial morphology through proteolytic cleavage of OPA1. *EMBO J.* **2006**, *25*, 2966–2977.

39. Anand, R.; Wai, T.; Baker, M.J.; Kladt, N.; Schauss, A.C.; Rugarli, E.; Langer, T. The i-AAA protease YME1L and OMA1 cleave OPA1 to balance mitochondrial fusion and fission. *J. Cell Biol.* **2014**, *204*, 919–929.

40. Iijima, T. Mitochondrial membrane potential and ischemic neuronal death. *Neurosci. Res.* **2006**, *55*, 234–243.

41. Azzopardi, D.; Wyatt, J.S.; Hamilton, P.A.; Cady, E.B.; Delpy, D.T.; Hope, P.L.; Reynolds, E.O. Phosphorus metabolites and intracellular pH in the brains of normal and small for gestational age infants investigated by magnetic resonance spectroscopy. *Pediatr. Res.* **1989**, *25*, 440–444.

42. Rainbolt, T.K.; Saunders, J.M.; Wiseman, R.L. YME1L degradation reduces mitochondrial proteolytic capacity during oxidative stress. *EMBO Rep.* **2015**, *16*, 97–106.

43. Stiburek, L.; Cesnekova, J.; Kostkova, O.; Fornuskova, D.; Vinsova, K.; Wenchich, L.; Houstek, J.; Zeman, J. YME1L controls the accumulation of respiratory chain subunits and is required for apoptotic resistance, cristae morphogenesis, and cell proliferation. *Mol. Biol. Cell* **2012**, *23*, 1010–1023.

44. Nijboer, C.H.; Heijnen, C.J.; van der Kooij, M.A.; Zijlstra, J.; van Velthoven, C.T.; Culmsee, C.; van Bel, F.; Hagberg, H.; Kavelaars, A. Targeting the p53 pathway to protect the neonatal ischemic brain. *Ann. Neurol.* **2011**, *70*, 255–264.

45. Zhu, C.; Qiu, L.; Wang, X.; Hallin, U.; Cande, C.; Kroemer, G.; Hagberg, H.; Blomgren, K. Involvement of apoptosis-inducing factor in neuronal death after hypoxia-ischemia in the neonatal rat brain. *J. Neurochem.* **2003**, *86*, 306–317.

46. Zhu, C.; Xu, F.; Fukuda, A.; Wang, X.; Fukuda, H.; Korhonen, L.; Hagberg, H.; Lannering, B.; Nilsson, M.; Eriksson, P.S.; *et al.* X chromosome-linked inhibitor of apoptosis protein reduces oxidative stress after cerebral irradiation or hypoxia-ischemia through up-regulation of mitochondrial antioxidants. *Eur. J. Neurosci.* **2007**, *26*, 3402–3410.

47. Sanderson, T.H.; Raghunayakula, S.; Kumar, R. Neuronal hypoxia disrupts mitochondrial fusion. *Neuroscience* **2015**, *301*, 71–78.

48. Thornton, C.; Bright, N.J.; Sastre, M.; Muckett, P.J.; Carling, D. AMP-activated protein kinase (AMPK) is a tau kinase, activated in response to amyloid beta-peptide exposure. *Biochem. J.* **2011**, *434*, 503–512.

49. Fleiss, B.; Chhor, V.; Rajudin, N.; Lebon, S.; Hagberg, H.; Gressens, P.; Thornton, C. The anti-inflammatory effects of the small molecule Pifithrin-μ on BV2 microglia. *Dev. Neurosci.* **2015**, *37*, 363–375.

50. Livak, K.J.; Schmittgen, T.D. Analysis of relative gene expression data using real-time quantitative PCR and the $2^{-\Delta\Delta Ct}$ method. *Methods* **2001**, *25*, 402–408.

51. Rizk, A.; Paul, G.; Incardona, P.; Bugarski, M.; Mansouri, M.; Niemann, A.; Ziegler, U.; Berger, P.; Sbalzarini, I.F. Segmentation and quantification of subcellular structures in fluorescence microscopy images using Squassh. *Nat. Protoc.* **2014**, *9*, 586–596.

Permissions

All chapters in this book were first published by MDPI; hereby published with permission under the Creative Commons Attribution License or equivalent. Every chapter published in this book has been scrutinized by our experts. Their significance has been extensively debated. The topics covered herein carry significant findings which will fuel the growth of the discipline. They may even be implemented as practical applications or may be referred to as a beginning point for another development.

The contributors of this book come from diverse backgrounds, making this book a truly international effort. This book will bring forth new frontiers with its revolutionizing research information and detailed analysis of the nascent developments around the world.

We would like to thank all the contributing authors for lending their expertise to make the book truly unique. They have played a crucial role in the development of this book. Without their invaluable contributions this book wouldn't have been possible. They have made vital efforts to compile up to date information on the varied aspects of this subject to make this book a valuable addition to the collection of many professionals and students.

This book was conceptualized with the vision of imparting up-to-date information and advanced data in this field. To ensure the same, a matchless editorial board was set up. Every individual on the board went through rigorous rounds of assessment to prove their worth. After which they invested a large part of their time researching and compiling the most relevant data for our readers.

The editorial board has been involved in producing this book since its inception. They have spent rigorous hours researching and exploring the diverse topics which have resulted in the successful publishing of this book. They have passed on their knowledge of decades through this book. To expedite this challenging task, the publisher supported the team at every step. A small team of assistant editors was also appointed to further simplify the editing procedure and attain best results for the readers.

Apart from the editorial board, the designing team has also invested a significant amount of their time in understanding the subject and creating the most relevant covers. They scrutinized every image to scout for the most suitable representation of the subject and create an appropriate cover for the book.

The publishing team has been an ardent support to the editorial, designing and production team. Their endless efforts to recruit the best for this project, has resulted in the accomplishment of this book. They are a veteran in the field of academics and their pool of knowledge is as vast as their experience in printing. Their expertise and guidance has proved useful at every step. Their uncompromising quality standards have made this book an exceptional effort. Their encouragement from time to time has been an inspiration for everyone.

The publisher and the editorial board hope that this book will prove to be a valuable piece of knowledge for researchers, students, practitioners and scholars across the globe.

List of Contributors

Heng Du
Department of Surgery, Physicians & Surgeons College of Columbia University, New York, NY 10032, USA

Shirley ShiDu Yan
Department of Surgery, Physicians & Surgeons College of Columbia University, New York, NY 10032, USA
Department of Pathology & Cell Biology, Physicians & Surgeons College of Columbia University, New York, NY 10032, USA
The Taub institute for Research on Alzheimer's Disease and the Aging Brain, Columbia University, New York, NY 10032, USA

Zhicheng Wang, Jie Wang, Ruilai Liu and Yuan Lu
Department of Laboratory Medicine, Huashan Hospital, Shanghai Medical College, Fudan University, Shanghai 200040, China

Rufeng Xie
Blood Engineering Laboratory, Shanghai Blood Center, Shanghai 200051, China

Jaime M. Ross, Lars Olson and Giuseppe Coppotelli
Department of Neuroscience, Karolinska Institutet, Retzius väg 8, Stockholm 171 77, Sweden

Seok-Jo Kim, Paul Cheresh, Renea P. Jablonski, David B. Williams and David W. Kamp
Department of Medicine, Division of Pulmonary and Critical Care Medicine Jesse Brown VA Medical Center, Chicago, IL 60612, USA
Division of Pulmonary & Critical Care Medicine, Northwestern University Feinberg School of Medicine, Chicago, IL 60611, USA

Yuliya Mikhed and Andreas Daiber
2nd Medical Clinic, Medical Center of the Johannes Gutenberg-University, Mainz 55131, Germany

Sebastian Steven
2nd Medical Clinic, Medical Center of the Johannes Gutenberg-University, Mainz 55131, Germany
Center for Thrombosis and Hemostasis, Medical Center of the Johannes Gutenberg-University, Mainz 55131, Germany

Lin Ding and Yilun Liu
Department of Radiation Biology, Beckman Research Institute, City of Hope, Duarte, CA 91010-3000, USA

Josephine S. Modica-Napolitano
Department of Biology, Merrimack College, North Andover, MA 01845, USA

Volkmar Weissig
Department of Pharmaceutical Sciences, Midwestern University, College of Pharmacy, Glendale, AZ 85308, USA

Janina A. Vaitkus, Jared S. Farrar and Francesco S. Celi
Division of Endocrinology and Metabolism, Department of Internal Medicine, Virginia Commonwealth University School of Medicine, Richmond, VA 23298, USA

Francesca Forini and Giorgio Iervasi
CNR Institute of Clinical Physiology, Via G. Moruzzi 1, Pisa 56124, Italy

Giuseppina Nicolini
Tuscany Region G. Monasterio Foundation, Via G. Moruzzi 1, Pisa 56124, Italy

Paola Maura Tricarico
Department of Medicine, Surgery and Health Sciences, University of Trieste, Piazzale Europa 1, 34128 Trieste, Italy

Fulvio Celsi
Institute for Maternal and Child Health "Burlo Garofolo", via dell'Istria 65/1, 34137 Trieste, Italy

Sergio Crovella
Department of Medicine, Surgery and Health Sciences, University of Trieste, Piazzale Europa 1, 34128 Trieste, Italy
Institute for Maternal and Child Health "Burlo Garofolo", via dell'Istria 65/1, 34137 Trieste, Italy

Ana A. Baburamani, Chloe Hurling, Helen Stolp and Claire Thornton
Centre for the Developing Brain, Division of Imaging Sciences and Biomedical Engineering, King's College London, St. Thomas' Hospital, SE1 7EH London, UK

Kristina Sobotka
Perinatal Center, Institute for Clinical Sciences and Physiology & Neuroscience, Sahlgrenska Academy, University of Gothenburg, 41685 Gothenburg, Sweden

Henrik Hagberg
Centre for the Developing Brain, Division of Imaging
Sciences and Biomedical Engineering, King's College
London, St. Thomas' Hospital, SE1 7EH London, UK
Perinatal Center, Institute for Clinical Sciences and
Physiology & Neuroscience, Sahlgrenska Academy,
University of Gothenburg, 41685 Gothenburg,
Sweden

Pierre Gressens
Centre for the Developing Brain, Division of Imaging
Sciences and Biomedical Engineering, King's College
London, St. Thomas' Hospital, SE1 7EH London, UK
Inserm, U 1141, 75019 Paris, France
University Paris Diderot, Sorbonne Paris Cité, UMRS
1141, 75019 Paris, France

Index

Printed in the USA
CPSIA information can be obtained
at www.ICGtesting.com
JSHW061340150424
61201JS00005B/83

9 781646 465590